Maternity, Newborn and Women's Health: A Case-Based Approach

Maternity, Newborn and Women's Health: A Case-Based Approach

Edited by Nicole McConnell

AMERICAN
MEDICAL PUBLISHERS
www.americanmedicalpublishers.com

American Medical Publishers,
41 Flatbush Avenue,
1st Floor, New York,
NY 11217, USA

Visit us on the World Wide Web at:
www.americanmedicalpublishers.com

ISBN: 978-1-63927-156-6

Cataloging-in-Publication Data

Maternity, newborn and women's health : a case-based approach / edited by Nicole McConnell.
p. cm.
Includes bibliographical references and index.
ISBN 978-1-63927-156-6
1. Maternal health services. 2. Newborn infants--Health and hygiene. 3. Women—Health and hygiene.
4. Women's health services. 5. Maternal and infant welfare. 6. Obstetrics.
7. Neonatology. I. McConnell, Nicole.
RG940 .M38 2022
618.24--dc23

Table of Contents

Preface

Maternity is a period during pregnancy and shortly after childbirth. During birth, the newborns may have complications like lack of oxygen, birth trauma and infections. They are also at a high risk of getting infected by diseases like neonatal jaundice, infant respiratory distress syndrome, neonatal conjunctivitis, neonatal sepsis, etc. The period after childbirth is known as the postpartum period, and in this period the mother's body, its hormone levels and uterus size, return to non-pregnant size. It can be divided into three distinct stages; the initial or acute phase, the subacute postpartum period, and the delayed postpartum period. During this time period, the mother may face various health issues such as postpartum bleeding, deep vein thrombosis, postpartum depression, posttraumatic stress disorder, etc. There are various measures taken to avoid such health issues affecting the child and the mother. The objective of this book is to give a general view of the different areas of maternity, newborn and women's health. It will also provide interesting topics for research which interested readers can take up. Coherent flow of topics, student-friendly language and extensive use of examples make this book an invaluable source of knowledge.

The information shared in this book is based on empirical researches made by veterans in this field of study. The elaborative information provided in this book will help the readers further their scope of knowledge leading to advancements in this field.

Finally, I would like to thank my fellow researchers who gave constructive feedback and my family members who supported me at every step of my research.

Editor

1

The status of maternal and newborn health care services in Zanzibar

Bakar Fakih[1], Azzah A. S. Nofly[2], Ali O. Ali[2], Abdallah Mkopi[1], Ali Hassan[4], Ali M. Ali[1], Kate Ramsey[1,3], Theopista John Kabuteni[5], Godfrey Mbaruku[1] and Mwifadhi Mrisho[1*]

Abstract

Background: It is estimated that 287,000 women worldwide die annually from pregnancy and childbirth-related conditions, and 6.9 million under-five children die each year, of which about 3 million are newborns. Most of these deaths occur in sub-Saharan Africa. The maternal health situation in Tanzania mainland and Zanzibar is similar to other sub-Saharan countries. This study assessed the availability, accessibility and quality of emergency obstetric care services and essential resources available for maternal and child health services in Zanzibar.

Methods: From October and November 2012, a cross-sectional health facility survey was conducted in 79 health facilities in Zanzibar. The health facility tools developed by the Averting Maternal Death and Disability program were adapted for local use.

Results: Only 7.6 % of the health facilities qualified as functioning basic EmONC (Emergency Obstetric and Neonatal Care) facilities and 9 % were comprehensive EmONC facilities. Twenty-eight percent were partially performing basic EmONC and the remaining 55.7 % were not providing EmONC. Neonatal resuscitation was performed in 80 % of the hospitals and only 17.4 % of the other health facilities that were surveyed. Based on World Health Organisation (WHO) criteria, the study revealed a gap of 20 % for minimum provision of EmONC facilities per 500,000 population. The met need at national level (proportion of women with major direct obstetric complications treated in a health facility providing EmONC) was only 33.1 % in the 12 months preceding the survey. The study found that there was limited availability of human resources in all visited health facilities, particularly for the higher cadres, as per Zanzibar minimum staff requirements.

Conclusion: There is a need to strengthen human resource capacity at primary health facilities through training of health care providers to improve EmONC services, as well as provision of necessary equipment and supplies to reduce workload at the higher referral health facilities and increase geographic access.

Keywords: Zanzibar, Emergency obstetric and newborn care, Signal functions

Background

Despite the high priority given to maternal and child health, it is now clear that the realization of Millennium Development Goals (MDGs) by 2015 is unrealistic. Annually, it is estimated that 287,000 women worldwide die from pregnancy and childbirth-related conditions, and 6.9 million under-five children die each year, of which about 3 million are newborns. Most of these deaths occur in sub-Saharan Africa [1, 2].

* Correspondence: mwifadhi.mrisho@gmail.com
[1]Ifakara Health Institute, P.O. Box 78373, Dar es Salaam, Tanzania
Full list of author information is available at the end of the article

The maternal health situation in Tanzania mainland and Zanzibar is similar to other sub-Saharan countries [3]. A significant proportion of maternal deaths occur as a result of direct and indirect obstetric complications between the third trimester and the first week after delivery [4–7]. Since many of the obstetric complications cannot be predicted, skilled delivery and access to emergency obstetric care continue to be the most important strategies to reduce maternal and perinatal mortality [8–14].

In Tanzania, estimates of maternal mortality vary based on the sources, but all have wide confidence intervals. For example the Tanzania Demographic Health

Survey, (TDHS) [3] estimates 454 maternal deaths per 100,000 live births [3] while the UN estimates 790 maternal deaths per 100,000 live births in the same year [15]. Although separate estimates for Zanzibar are not available from the TDHS, a study of facility-based maternal deaths from 2005 to 2007 in Zanzibar showed a surprisingly high maternal mortality ratio among women who delivered in facilities [16]. Significant declines in child mortality have been observed in the Tanzania Mainland and Zanzibar, but with insufficient progress in reducing neonatal deaths [3, 17].

In committing to MDGs 4 and 5, the Government agreed to reduce the under-five mortality rate by two-thirds and reduce the maternal mortality ratio by three-quarters, by 2015 from 1990 levels. Many countries have been embarking on Emergency Obstetric and Newborn Care (EmONC) needs assessments in order to obtain the data necessary to improve maternal health services [18, 19]. As part of the government of Zanzibar's efforts to improve maternal and newborn care, we undertook an assessment of the availability, accessibility and quality of maternal and newborn services in public and private health facilities in Zanzibar.

Methods

Design and Study area

A cross-sectional health facility survey was conducted in Unguja and Pemba Islands of Zanzibar between October and November, 2012.

Description of the facilities

The study involved public, private for profit, and non-governmental organization health facilities providing maternal and child health (MCH) services. There were 224 health facilities in Zanzibar at the time of the survey. Sixty four percent of these facilities were government owned; 34 % were privately owned, while 2 % were parastatal. The health sector in Zanzibar includes three levels of care and corresponding facilities as follows: a) Primary level: Health Care Units and Centres (PHCUs, PHCU+ and Primary Health Care Centres-PHCCs) b) Secondary level: District Hospitals c) Tertiary level: Mnazi Mmoja National Hospital. PHCUs provide Primary health care services, PHCU+ are selected to provide additional services such as delivery, dental, laboratory and pharmacy services. PHCCs provide the same services as PHCU+ with the addition of inpatient and X-ray services. District hospitals provide second line referral services, including basic surgery and the tertiary hospital (Mnazi Mmoja Hospital) provides referral services.

Sample size

A measure of relative variance was applied to determine the sample number of health facilities required [20]. All secondary and tertiary health facilities (43 facilities) offer maternity services and thus were included in the sample. A stratified random sampling procedure was applied to sample first line PHCUs. The targeted health facilities were divided into two strata. The first stratum was comprised of first line Primary Health Care Units (PHCUs) and the second stratum of PHCU+ and PHCC facilities.

All higher secondary and tertiary health facilities (43 facilities) were included in the sample as they offer maternity health services. The random sampling procedure was applied to get the remaining sample of the first line PHCUs. The sampling frame included 100 PHCUs in all districts. STATA 12.0 software was used to conduct random sampling required sample size (38 of 100 PHCUs). Our initial sample was 80 health facilities; however, one health facility was dropped due to unavailability of staff to participate in the study.

Procedure

The assessment methods and modules developed by the Averting Maternal Death and Disability (AMDD) program (www.mailman.columbia.edu/research/averting-maternal-death-and-disability-amdd) at Columbia University, New York, USA, and United Nations (UN) Partners were adapted for local use. Methods included key informant interviews, observations, and data extraction. A workshop with the Zanzibar Ministry of Health (ZMOH) and other stakeholders was held to make the relevant adaptations to the Zanzibar context [21]. In order to ensure that the wording of the questions was correct and understood by both, interviewer and interviewee, study instruments were translated into Swahili and pilot-tested in Kivunge, Chukwani, Kitope, Jambiani and Mwera health facilities.

A total of 5 teams, each of which included a supervisor, data entry clerk and three research assistants (RAs), were recruited, ensuring at least one midwife per team. All interviewers had completed at least secondary school education. Research assistants and supervisors were trained for three days to ensure that they understood the objectives of the survey, the study methods and the content of the modules. During the training, roles of supervisors, research assistants and other study team members were also explained. A training manual was prepared to enhance the effectiveness of training and was also used as a reference for data collectors during the survey.

Teams were assigned to move around the districts ensuring data collection from all sampled facilities. With exception of hospitals, data collection required approximately one day per health facility. Supervisors contacted the health facility in-charge, assigned work to RAs, maintained continuous progress in data collection and reviewed the completed questionnaires for errors and omissions on a daily basis. Interviews were conducted with health facility in-charges or midwives at the PHCUs and PHCUs + and in-charges of the maternity wards, pharmacy, laboratory and human resource for PHCC and hospital levels.

Data analysis

Data cleaning and consistency checks were conducted after the survey. Data were analyzed using STATA (version 12.0, College Station, Texas, USA). Analyses were conducted in accordance with UN guidelines for monitoring obstetric services [22], including performance of signal functions and the calculation of the EmONC indicators.

The World Health Organisation (WHO) handbook on monitoring emergency obstetric and neonatal care EmONC defines the signal functions as 1) administration of parenteral antibiotics, 2) administration of parenteral uterotonics, 3) administration of parenteral anticonvulsants; 4) manual removal of the placenta (MRP); 5) removal of retained products; 6) Assisted Vaginal Delivery (AVD); 7) neonatal resuscitation; 8) blood transfusion; and 9) obstetric surgery. The handbook classifies health facilities that have performed the first seven signal functions in the last three months as basic EmONC (BEmONC) facilities and those providing all nine signal functions are classified as comprehensive EmONC (CEmONC) facilities [22]. Furthermore, any facility providing at least one of the first seven signal functions was considered as partially functioning. A non-EmONC facility was defined as a facility which never provided any of the seven basic signal functions in the three-month period before the assessment.

Results

Availability of EmONC services

The availability of EmONC services was measured by determining the number of facilities that performed the complete set of required signal functions in the three-month period prior to the assessment. Only 7.6 % (6/79) of the visited health facilities qualified as fully functioning Basic Emergency Obstetric and Neonatal Care (BEmONC) facilities and 9 % (7/79) were comprehensive EmONC facilities. Twenty eight percent (22/79) of the visited health facilities were classified as partially performing BEmONC and 55.7 % (44/79) were considered non-EmONC facilities (Table 1).

Figure 1 below shows the distribution pattern of health facilities in which each of the 7 signal functions were performed during the 3 months prior to the survey.

The WHO handbook on monitoring emergency obstetric care recommends the minimum acceptable number of EmONC facilities as 5 EmONC with at least one CEmONC per 500,000 population [22]. According to these criteria there are 20 % fewer EmONC facilities in Zanzibar than required. Yet, the number of CEmONC facilities surpassed the required minimum (133 %) (Table 2). Overall, minimum recommended level of EmONC services in Zanzibar has been met by 87 %.

Geographic distribution of EmONC facilities

The distribution of BEmONC and CEmONC varied across Zanzibar. Basic EmONC facilities were mainly available in North Pemba and South Pemba regions, as well as West Urban regions, as shown in Fig. 2. CEmONC facilities were mainly concentrated in Urban West (Unguja); North Pemba and South Pemba regions.

Proportion of all births in EmONC facilities

Overall, 47 % (25,560/54,057) of all births occurred in EmONC health facilities. The proportion of health facility delivery was slightly higher in Unguja zone as compared to Pemba. The highest proportion of births in health facilities were noted in Chake Chake and South Unguja. South District had the highest proportion of births occurring in EmONC facilities followed by Chake Chake. North B District had a higher proportion of

Table 1 Facilities with Comprehensive Emergency Obstetric Neonatal Care (CEmONC) & BEmONC (*N* = 79)

	Health facility status			
	CEmONC % (*n*)	BEmONC % (*n*)	Partially BEmONC % (*n*)	Non-EmONC % (*n*)
OVERALL	9	7.6	27.9	55.7
Number of health facilities	7	6	22	44
Health facility type				
National Hospital	1.3 (1)	0 (0)	0 % (0)	0 (0)
District hospital	3.8 (3)	0 (0)	0 (0)	0 (0)
Cottage Hospital (PHCC)	1.3 (1)	2.5 (2)	1.3 (1)	0 (0)
PHCU+	0 (0)	5.1 (4)	21.5 (17)	16.5 (13)
PHCU	0 (0)	0 (0)	5.1 (4)	39.2 (31)
Maternity hospital	1.3 (1)	0 (0)	0 (0)	0 (0)
Private hospital	1.3 (1)	0 (0)	0 (0)	0 (0)

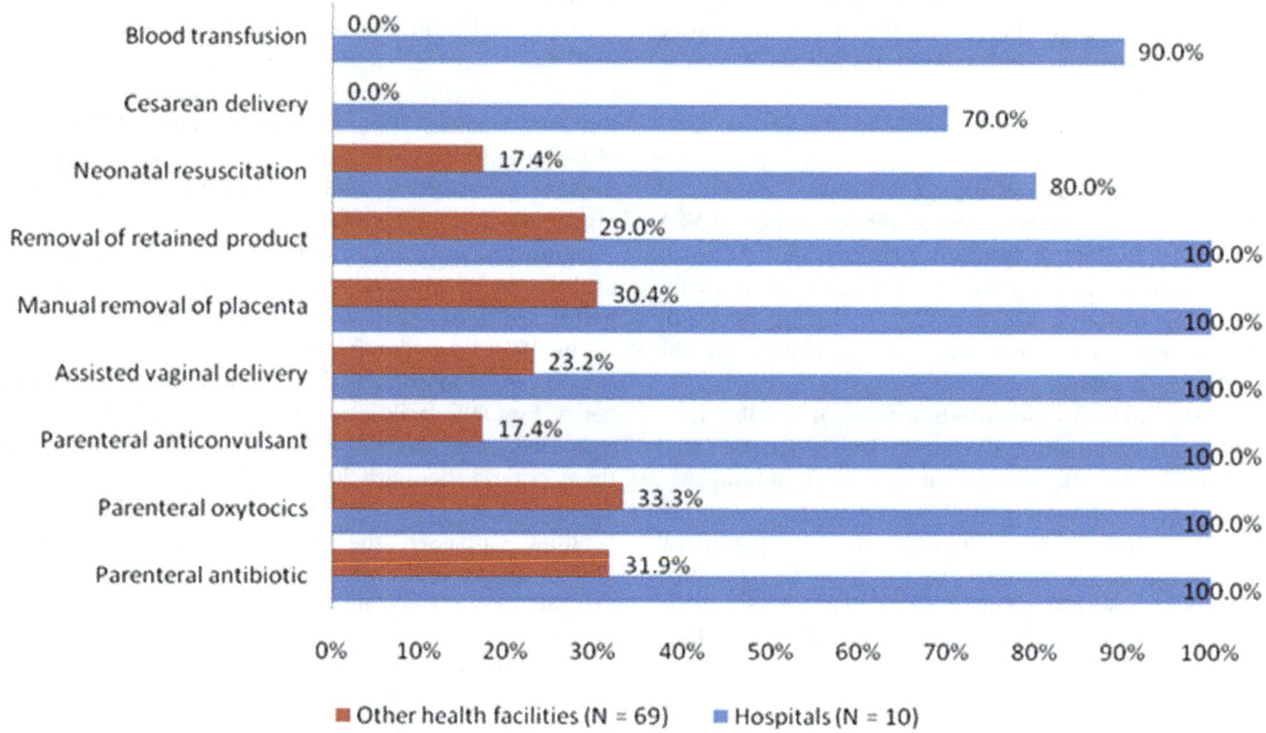

Fig. 1 Proportion of health facilities in which each signal function was performed during the past 3 months, Zanzibar 2012

Table 2 Distribution of Basic and Comprehensive EmONC in visited districts ($N = 79$)

	Total population*	Surveyed facilities (all)	Existing Basic EmOC	Existing Comprehensive	Min number of comprehensive required	overall minimum number of facilities required (Basic + Comprehensive)[a]	% of the facility available (Basic + Comprehensive)	% of comprehensive facility available
OVERALL	1460987	79	6	7	3	15	87	233.3
By Zones								
Pemba	461417	33	4	3	1	5	140	300
Unguja	999570	46	2	4	2	10	60	200
By district								
ChakeChake	104461	7	1	1	1	5	40	100
Mkoani	115228	9	1	1	1	5	40	100
Wete	125907	9	0	1	1	5	20	100
Micheweni	115820	8	2	0	1	5	40	0
Kaskazini A	106972	7	1	0	1	5	20	0
Kaskazini B	65148	6	0	0	1	5	0	0
Kati	78525	9	0	0	1	5	0	0
Kusini	37756	7	0	1	1	5	20	100
Magharibi	462221	8	1	0	1	5	20	0
Mjini	248948	9	0	3	1	5	60	300

*National Bureau of Statistics (2002 census), Population projection 2012

[a]A product of multiplication minimum number of comprehensive required by 5

births occurring in non-EmONC facilities as compared to other districts. In the urban districts, women from the outside the catchment areas were often delivering at Mnazi Mmoja National Hospital (MMNH). There were few deliveries occurring in health facilities in Central and West districts and neither had functioning EmONC facilities.

Met need for EmONC services

According to the WHO handbook on monitoring emergency obstetric care, 'Met need' estimates the proportion of all women with major direct obstetric complications who are treated in a health facility providing EmONC services [22]. The international minimum standard is 100 %. Findings from this study indicated that the national met need for EmONC was only 33.1 % (2519/7354) in the 12 months preceding the survey. Unguja zone had a higher met need of 33.7 % (1396/4137) as compared to Pemba zone 22.7 % (930/4100). Urban District had the highest met need at 55.2 % (1315/2383) (Table 3).

Caesarean deliveries as a percentage of all births

This indicator calculates caesarean deliveries as a proportion of expected live births in the population in a specified period [18]. It is a measure of accessibility and utilization of critical services [22]. While there are debates about optimal rates, the EmONC indicators recommend a rate between 5 and 15 %. In the 12 months preceding the survey, 4.4 % of expected births in Zanzibar were cesarean deliveries. Unguja zone had a slightly higher caesarean delivery rate as compared to Pemba. The highest caesarean rate was in Urban District at 23.9 %.

Table 3 Met need for EmONC

	All HF % (n/N)	EmOC % (n/N)	Non-EmOC % (n/N)
OVERALL	34.3 (2519/7354)	33.1 (2435/7354)	1.1 (84/7354)
Zone			
Unguja	37.2 (1537/4137)	33.7 (1396/4137)	3.4 (141/4137)
Pemba	24.0 (982/4100)	22.7 (930/4100)	1.3 (52/4100)
District			
ChakeChake	15.8 (319/2016)	15.4 (310/2016)	0.4 (9/2016)
Mkoani	5.8 (116/2016)	4.7 (95/2016)	1.0 (21/2016)
Wete	11.5 (239/2085)	11.3 (236/2085)	0.1 (3/2085)
Micheweni	14.8 (308/2085)	13.9 (289/2085)	0.9 (19/2085)
North A	9.2 (112/1220)	8.9 (109/1220)	0.2 (3/1220)
North B	0.6 (7/1220)	0 (0/1220)	0.6 (7/1220)
Central	0.7 (4/535)	0 (0/535)	0.7 (4/535)
South	71/535 (13.3)	11.8 (63/535)	1.5 (8/535)
West	1.1 (26/2383)	0.8 (18/2383)	0.3 (8/2383)
Urban	1317/2383 (55.3)	55.2 (1315/2383)	0.1 (2/2383)

n = number of women treated for direct obstetric complications
N = expected number of women who would have major obstetric complications

Direct obstetric Case Fatality Rate (CFR)

This indicator provides an indication of quality of care in health facilities. According to the WHO handbook on monitoring emergency obstetric care the maximum acceptable level of CFR is less than one percent [22]. Although there was substantial geographical variation between the districts, the overall direct obstetric case fatality rate was 2.5 % for all health facilities surveyed and 2.2 % in EmONC facilities in the 12 months preceding the survey. The highest CFRs were noted in Wete followed Mkoani and Chake Chake districts in Pemba Island.

Intrapartum and very early neonatal death

Quality of intrapartum and newborn care was also assessed through facility-based perinatal mortality. The WHO handbook on monitoring emergency obstetric care defines the intrapartum and very early neonatal death rate as the proportion of births that result in a very early neonatal death or an intrapartum death (fresh stillbirth) in an EmONC facility. The numerator for this indicator is the sum of intrapartum and very early neonatal deaths within the first 24 h of life and the denominator was all deliveries in the facilities during the same period [22]. The intrapartum and very early neonatal death rate was 2 % ($n = 553$) in all health facilities visited in the 12 months preceding the survey. The district variation was noted for this indicator, the highest being in South and Urban districts with 5.8 % ($n = 46$) and 2.4 % ($n = 377$) respectively.

Availability of 24-hour daily services

Health facilities' in-charges were asked if the facilities provide obstetric and neonatal care services 24 h a day and 7 days a week. Of the visited health facilities, only 18 % (14/79) provide obstetric and neonatal care continuously on a daily basis.

Cesarean Review

Reviews of three randomly selected Cesarean deliveries from birth registers performed in the last 12 months were conducted at seven health facilities offering Cesarean delivery services, with a total of 21 cases analyzed. Eighteen cesarean cases were classified in the register as emergency and two were elective. The main documented reasons for cesarean delivery were obstructed labour (4 cases), followed by fetal distress (3 cases). However, there was no documentation of the indications for most (14 cases) of the caesarean deliveries reviewed. With regard to the timely management, on average, 67 min elapsed from a decision to the actual performance of

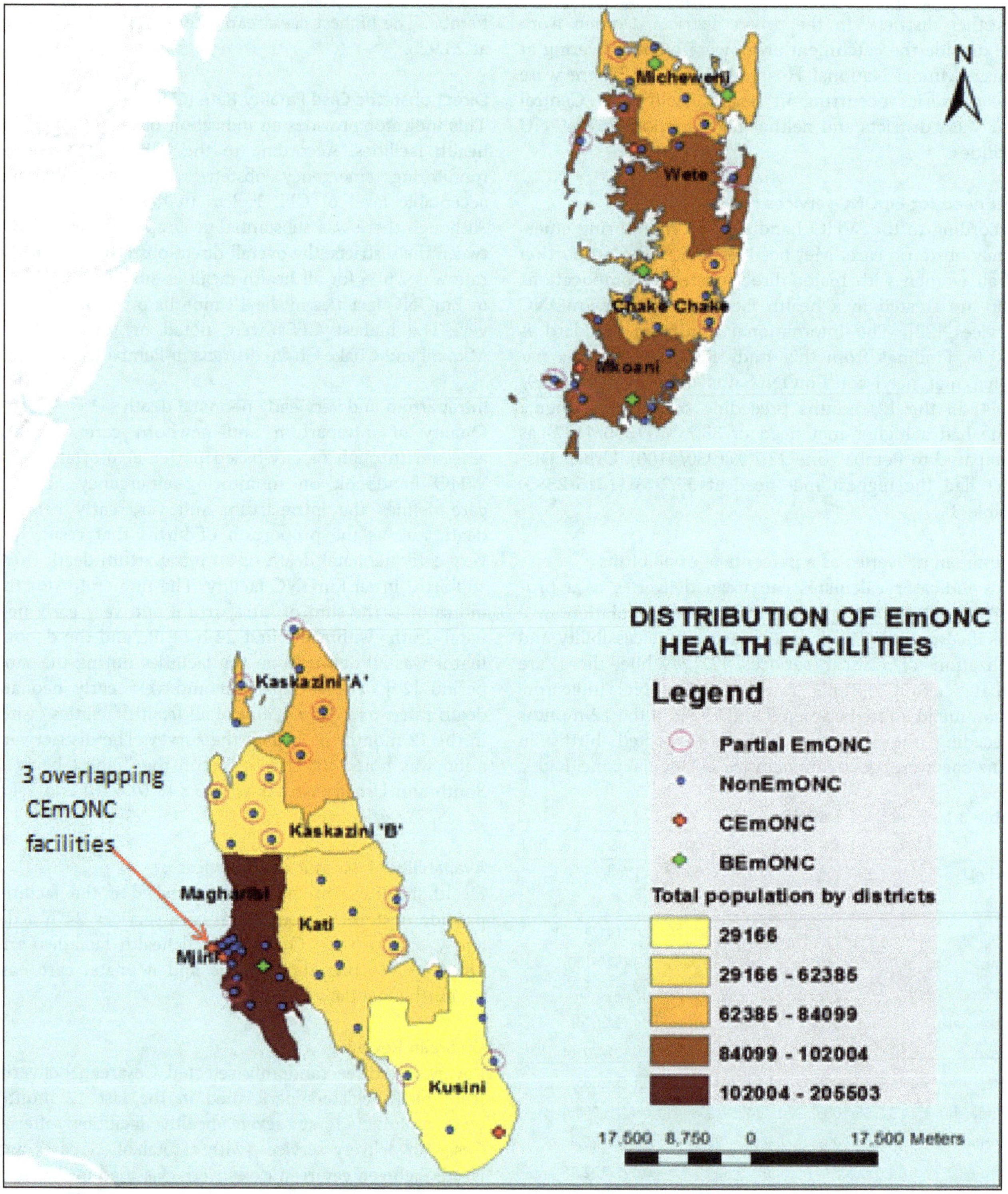

Fig. 2 District Populations and distribution of EmONC facilities in Zanzibar, 2012

cesarean section. The minimum time taken was 30 min and the maximum was 86 min in Mwembeladu and district hospitals respectively. About half (10 cases) of cesarean deliveries were performed by obstetrician/gynecologists, mainly based in the district and private hospitals, while 7 cesareans were conducted by trained Assistant Medical Officers (AMOs) and 4 cases by Medical doctors (MDs). AMOs receive training on emergency obstetric and neonatal care during their pre-service training, but also undergo special three-month competency-based training on cesarean sections and provision of quality EmONC services, while MDs are trained during their pre-service study period and internship.

Availability of qualified staff to perform EmONC services

The provision of health services depend to a large extent, on the availability of both human resources and properly equipped health facilities. The study found that there was limited supply of human resources in all visited health facilities, particularly for the higher cadres, in relation to Zanzibar minimum staff requirements For example, at MMNH there was a 50 % gap between the planned versus actual number of medical doctors. The met need for nurses (excluding midwives) was only 22.7 %. However, the planned need of midwives surpassed the required number in most of the visited health facilities. At district level, the human resource situation was similar to that in Mnazi Mmoja Hospital. Medical doctors and general surgeons were not available at any of the district hospitals where six are required by policy. Obstretrician-Gynecologists were only available 33.3 % of staffing establishment at the time of the survey. With regard to the availability of trained AMOs, the study found that only 10.0 % of the AMOs and 11.1 % of anesthesiologists were available at PHCCs. There was also insufficient numbers of the most important cadres to perform duties at PHCU+ level. At private hospitals the availability of human resources was quite similar with exception of greater availability of MDs and Anesthesiologists (MD).

Infrastructure, communication, drugs, equipment, and supplies

The survey team inspected the infrastructure of 35 health facilities offering delivery services to see if they were convenient for both staff and patients. Overall, 91 % (32/35) of the facilities had good infrastructure and nearly all had sufficient light source to perform tasks during the day and night. More than 85 % of health facilities' toilets were in good condition and well-functioning. Water was available in 86 % (30/35) of the visited facilities offering delivery services. Privacy was well guaranteed with presence of curtains in 86 % (30/35) of facilities.

With regard to communication, the study found that 30.4 % (24/79) of all the visited health facilities had a functional mobile phone owned by the facility. Every health facility had individual health providers who had personal, functional mobile phones and 78.5 % (62/79) of the staffs used their own mobile phones to refer patients to the next level of care.

Oxytocics and prostaglandins drugs were available at 39 % (31/79) of all health facilities visited. Among those facilities reported to have oxytocics and prostaglandins, oxytocin was highly available at 90 % (28/31) followed by misoprostol at 71 % (22/31). Anticonvulsants drugs were available at 43 % (34/79) in visited health facilities.

Overall, general equipment and supplies needed for labor and delivery services were available at 60 % (21/35) of facilities offering delivery services. Fetal stethoscope and kidney basins were equally available at 97.1 % (34/35). The supplies which were reasonably found in all health facilities offering delivery services included: IV cannulae 71.4 % (25/35), clinical oral thermometer 68.6 % (24/35), suture needles/suture materials 65.7 % (23/35) and examination table 77.1 % (27/35). Labor/delivery tables with and without stirrups were available at 45.7 % (16/35). Partographs were available at 51.4 % (18/35) while adult ventilator bags and mask were available at 25.7 % (9/35). Ultrasounds were available at 23 % (8/35).

Discussion

For every 500,000 population, the minimum acceptable level is five EmONC facilities with at least one of which provides comprehensive care [22]. This study has shown that the minimum acceptable level of EmONC services in Zanzibar overall has been met, although, urban district facilities are overloaded with deliveries which poses rising concerns regarding ability to provide high quality care. While the minimum has been met overall, distribution of facilities is not equitable. The assessment revealed that there was a gap of 50 % of EmONC facilities in Unguja, while Pemba zone surpassed the minimum by 40 %. Most of the CEmONC services were largely found in the urban districts, raising concern about accessibility for some parts of the islands. Similar findings have been reported in other low-income countries [18, 24]. Furthermore, in some situations where the population is widely dispersed and travel is difficult; EmONC facilities will likely need to exceed the minimum acceptable level for more equitable geographic distribution [22].

Although most facility-based deliveries are taking place in EmONC health facilities, few deliveries were noted in Central, North B and West districts. Furthermore, the study found that there was a high volume of deliveries in the urban district. These deliveries might have been conducted in lower health facilities like PHCU + s and PHCCs, hence reducing the workload at tertiary level. Human resource and infrastructural capacity would be needed to ensure quality delivery services at lower level health facilities. Unlike Unguja, Pemba has a relatively even distribution of EmONC facilities; however, most of these EmONC facilities are underutilized for delivery services. Specialists perform most of the caesarean sections as compared to the trained AMO's. Yet, most of these Caesarean sections are performed in the district and private hospitals. Ideally, specialists at MMNH referral hospital should have attended most of the complicated cases but this was not the case. In comparison, to the mainland, 80 % of Caesarean sections are performed by trained AMO's [25, 26].

Met need for EmONC is another indicator that reflects a health system's capacity to respond to women's obstetric needs when complications develop [18]. The met need has reached only half the acceptable level, meaning that a large proportion of women who experienced complications did not receive the medical care they needed.

The majority of the caesarean sections were for emergencies, which show that these occur at a large extent due to (assumed) poor monitoring of pregnancies, given the types of 'expected' common complications. In fact, the issue of delays corroborates these findings as specialists are few but also it seems that even AMOs are too few on the islands. Generally, human resource data found in the survey suggests that there is a gap of specialists in CEmONC health facilities in particular among the higher cadres.

Although the WHO handbook on monitoring emergency obstetric care recommends 5 %–15 % of pregnancies are expected to require Cesarean delivery [22], what matters most is for all women who need this service to receive it. The highest caesarean rate (23.9 %) in Urban district is worrying and needs a careful interpretation. Most of these caesareans are happening at MMNH, which is a referral hospital that serves all six districts in Unguja zone. However, if the caesarean rate is included in the overall served six districts of Unguja zone, it is reduced to 3.6 %.

The maximum acceptable level of direct obstetric case fatality rate can sometimes be misinterpreted due to the lack of comparability among health facilities. For example, women with the most serious complications may be referred from the PHCCs and die at MMNH referral hospital, hence increasing the direct obstetric case fatality rate in the hospital. The high overall CFR suggests poor quality of care in the respective health facilities, which may include delayed and inappropriate referrals. Inadequate human resources, limited availability of equipment and supplies might have contributed to the higher CFR. The study did not capture specific reasons for the alarming high CFR in Wete, Mkoani and Chake Chake districts and deeper understanding of quality of care should therefore be sought.

There was also district variation with regard to the intrapartum and very early neonatal deaths, with the highest rates in South, Wete and Urban districts. Poor monitoring of progress of labour and delay in management of complications may be at the root of many of these deaths. Manual vacuum aspiration/dilation and curettage, and AVD were the least performed signal functions in PHCU + s. This reflects both the need for training and improving utilization of services. Similar findings have been reported in other low-income countries [17, 18].

This study has limitations and strengths that should be borne in mind. For instance, if the direct obstetric case fatality rate is acceptable, but EmONC coverage or met need is insufficient, the implication is that women who deliver in EmONC facilities are likely to survive but maternal death outside health facilities might still be common as only half of women deliver in facilities [22]. Hence, community studies are important to explore the reasons for underutilization of healthcare services. In general, the number of deliveries reviewed here were few; therefore the percentages should be interpreted with caution. It would be useful to learn from health care providers in the facilities as to why particular signal functions are not performed. The interpretation of caesarean section review should also be taken with precaution as the very low number of the reviews meant that findings could not be expressed in percentages. The small sample was a result of the low numbers of health facilities providing caesarean deliveries in Zanzibar. Additionally, we noted that there was inadequate documentation of obstetric emergencies in the delivery record books, which may partially explain the low met need for EmONC. For example, fresh stillbirths are quite often documented as macerated stillbirths and obstetric emergencies are sometimes not indicated in the delivery record books especially after treatment. Thus, despite these potential concerns, our findings can inform the development of intervention strategies aimed at saving the lives of mothers and newborn babies.

Conclusions

Despite Zanzibar having met the minimum standards for EmONC availability per population, the met need is still quite low. With only 50 % delivering in health facilities it will be very hard to reach this without increase in utilization. Evidence about quality of care and availability of human resources and supplies, as well as geographic distribution, might explain why these numbers are still low. Yet it will be essential to also make sure that women seek care in order to make real change in this coverage. In order to improve quality of care it is important to consider other important issues like effective training, and monitor the success through supportive supervision and good leadership by senior physicians, which may also encourage women to use services. The use of evidence-based practices should highly be encouraged at all levels. Audit within medical institutions are needed to review patient charts and determine whether the indications for cesarean delivery are appropriate and to determine the causes behind the high case fatality rates found in this survey [27].

Abbreviations

AMDD, Averting Maternal Death and Disability; AMOs, Assistant Medical Officers; AVD, Assisted Vaginal Delivery; BEmONC, Basic Emergency Obstetric Neonatal Care; CeMONC, Comprehensive Emergency Obstetric Neonatal Care; CFR, case fatality rate; DANIDA, Danish International Development Agency; MCH, Maternal and child health; MD, Medical doctor; MDGs, Millennium Development Goals; MMNH, Mnazi Mmoja National Hospital; MRP, manual removal of the placenta; PHCC, Primary Health Care Centers; PHCUs, Primary Health Care Units; RA, Research Assistance; TDHS, Tanzania Demographic Health Survey; UN, United Nations; WHO, World Health Organisation; ZMOH, Zanzibar Ministry of Health

Acknowledgements

The authors wish to acknowledge the immense technical support and advice provided by WHO Zanzibar office as well as the office of Principal Secretary of ZMOH. The study would not have been successful without support from IHI and the Zanzibar Revolutionary Government Authority in the 10 districts as well as all health facility in-charges and health care providers interviewed. This study was funded by World Health Organization through Zanzibar Ministry of Health.

Authors' contributions

MM, KR, BF, AM and GM devised the study design and objectives; MM, BF, GM, AASN, AOA, AM, AH, AMA and TJK contributed to data collection, analysis and interpretation; MM & BF wrote the first draft of the manuscript. All authors read, commented on and approved the final manuscript.

Competing interests

The authors declare that they have no competing interests.

Consent for publication

Not applicable.

Ethics approval and consent to participate

The study complied with the International Ethical Guidelines for Biomedical Research Involving Human subjects [23]. Ethical approval was received from the Zanzibar Medical Research Ethical Committee (ZAMREC) (Certificate ZAMREC/0005/June/012 of 21st August 2012) and from the ethical committee of Ifakara Health Institute (IHI) Certificate IHI/IRB/No: 30-2012 of 4th September 2012. Written informed consent was obtained in local language from all participants taking part in the study. No names were used in any analysis or reporting, and codes were assigned to ensure confidentiality. Respondents were asked if they had any questions and whether they agree to take part in the study. Furthermore, the modules collect only aggregated utilization data and interviews are directed to general questions about the health facility and do not include personal information.

Author details

[1]Ifakara Health Institute, P.O. Box 78373, Dar es Salaam, Tanzania. [2]Intergrated Reproductive and Child Health Program - Zanzibar Ministry of Health, P.O Box 236, Zanzibar, Tanzania. [3]Columbia University Mailman School of Public Health, 722 W 168th St, New York, NY 10032, USA. [4]Ministry of Health, Health Sector Program Support, DANIDA-Zanzibar, P.O.Box 236, Zanzibar, Tanzania. [5]Maternal, Newborn and Child Health, World Health Organisation, P.O.Box 9292, Dar es Salaam, Tanzania.

References

1. WHO, UNICEF, UNFPA, World Bank. Trends in maternal mortality: 1990 – 2008. Geneva: The World Health Organization; 2010.
2. You D, Wardlaw T, Salama P, Jones G. Levels and trends in under-5 mortality, 1990–2008. Lancet. 2010;375:100–3.
3. NBS [Tanzania] and ORC Macro. Tanzania Demographic and Health Survey 2010 - Key Findings. National Bureau of Statistics, Dar es Salaam and ORC Macro, Calverton, MD. 2010.
4. United Nations. The Millenium Development Goals Report 2010. New York: United Nations; 2010.
5. Khan KS, Wojdyla D, Say L, Gulmezoglu AM, Van Look PF. WHO analysis of causes of maternal death: a systematic review. Lancet. 2006;367:1066–74.
6. Ronsmans C, Graham WJ. Maternal mortality. who, when, where, and why. Lancet. 2006;368:1189–200.
7. WHO, Make Every Mother and Child Count. The World Health Report. Geneva: World Health Organization; 2005.
8. Adegoke AA, van den Broek N. Skilled birth attendance – lessons learnt. BJOG. 2009;116 Suppl 1:33–40.
9. Campbell OM, Graham WJ. Strategies for reducing maternal mortality: getting on with what works. Lancet. 2006;368:1284–99.
10. Filippi V, Ronsmans C, Campbell OM, Graham WJ, Mills A, Borghi J, et al. *Maternal health in poor* countries: the broader context and a call for action. Lancet. 2006;368:1535–41.
11. Koblinsky M, Matthews Z, Hussein J, Mavalankar D, Mridha MK, Anwar I, et al. Going to scale with professional skilled care. Lancet. 2006;368:1377–86.
12. Paxton A, Maine D, Freedman L, Fry D, Lobis S. The evidence for emergency obstetric care. Int J Gynaecol Obstet. 2005;88:181–93.
13. Scott S, Ronsmans C. The relationship between birth with a health professional and maternal mortality in observational studies: a review of the literature. Trop Med Int Health. 2009;14:1523–33.
14. Lund S, Hemed M, Nielsen B, Said A, Said K, Makungu M, Rasch V. Mobile phones as a health communication tool to improve skilled attendance at delivery in Zanzibar: a cluster-randomised controlled trial. BJOG. 2012;119: 1256–64.
15. The State of the World's Midwifery 2011 available at: (http://www.unfpa.org/sites/default/files/pub-pdf/en_SOWMR_Full.pdf) Accessed on 17th Dec 2013.
16. Lund S, Said AA, Hemed M, Khamis RK, Jiddawi N. Facility based maternal mortality in Zanzibar 2005-2007. Unpublished (Available at http://www.bibalex.org/search4dev/files/428882/455710.pdf) Accessed 3 Jul 2016.
17. Bureau of Statistics (Tanzania), Macro International Inc,. Tanzania Demographic and Health Survey. Macro International, Inc. 1999.
18. Oyerinde K, Harding Y, Amara P, Kanu R, Shoo R, Daoh K. Averting Maternal Death and Disability, The status of Maternal and Newborn Care in Searra Leone 8 years After Ceasefire. Int J Gynaecol Obstet. 2001;114(2011):168–73.
19. Manji K. *Situation analysis of newborn health in Tanzania: Current situation, existing plans and* strategic next steps for newborn health. Dar es Salaam: Ministry of Health and Social Welfare, Save the Children; 2009.
20. Sampling Manual for Facility Surveys for Population, Maternal Health, Child Health and STD Programs in Developing Countries. MEASURE Evaluation Manual Series, No. 3. MEASURE Evaluation. Carolina Population Center, University of North Carolina at Chapel Hill. July 2001.
21. The revolutionary government of Zanzibar. Assesment of the Availability of Health Services in terms of accessibility and quality of health care. Draft report, 2010.
22. WHO, UNFPA, UNICEF & AMDD. A Handbook 2009: Monitoring emergency obstetric care. 2009.
23. Council for International Organizations of Medical Sciences (IOMS). "International ethical guidelines for biomedical research involving human subjects." Bulletin of medical ethics 182, 2002:17.
24. Unicef Somalia. Report on Findings Emergency Obstetric and Neonatal Care (EmONC) needs Assessment in Selected Health Facilities in NEZ, Puntland. 2011.
25. Pereira C, Mbaruku G, et al. Emergency Obstetric Surgery by non-physician clinicians in Tanzania. Int J Gynaecol Obstet. 2011;114(2):180–3.
26. Nyamtema A, Pemba S, Mbaruku G, et al. Tanzania lessons in using non-physician clinicians to scale up comprehensive emegence obstetric care in remote and rural areas. Hum Resour Health. 2011;9:28. doi 101186/147-4491-928.
27. Chin-Yuan HSU, Lo JC, Chang JH, Chen CP, Yu S, Huang FY. Cesarean births in Taiwan. Int J Gynaecol Obstet. 2007;96:57–61.

2

Using a quality improvement model to enhance providers' performance in maternal and newborn health care: a post-only intervention and comparison design

Firew Ayalew[1*], Gizachew Eyassu[1], Negash Seyoum[1], Jos van Roosmalen[2], Eva Bazant[3], Young Mi Kim[3], Alemnesh Tekleberhan[1], Hannah Gibson[1], Ephrem Daniel[1] and Jelle Stekelenburg[4,5]

Abstract

Background: The Standards Based Management and Recognition (SBM-R©) approach to quality improvement has been implemented in Ethiopia to strengthen routine maternal and newborn health (MNH) services. This evaluation assessed the effect of the intervention on MNH providers' performance of routine antenatal care (ANC), uncomplicated labor and delivery and immediate postnatal care (PNC) services.

Methods: A post-only evaluation design was conducted at three hospitals and eight health centers implementing SBM-R and the same number of comparison health facilities. Structured checklists were used to observe MNH providers' performance on ANC (236 provider-client interactions), uncomplicated labor and delivery (226 provider-client interactions), and immediate PNC services in the six hours after delivery (232 provider-client interactions); observations were divided equally between intervention and comparison groups. Main outcomes were provider performance scores, calculated as the percentage of essential tasks in each service area completed by providers. Multilevel analysis was used to calculate adjusted mean percentage performance scores and standard errors to compare intervention and comparison groups.

Results: There was no statistically significant difference between intervention and comparison facilities in overall mean performance scores for ANC services (63.4% at intervention facilities versus 61.0% at comparison facilities, $p = 0.650$) or in any specific ANC skill area. MNH providers' overall mean performance score for uncomplicated labor and delivery care was 11.9 percentage points higher in the intervention than in the comparison group (77.5% versus 65.6%; $p = 0.002$). Overall mean performance scores for immediate PNC were 22.2 percentage points higher at intervention than at comparison facilities (72.8% versus 50.6%; $p = 0.001$); and there was a significant difference of 22 percentage points between intervention and comparison facilities for each PNC skill area: care for the newborn and health check for the mother.

Conclusions: The SBM-R quality improvement intervention made a significant positive impact on MNH providers' performance during labor and delivery and immediate PNC services, but not during ANC services. Scaling up the intervention to other facilities and regions may increase the availability of good quality MNH services across Ethiopia. The findings will also guide implementation of the government's five-year (2015–2020) health sector transformation plan and health care quality strategies needed to meet the country's MNH goals.

Keywords: SBM-R, Ethiopia, Antenatal care, Postnatal care, Labor and delivery, Provider performance, Quality improvement, Maternal health, Newborn health

* Correspondence: Firew.Ayalew@Jhpiego.org
[1]Jhpiego Ethiopia, Addis Ababa, Ethiopia
Full list of author information is available at the end of the article

Background

Maternal and child mortality have declined over the past 20 years in Ethiopia. However, 2015 estimates show that mortality remains high in the months before and after childbirth, with 420 mothers dying per 100,000 live births, 41 infants dying per 1000 live births, 28 neonates dying per 1000 live births and neonatal deaths accounting for 47% of all under-five mortality [1]. In line with Sustainable Development Goals, by 2020 Ethiopia aims to reduce the maternal mortality ratio to 199 per 100,000 live births, the infant mortality rate to 20 per 1000 live births and the neonatal mortality rate to 10 per 1000 live births [2].

Achieving these goals will require improvements in the quality of maternal and newborn care services. The World Health Organization (WHO) defines eight standards for improving the quality of maternal and newborn care, one of which calls for "competent, motivated staff to be consistently available to provide routine care and manage complications" [3]. Multiple factors influence health workers' performance, including health workers' knowledge and skills gaps, caseload, patient demand, clinical practices, educational opportunities, availability of supplies and equipment and also the presence of a quality improvement process [4].

Various quality improvement models have been implemented in low, middle and high-income countries to improve healthcare providers' performance and quality of services [5, 6]. WHO has concluded that any of these strategies can help to ensure high quality antenatal, intrapartum, and postnatal care [3].

Multifaceted interventions that include supervision, training, audit and feedback have been shown to have a greater impact than single interventions on the quality of health workers' performance [5, 7]. One such approach is Standards-Based Management and Recognition (SBM-R©), which includes four stages to improve performance and quality of health services [8].

In Ethiopia, the Ministry of Health (MOH) began implementing the SBM-R quality improvement model in 2003 to improve HIV/AIDS and maternal and newborn health (MNH) services. However, the effect of SBM-R on healthcare providers' performance and the quality of MNH services has not been evaluated in Ethiopia. This study seeks to address gaps in the literature regarding the effectiveness of MNH quality improvement interventions [3, 9] on providers' performance by evaluating the impact of the SBM-R intervention in Ethiopia.

The evaluation asked: Do MNH providers in facilities that have implemented SBM-R perform better than providers at comparison facilities during routine delivery of antenatal care (ANC), uncomplicated labor and delivery, and immediate postnatal care (PNC) services within the first six hours after delivery [10]?

Methods

Study design and setting

This study employed a post-only intervention and comparison evaluation design to assess the impact of the SBM-R intervention on provider performance at public health facilities located in four major regions of Ethiopia: Tigray, Amhara, Oromia and Southern Nations, Nationalities and Peoples' (SNNP). An SBM-R process to improve the performance and quality of MNH services was introduced at 116 government health facilities (15 hospitals and 101 health centers) from March 2011 to June 2014 with a phased-in approach. This study focuses on the 21 health facilities (15 health centers and 6 hospitals) in the first phase. All of these facilities had proceeded through the entire SBM-R process within three years of implementation and were ready for external assessment.

Description of SBM-R intervention

Guided by national MNH policies and guidelines, performance standards in 10 technical areas were developed for providing quality MNH services, including 80 standards for health centers and 79 standards for hospitals. Technical areas included: routine ANC, uncomplicated labor and delivery care and post-partum care; management of antenatal, intrapartum, and postpartum complications; infection prevention; laboratory; pharmacy; human, physical and materials resources; information, education, communication and community participation; and management system. Each standard comprised a series of specific items that could be scored as a measure of achievement. After authorities endorsed the standards, they were introduced in each health facility. Health managers and providers received three rounds of SBM-R modular trainings focusing on how to use and implement the standards, measure progress, and recognize performance.

After completing the first round of SBM-R training, each facility established a quality improvement team to implement the intervention. This team conducted a baseline assessment of services at the facility using standard tools to identify performance gaps and analyze root causes. Commonly identified performance gaps included deficits in health providers' skills and knowledge as well as shortages of supplies and equipment. Based on the initial gap assessment, intervention facilities received essential equipment and supplies (such as newborn weighing scales, autoclaves, examination beds, delivery beds, baby towels and hats, and infection prevention supplies), training on Basic Emergency Obstetric Newborn Care (BEmONC) for providers, and regular follow-up from regional health bureaus and partners, including site mentoring, review meetings and quarterly supportive supervision. Quality improvement teams at each facility conducted assessments every six months to track performance using direct structured observations, document review and provider interviews. Based on the results, the teams developed action plans to address remaining performance gaps. All target facilities completed the four stages of SBM-R and were eligible for external assessments verifying that they had achieved at least 80% of the standards.

Sampling and sample selection procedure

Sample sizes were calculated for observations of providers' performance in each of three service areas (ANC, labor and delivery, and immediate PNC) based on 95% level of statistical confidence, 80% statistical power, 20% expected difference in health providers' performance between intervention and comparison groups and the recommended value of 1% intraclass correlation coefficient for median value of primary health care research [11]. The intraclass correlation coefficient is the correlation between responses given by randomly selected respondents within clusters or facilities to measure degree of similarity [12].

Health providers' mean performance scores from a 2010 quality of care study in Ethiopia [13] informed the reference values used to calculate the three sample sizes. For ANC, a mean percentage performance score of 38% for preventive treatments, including the administration of tetanus toxoid and prescription or provision of iron/folic acid was used. For uncomplicated labor and delivery care, a mean percentage performance score of 29% on active management of the third stage of labor was used. For immediate PNC, a mean percentage performance score of 47% on immediate newborn care services was used. Based on these, we calculated sample sizes of 236 provider-client interactions (observations) for ANC, 226 for uncomplicated labor and delivery care, and 232 for immediate PNC. Each sample was divided equally between intervention and comparison groups.

A total of six hospitals and 15 health centers had completed all stages of SBM-R. Half (three hospitals and eight health centers) were randomly selected for the study sample. Comparison facilities that had not implemented SBM-R (three hospitals and eight health centers) were selected from the same region and zone as the intervention facilities, but from different districts. Comparison facilities were matched with intervention facilities on staff size and client volume, including the number of first ANC visits and deliveries attended by skilled birth attendants.

The estimated number of MNH providers (those who offer ANC, labor and delivery, and/or PNC services) at each facility was 12 per hospital and five per health center, for a total of 152 across all intervention and comparison facilities in the sample. Because the number of MNH providers at each facility was small, all of them were invited to participate in the study. Women who sought ANC or labor and delivery followed by immediate PNC at these facilities during the study period were invited to participate.

Observation tool

Observations of service delivery using structured checklists were conducted to measure provider performance in ANC, uncomplicated labor and delivery care, and immediate PNC. The clinical observation tool listed essential maternity and newborn care tasks and was adapted from an earlier quality of care study in Ethiopia [13], national BEmONC training guidelines [10], and SBM-R tools. The ANC portion of the tool consisted of 53 tasks in eight skill areas; the labor and delivery portion consisted of 105 tasks in 10 skill areas; and the PNC portion included nine tasks in two skill areas. Observers coded each task as "Yes, task performed" or "No, task not performed." The tool also captured basic characteristics of health providers.

Data collection

Data were collected from July 7 to August 3, 2014 by 20 experienced assessors. Assessors consisted of midwives and health officers with at least a Bachelor of Science degree and national BEmONC master trainers. The assessors attended a four-day training on consent, study instruments, observation techniques, and data quality, and demonstrated their competency through role plays on consents and observation checklists before deployment. A team of two assessors conducted observations at each facility. Five supervisors and one study coordinator supervised them. To minimize observer's bias, assessors were not assigned to health facilities where they worked.

Assessors collected information on providers' sociodemographic characteristics and conducted observations while providers performed each step of routine ANC services, all stages of uncomplicated labor and delivery care, and/or the full range of immediate PNC services within the first six hours after delivery. Assessors stayed overnight at facilities to conduct observations, remaining up to five days at each facility until they observed at least one provider-client interaction per facility. Providers could be observed with more than one patient during this time. If no delivery took place in the facility during the assessors' visit, the study coordinator instructed assessors to move to the next sample facility and observe more providers to compensate. Before traveling to the next sample facility, assessors and supervisors checked the completed observation tools for completeness and consistency.

Data management and analysis

Data was cleaned and entered into CSPro V 5.0 and exported to STATA V 13.1 for statistical analysis. Descriptive statistics, including frequency and percentages, were computed to identify outliers and missing values. Data were nested in three levels: clients (first level) were clustered by provider (second level), and providers were clustered by facility (third level); this nesting structure creates dependency of data. The analysis examined three outcome variables: provider performance scores on ANC, uncomplicated labor and delivery care, and immediate PNC, calculated as the percentage of essential tasks in each service area completed by providers. For this study, health providers' performance is defined as the extent to which actual work practices reflect the skills and knowledge taught in training using standardized operating procedures [14].

Multilevel analysis was used to calculate adjusted mean percentage performance scores and standard errors to compare intervention and comparison groups. The multilevel model is appropriate to generate adjusted standard errors of the estimates and test statistics or p-values for clustered data, instead of conventional linear models that overestimate test statistics and lead to misleading inferences [15, 16]. Mean performance scores ranged from 0 to 1. The mean percentage performance score was calculated by dividing mean performance scores by the maximum mean score and multiplying by 100.

Interclass correlation coefficients (ICC) were computed to assess variations explained by facility and health provider clustering effects on three outcome variables: health provider performance on ANC, uncomplicated labor and delivery care, and immediate PNC. ICC ranges from 0 to 1 and is used to estimate the degree of providers' performance similarity within and among clusters, where an ICC value close to 1 indicates similarities between individual's performance within clusters and an ICC value close to 0 shows independence of individual's performance within clusters and/or an indication to use single level analysis [17]. ICC values suggest the use of multilevel analysis even if they are close to 0.05 [18].

A Chi-square test was used to assess associations of study participants and facility characteristics among intervention and comparison groups. A p-value of less than 0.05 was used for all statistical tests. We computed adjusted standard errors of the mean performance scores to calculate 95% of confidence interval of the mean.

Ethical considerations

Study approvals were obtained from the Ethiopian Ministry of Science and Technology National Research Ethics Review Committee and the Johns Hopkins Bloomberg School of Public Health Institutional Review Board. Trained assessors informed health providers and women sought MNH services about the study and asked for their written consent to be observed. Woman was asked to allow trained assessor to observe only her labor and delivery services with the provider however, assessors did not collect data on her name, identification number and pregnancy history. For those women who arrived to the facility with labor pain, her next of kin was asked for written consent for observation. If a woman had complication, assessors did not ask written consent from a woman or her next of kin; and they waited another women who came for labor and delivery services to use for providers observations.

Results

Sample characteristics

The sample consisted of 147 MNH providers (79 in the SBM-R intervention group and 68 in the comparison group). Most providers were female in both intervention (77.2%) and comparison (70.6%) groups, and one-third were over age 30 (Table 1). A large majority were midwives and nurses, and about half worked at hospitals and half at health centers. Almost half had fewer than five years of work experience in both intervention (48.1%) and comparison (45.6%) groups. There were no significant differences in provider or facility characteristics between intervention and comparison groups.

Degree of similarity of MNH providers' performance at facility and provider levels

As shown in Table 2, assessors observed 232 ANC clients who were attended by 63 different health providers, 226 labor and delivery clients who were observed with 117 different providers and 229 PNC clients who were observed with 109 providers. ICC values vary, but are higher in the intervention than in the comparison group with one exception (PNC services at the facility level). This suggests that the quality of services offered was more uniform at intervention than comparison facilities. The greatest differences between intervention and comparison groups were seen in labor and delivery services: provider performance was more similar within each facility in intervention (ICC = 0.775) than in comparison facilities (ICC = 0.454), and performance was also more similar for multiple observations of the same provider in intervention (ICC = 0.632) than in comparison facilities (ICC = 0.474).

Health provider performance

ANC services

Average overall performance scores for ANC services were 63.4% in the intervention and 61.0% in the comparison group ($p = 0.650$). There were no significant differences between study groups in any of the eight skill

Table 1 Characteristics of providers observed

Demographic and work-related characteristics	Intervention group ($n = 79$)		Comparison group ($n = 68$)		p-value (Chi square test)
	n	%	n	%	
Gender					
Female	61	77.2	48	70.6	0.360
Male	18	22.8	20	29.4	
Age					
< 25 years	23	29.1	27	39.7	0.337
25–30 years	28	35.5	18	26.5	
Over 30 years	28	35.4	23	33.8	
Qualification					
Nurse	29	36.7	28	41.2	0.746
Midwife	41	51.9	31	45.6	
Other (doctor, health officer)	9	11.4	9	13.2	
Years of work experience in the health care system (private and public)					
< 5 years	38	48.1	31	45.6	0.856
5 to 10 years	20	25.3	20	29.4	
> 10 years	21	26.6	17	25.0	
Type of facility					
Hospital	40	50.6	36	52.9	0.780
Health center	39	49.4	32	47.1	
Region					
Amhara	16	20.3	15	22.1	0.529
Oromia	25	31.7	24	35.3	
SNNP	22	27.8	12	17.6	
Tigray	16	20.2	17	25.0	

areas, although performance scores were higher by over 10 percentage points for rapid initial assessment, preventive treatment and counseling on danger signs in intervention as compared to comparison facilities. Health providers' strengths and weaknesses, as evidenced by higher and lower scores in the various skill areas, were similar in both study groups (Table 3).

Uncomplicated labor and delivery services

Average overall performance scores for uncomplicated labor and delivery services were significantly higher in the intervention than in the comparison group (77.5% versus 65.6%, $p = 0.002$). MNH providers at intervention facilities significantly outperformed those at comparison facilities in 7 of 10 skill areas. Differences between the study groups were greatest for rapid initial assessment (60.6% versus 42.8%, $p = 0.019$), care during labor (81.1% versus 66.0%, $p = 0.001$), and immediate newborn care (76.9% versus 61.9%, $p = 0.013$). Differences between the study groups were smallest (less than 10 percentage points) and not significant for quality utilization of partograph and infection prevention (Table 3).

Table 2 Number of MNH providers and provider-client interactions observed, and intraclass correlation coefficients

Service area	Number of MNH providers observed			Number of provider-client interactions observed			Intraclass Correlation Coefficient (ICC)		
	Total	Inter-vention group	Com-parison group	Total	Inter-vention group	Com-parison group	Cluster level	Inter-vention group	Com-parison group
ANC	63	29	34	232	118	114	Facility	0.551	0.458
							Provider	0.763	0.667
Labor & delivery	117	57	60	226	123	123	Facility	0.632	0.474
							Provider	0.775	0.454
PNC	109	57	52	229	119	110	Facility	0.530	0.573
							Provider	0.658	0.574

Table 3 Adjusted mean provider performance scores, by service area and study group

Skill areas	Number of items	Intervention group		Comparison group		% point difference between study groups	*p*-value[a]
		Mean score	Standard error	Mean score	Standard error		
Antenatal care (*n* = 124 for intervention group; *n* = 120 for comparison group)							
Rapid initial assessment	6	56.5	0.07	40.8	0.07	+15.7	0.099
Preventive treatment	3	58.8	0.05	47.7	0.06	+11.1	0.140
Counseling on danger signs	6	69.7	0.06	59.1	0.05	+10.6	0.174
Friendly reception for women	2	58.6	0.07	50.0	0.07	+8.6	0.346
Obstetrical history taking	11	81.8	0.07	77.4	0.07	+4.4	0.651
Laboratory screening tests	3	82.6	0.10	79.0	0.10	+3.6	0.783
Physical examination	11	73.8	0.03	70.4	0.03	+3.4	0.380
Birth preparedness	11	45.2	0 .07	43.5	0.07	+1.7	0.858
Overall (composite) score	*53*	*63.4*	*0.04*	*61.0*	*0.04*	*+2.4*	*0.650*
Labor and delivery (*n* = 123 for intervention group; *n* = 117 for comparison group)							
Rapid initial assessment	12	60.6	0.05	42.8	0.05	+17.8	**0.019**
Care during labor	10	81.1	0.03	66.0	0.03	+15.9	**0.001**
Assisting women to have safe and clean birth	13	58.9	0.04	43.7	0.04	+15.2	**0.003**
Immediate newborn care	4	76.9	0.04	61.9	0.04	+15.0	**0.013**
Preparation of supplies and equipment	13	81.7	0.03	67.8	0.03	+13.9	**0.001**
Physical and vaginal exam	18	78.1	0.04	65.2	0.04	+12.9	**0.013**
AMTSL[b]	7	82.9	0.03	71.7	0.03	+11.2	**0.005**
Obstetrical history taking	8	84.9	0.06	74.6	0.06	+10.3	0.240
Quality utilization of partograph	14	77.1	0.04	70.7	0.04	+6.4	0.256
Infection prevention steps	6	92.6	0 .02	87.1	0.02	+5.5	0.104
Overall (composite) score	*105*	*77.5*	*0.03*	*65.6*	*0.03*	*+ 11.9*	***0.002***
Immediate postnatal care (*n* = 119 for intervention group; *n* = 110 for comparison group)							
Care for the newborn within first hour after birth	5	79.3	0.04	57.0	0.04	+22.3	**0.001**
Check mother's health after birth	4	66.2	0 .06	44 .2	0.06	+22.0	**0.012**
Overall (Composite) score	*9*	*72.8*	*0.05*	*50.6*	*0.03*	*+ 22.2*	***0.001***

[a]Results after adjusting for clustering effects
[b]*AMTSL* Active management of third stage of labor

Immediate PNC services

Average overall performance scores for immediate PNC services were significantly higher at intervention than at comparison facilities (72.8% versus 50.6%, $p = 0.001$). There was a significant difference of 22 percentage points between study groups in both skill areas: care for the newborn and health check for the mother (Table 3).

Discussion

This evaluation found that the SBM-R quality improvement intervention in Ethiopia had a positive impact on MNH providers' performance in two out of three service areas: uncomplicated labor and delivery care and immediate PNC. Notably, significant and positive impacts on certain important skills that can save the lives of mothers and newborns were found. Rapid initial assessment determines whether pregnant women need emergency care, while immediate newborn care can identify and address potentially life-threatening conditions for newborns. Similarly, active management of the third stage of labor is a proven obstetric intervention for the prevention and management of postpartum hemorrhage [19]. SBM-R also contributed to substantial improvements on postnatal health checks for mother and baby after delivery, which are important to avert key causes of maternal and newborn deaths such as asphyxia, bleeding and severe infection [20].

Several factors likely contributed to these improvements. First is BEmONC training conducted in response to initial results of the SBM-R facility assessments, which primarily targeted midwives working in labor and delivery rooms. Training emphasized clinical competencies of labor and delivery care and immediate PNC services and utilized both simulated and clinical settings. Second is the low percentage of institutional deliveries in Ethiopia at the time of the study [21]; the lighter workload may have allowed midwives to take time needed to properly follow SBM-R standards before, during and after delivery. Third, the SBM-R intervention facilitated mobilization of resources within and outside facilities to address performance gaps. Also, intervention facilities received medical equipment and supplies to improve quality of intra- and postpartum care; this likely increased providers' confidence in their clinical skills.

Findings on labor and delivery care and PNC are generally consistent with evidence from other SBM-R quality improvement interventions directed at MNH services. For example, studies in Malawi and Tanzania showed significant improvements in PNC performance, such as essential newborn care, at sites that implemented SBM-R [8, 22, 23]. Assessments conducted in 11 low-resource countries in Africa and Latin America found evidence that SBM-R interventions not only caused substantial improvement in labor and delivery service delivery practices such as partograph use and active management of the third stage of labor, but also contributed to positive intermediate and long-term health outcomes, such as lower rates of episiotomy and postpartum hemorrhage and reductions in maternal complications and maternal, neonatal and under five mortality [8, 24–27]. However, systematic evaluations of SBM-R in Malawi and Afghanistan found no significant differences in providers' performance in labor and delivery care between intervention and comparison facilities [8, 22].

In contrast to labor and delivery care and PNC, the intervention did not show a significant improvement in providers' performance on ANC. Anecdotal evidence suggests that the lesser impact of the intervention on the quality of ANC performance could be related to providers' qualifications. Unpublished supervision reports from the SBM-R roll-out in Ethiopia indicate that routine ANC is often provided by nurses because the number of midwives at public health facilities is limited. These nurses were trained on general nursing during their pre-service education and did not specialize in MNH. They also did not have the opportunity to receive BEmONC training informed by SBM-R standards. In addition, ANC was often provided to multiple women at the same time, which may have prevented nurses and midwives from meeting SBM-R standards. It is important moving forward to provide refresher training on ANC tasks to all providers who offer these services, including nurses.

Previous studies of the impact of SBM-R interventions on ANC performance have shown mixed results. For example, after SBM-R was introduced at Zambian Defence Force facilities, overall ANC performance increased at intervention sites compared to control sites, but the difference was not statistically significant [28]. Exactly the same pattern was shown in this study, suggesting that SBM-R intervention likely contributed to the wellbeing of maternal, fetal and neonatal health. Other evaluations found that SBM-R interventions improved providers' performance in ANC services in Afghanistan, but not in Zambia and Malawi [8, 22]. Another study in Kenya and Afghanistan indicated that quality improvement interventions enhanced ANC services [19, 25].

As noted above, many of the practices targeted by this intervention have the potential to save lives. Findings from systematic reviews in low- and middle-income countries confirm that quality improvement interventions focusing on healthcare providers' skills can have a direct impact on health outcomes [8]. For example, SBM-R interventions in West African countries have contributed to decreases in institutional rates of postpartum hemorrhage and maternal and neonatal deaths [27, 29]. This suggests that scaling up SBM-R could contribute to achieving national goals for the reduction of maternal and newborn mortality rates. This quality model could also contribute to achieving the Ethiopia MOH's 2020 strategic aims to improve intermediate and long-term health outcomes, such as increasing coverage of four ANC visits from 68 to 95%, births attended by skilled health personnel from 60 to 90%, and postnatal coverage from 90 to 95% [2].

With regard to sustainability, officials who offered supportive supervision and monitored the SBM-R intervention helped in building local ownership of quality improvement strategies at the district and facility levels. Results of the analysis of ICC values suggest that SBM-R contributed to standardization of provider skills in delivering ANC, labor and delivery care and immediate PNC services within and among facilities. Additional activities, such as ongoing mentorship at each facility, may be needed to reinforce and sustain these gains in providers' MNH skills and performance over time.

Strengths and limitations

Strengths of the study included its reliance on direct observations of routine services by experienced assessors using comprehensive and verifiable tools to assess quality of care by comparing intervention and comparison groups. The biggest limitation is the lack of baseline information on provider performance, which makes it impossible to compare changes in provider performance over time between study groups. In future, pre-post study designs are needed to examine the full effects of SBM-R quality improvement tools. In addition, qualitative interview data that could provide a deeper understanding of providers' performance and clients' perspective on the quality of services are lacking. Findings cannot be generalized to all facilities across all regions, and it is possible that other quality improvement approaches fielded by international non-governmental organizations may have contaminated effects in comparison sites. Finally, the study may have introduced the Hawthorne effect, in which providers perform better than usual in response to being observed by external assessors; however, this would have affected both study groups equally.

Conclusions

The SBM-R quality improvement intervention led to significant improvements in health providers' performance in delivering uncomplicated labor and delivery care and immediate PNC services in Ethiopia, a country with limited resources and a low density of healthcare providers. This substantial change contributed to increased availability of good quality MNH services at intervention hospitals and health centers. It also strengthened key skills that have the potential to save lives and reduce maternal and newborn mortality.

The Ministry of Health integrated the SBM-R approach within the existing MNH performance and quality improvement tool; and suggests to scale up across the remaining health facilities in all regions of the country, in order to improve healthcare providers' performance and the quality of care and to contribute to health system strengthening across Ethiopia. These findings will serve as input for implementation of the government's five-year (2015–2020) health sector transformation plan and health care quality strategies to meet the country's sustainable development goals.

Abbreviations

AMTSL: Active management of third stage of labor; ANC: Antenatal care; BEmONC: Basic emergency obstetric and newborn care; ICC: Intraclass correlation coefficient; MNH: Maternal and newborn health; MOH: Ministry of Health; PNC: Postnatal care; SBM-R: Standards-Based Management and Recognition; SNNP: Southern Nations, Nationalities and Peoples; USAID: United States Agency for International Development; WHO: World Health Organization

Acknowledgements

We acknowledge the Federal Ministry of Health of Ethiopia for giving permission to conduct the study and the United States Agency for International Development (USAID) for providing financial support. We are also grateful to Professor Judith T. Fullerton and Adrienne Kols for their critical reviews of the manuscript and Dr. Diwakar Mohan for providing guidance in data analysis. Finally, we would like to acknowledge the study participants, the data collectors and supervisors.

Funding

This study was made possible by the generous support of USAID under the terms of the Leader with Associates Cooperative Agreement GHS-A-00-08-00002-00 of the Maternal and Child Health Integrated Program (MCHIP). The contents are the responsibility of Jhpiego and do not necessarily reflect the views of USAID or the United States Government. USAID did not have any additional role in the study design, data collection and analysis, interpretation of the data, or preparation of the manuscript. Study participants did not receive financial incentives for their participation in the study.

Authors' contributions

FA contributed to the study design, managing data collection, performed the data analysis, interpretation of data and wrote the manuscript. NS, JVR, JS and HG contributed to interpretation of data, drafting and reviewing the manuscript. GE, EB and YMK contributed to the development of the study design and writing the manuscript. AT and ED contributed to the study design, participated in data collection, and writing the manuscript. All authors read and agreed to be accountable for the whole process of the manuscript development; and they approved the final manuscript.

Authors' information

FA: MSc, MA, PhD fellow, Research Team Lead, Jhpiego Ethiopia. GE: MPH, Maternal and Newborn Health Advisor, Jhpiego Ethiopia. NS: MD, MPH, Quality Improvement Advisor, Jhpiego Ethiopia. JVR: Professor, Athena Institute, VU University Amsterdam, the Netherlands. EB: DrPH, MPH, Research Team Lead, Jhpiego USA. YMK: EdD, Senior Research and Evaluation Associate, Jhpiego USA. AT: MPH, Technical Director, Jhpiego Ethiopia. HG: MIH, Registered Midwife, Jhpiego Ethiopia Country Director. ED: MA, Monitoring and Evaluation Team Lead, Jhpiego Ethiopia. JS: Professor, Department of Obstetrics and Gynecology, Leeuwarden Medical Centre and Department of Health Sciences, Global Health, University Medical Centre Groningen, University of Groningen, the Netherlands

Competing interests

The authors declare that they have no competing interests.

Author details

[1]Jhpiego Ethiopia, Addis Ababa, Ethiopia. [2]Athena Institute, VU University, Amsterdam, The Netherlands. [3]Jhpiego, 1615 Thames St # 200, Baltimore, MD 21231, USA. [4]Department of Health Sciences, Global Health, University Medical Centre Groningen, University of Groningen, Groningen, The Netherlands. [5]Department of Obstetrics and Gynecology, Leeuwarden Medical Centre, Leeuwarden, The Netherlands.

References

1. Countdown to 2015. A decade of tracking progress for maternal, newborn and child survival. The 2015 report. Geneva: UNICEF and World Health Organization; 2015. http://countdown2030.org/documents/2015Report/CDReport_2015_ex-profiles_final.pdf. Accessed 24 May 2016.
2. Federal Democratic Republic of Ethiopia Ministry of Health. Health Sector Transformation Plan: 2015/16-2019/20. Addis Ababa: Ethiopia Ministry of Health; 2015. http://www.moh.gov.et/documents/26765/0/Health+Sector+Transformation+Plan/5542a23a-9bc7-46a2-8c1f-8b32c2603208?version=1.0. Accessed 24 May 2016.
3. World Health Organization (WHO). Standards for improving quality of maternal and newborn care in health facilities. Geneva: WHO; 2016. http://apps.who.int/iris/bitstream/10665/249155/1/9789241511216-eng.pdf. Accessed 20 August, 2016.
4. Rowe AK, de Savigny D, Lanata CF, Victora CG. How can we achieve and maintain high-quality performance of health workers in low-resource settings? Lancet. 2005;366:1026–35.

5. Dettrick Z, Firth S, Jimenez Soto E. Do strategies to improve quality of maternal and child health care in lower and middle income countries lead to improved outcomes? A review of the evidence. PLoS One. 2013;8(12), e83070. doi:10.1371/journal.pone.0083070.
6. Tawfik Y, Segall M, Necochea E, Jacobs T. Finding common ground: harmonizing the application of different quality improvement models in maternal, newborn, and child health programs. Bethesda: University Research Co., LLC (URC); 2010. http://www.coregroup.org/storage/documents/ME/Finding_common_ground.pdf. Accessed 24 May 2016.
7. Althabe F, Bergel E, Cafferata ML, Gibbons L, Ciapponi A, Alemán A, et al. Strategies for improving the quality of health care in maternal and child health in low- and middle-income countries: an overview of systematic reviews. Paediatr Perinat Epidemiol. 2008;22 Suppl 1:42–60.
8. Necochea E, Tripathi V, Kim YM, Akram N, Hyjazi Y, da Luz Vaz M, et al. Implementation of the Standards-Based Management and Recognition approach to quality improvement in maternal, newborn, and child health programs in low-resource countries. Int J Gynaecol Obstet. 2015;130 Suppl 2:S17–24.
9. Lassi ZS, Musavi NB, Maliqi B, Mansoor N, de Francisco A, Toure K, Bhutta ZA. Systematic review on human resources for health interventions to improve maternal health outcomes: evidence from low- and middle-income countries. Human Resour Health. 2016;14:10.
10. Federal Democratic Republic of Ethiopia, Ministry of Health. Basic emergency obstetric & newborn care (BEmONC) training manual. Addis Ababa: Ethiopia Ministry of Health; 2013. http://pdf.usaid.gov/pdf_docs/PA00JX4F.pdf. Accessed 7 Nov 2016.
11. Adams G, Gulliford MC, Ukoumunne OC, Eldridge S, Chinn S, Campbell MJ. Patterns of intracluster correlation from primary care research to inform study design and analysis. J Clin Epidemiol. 2004;57:785–94.
12. Eldridge SM, Ukoumunne OC, Carlin JB. The intra-cluster correlation coefficient in cluster randomized trials: a review of definitions. Int Stat Rev. 2009;77:378–94.
13. Getachew A, Ricca J, Cantor D, Rawlins B, Rosen H, Tekleberhan A, et al. Quality of care for prevention and management of common maternal and newborn complications: a study of Ethiopia's hospitals. Baltimore: Jhpiego; 2011. http://www.healthynewbornnetwork.org/hnn-content/uploads/Ethiopia_QoC_formatted_final.pdf. Accessed 24 May 2016.
14. Scheffler RM, Bruckner T, Spetz J. The labor market for human resources for health in low and middle income countries. Human Resources for Health Observer No. 11. Geneva: World Health Organization; 2012. http://www.who.int/hrh/resources/Observer11_WEB.pdf. Accessed 7 Nov 2016.
15. Park S, Lake ET. Multilevel modeling of a clustered continuous outcome: nurses' work hours and burnout. Nurs Res. 2005;54:406–13.
16. Wears RL. Advanced statistics: statistical methods for analyzing cluster and randomized data. Acad Emerg Med. 2002;9:330–41.
17. Killip S, Mahfoud Z, Pearce K. What is an intracluster correlation coefficient? Crucial concepts for primary care researchers. Ann Fam Med. 2004;2:204–8.
18. Hayes FA. A primer on multilevel modeling. Hum Commun Res. 2006;32:385–410.
19. Tawfik Y, Bongiovanni A, Vaid S, Hermida J, Boucar M, Hill K. Taking every opportunity to save lives: the role of modern quality improvement in enhancing maternal, newborn, and child health programs. A synthesis of USAID Health Care Improvement Project field experience. Health Care Improvement Project Technical Report. Bethesda: University Research Co., LLC (URC); 2012. https://www.usaidassist.org/sites/assist/files/role_of_qi_in_enhancing_mnch_programs_june2012_0.pdf. Accessed 24 May 2016.
20. Matthews M, Severin VX, Jelka Z. WHO technical consultation on postpartum and postnatal care. Geneva: World Health Organization; 2010. https://www.usaidassist.org/sites/assist/files/role_of_qi_in_enhancing_mnch_programs_june2012_0.pdf. Accessed 20 Sep 2016.
21. Central Statistical Agency [Ethiopia] and ICF International. Ethiopia Demographic and Health Survey 2011. Addis Ababa: Ethiopia and Calverton, Maryland: Central Statistical Agency and ICF International; 2012.
22. Rawlins BJ, Kim YM, Bazant E, Rashidi T, Bandazi SN, Kachale F, et al. Reproductive health services in Malawi: an evaluation of a quality improvement intervention. Midwifery. 2013;29:53–9.
23. Makene CL, Plotkin M, Currie S, Bishanga D, Ugwi P, Louis H. Improvements in newborn care and newborn resuscitation following a quality improvement program at scale: results from a before and after study in Tanzania. BMC Pregnancy Childbirth. 2014;14:381.
24. Singh K, Brodish P, Speizer I, Barker P, Amenga-Etego I, Dasoberi I, et al. Can a quality improvement project impact maternal and child health outcomes at scale in northern Ghana? Health Res Policy Syst. 2016;14:45.
25. Zainullah P, Kim YM, Bazant E, Yari K. Raising the quality of care: an impact evaluation in Afghanistan. Presented at the ISQua 30th International Conference on Quality and Safety in Population Health and Healthcare. 2013. http://www.isqua.org/docs/default-source/edinburgh/abstract-15mins-edinburgh-2013.pdf?sfvrsn=2. Accessed 10 Feb 2016.
26. Kabo M, Otolorin E, Williams E, Orobaton O, Abdullahi H, Sadauki H, et al. Monitoring maternal and newborn health outcomes in Bauchi State, Nigeria: an evaluation of a standards-based quality improvement intervention. Int J Qual Health Care. 2016;28:566–72.
27. Rawlins B, Kim YM, Haver J, Rozario A, Kols A, Chiguvare H, et al. Case study: experience applying and tracking a quality improvement approach for maternal and newborn health services in Sub-Saharan Africa. World Health Popul. 2015;16(2):31–8.
28. Kim YM, Chilila M, Shasulwe H, Banda J, Kanjipite W, Sarkar S, et al. Evaluation of a quality improvement intervention to prevent mother-to-child transmission of HIV (PMTCT) at Zambia defence force facilities. BMC Health Serv Res. 2013;13:345.
29. Bhutta ZA, Darmstadt GL, Haws RA, Yakoob MY, Lawn JE. Delivering interventions to reduce the global burden of stillbirths: improving service supply and community demand. BMC Pregnancy Childbirth. 2009;9 Suppl 1:S7.

3

Principles and processes behind promoting awareness of rights for quality maternal care services: a synthesis of stakeholder experiences and implementation factors

Asha S. George[1,2*] and Casey Branchini[2]

Abstract

Background: Promoting awareness of rights is a value-based process that entails a different way of thinking and acting, which is at times misunderstood or deemed as aspirational.

Methods: Guided by the SURE framework, we undertook a secondary analysis of 26 documents identified by an earlier systematic review on promoting awareness of rights to increase use of maternity care services. We thematically analysed stakeholder experiences and implementation factors across the diverse initiatives to derive common elements to guide future efforts.

Results: Interventions that promote awareness of rights for maternal health varied in nature, methodological orientation, depth and quality. Materials included booklets, posters, pamphlets/ briefs and service standards/charters. Target populations included women, family members, communities, community structures, community-based and non governmental organizations, health providers and administrators, as well as elected representatives. While one initiative only focused on raising awareness, most were embedded within larger efforts to improve the accountability and responsiveness of service delivery through community monitoring and advocacy, with a few aiming to change policies and contest elections. Underlying these action oriented forms of promoting awareness of rights, was a critical consciousness and attitudinal change gained through iterative capacity-building for all stakeholders; materials and processes that supported group discussion and interaction; the formation or strengthening of community groups; situational analysis to ensure adaptation to local context; facilitation to ensure common ground and language across stakeholders; and strategic networking and alliance building across health system levels. While many positive experiences are discussed, few challenges or barriers to implementation are documented. The limited documentation and poor quality of information found indicate that while various examples of promoting awareness of rights for maternal health exists, research partnerships to systematically evaluate their processes, learning and effects are lacking.

Conclusion: Rather than being aspirational, several examples of promoting awareness of women's rights for quality maternity care services exist. More than mainly disseminate information, they aim to change stakeholder mindsets and relationships across health system levels. Due to their transformatory intent they require sustained investment, with strategic planning, concrete operationalization and political adeptness to manage dynamic stakeholder expectations and reactions overtime. More investment is also required in research partnerships that support such initiatives and better elucidate their context specific variations.

Keywords: Rights, Health promotion, Maternal health, Implementation, Context, Stakeholder perspectives

* Correspondence: asgeorge@uwc.ac.za
[1]South African Research Chair in Health Systems, Complexity and Social Change, School of Public Health, University of the Western Cape, Private Bag X17, Bellville 7535, South Africa
[2]Health Systems Program, Department of International Health, Johns Hopkins School of Public Health, 615 North Wolfe Street, Baltimore, MD 21205, USA

Background

Women's rights in pregnancy and childbirth were agreed to in 1994 at the International Conference on Population and Development [1]. Subsequently, these rights were endorsed by multiple United Nations agencies and bodies, donors and civil society [2–6]. Despite this affirmation, women still struggle to claim their sexual and reproductive rights, including those related to maternity care services. Notwithstanding overall declines in maternal mortality, skilled attendance at birth remains one of the most glaring inequalities in global health [7]. Even when women do access maternity care services, the disrespect and abuse they face in those services is an extreme violation of their rights [8].

In a previous systematic review, we assessed the effects of interventions that promote awareness of rights on the use of maternity care services in low and middle income countries (LMICs) [9]. We identified four studies promoting awareness of rights that reported health outcomes with clear research methods detailing increases in antenatal care [10–12] and facility births [11–13]. Improvements in human rights measures such as availability, acceptability, accessibility, quality of care, as well as the capacity of stakeholders were also reported to varying extents by these four studies.

Promoting awareness of rights is a value-based social process that often entails a different way of thinking and acting. Their efforts to transform health systems is at times misunderstood or seen as just aspirational. Shakespeare in Hamlet memorably stated 'though this be madness, yet there is method in it' [14]. We examine the diverse range of initiatives that promote awareness of rights to quality maternity care services to derive the common principles and processes related to stakeholder experiences and implementation factors to guide future efforts in this area.

Methods

We undertook a secondary analysis of the documents identified through the systematic review [9]. Documents were identified through a systematic mapping of maternal health literature published from 2000 to 2012 that focused on health system and community-based interventions for improving maternal health and for reducing maternal health inequities in low and middle-income countries (LMIC) (http://eppi.ioe.ac.uk/webdatabases4/Intro.aspx?ID=11). In addition, we conducted additional searches for studies in Pubmed from 2010 to 2014, an internet search and contact with experts. Inclusion and exclusion criteria were developed to find studies across all populations with participants defined as pregnant women or women in labor and with interventions aimed to improve awareness of rights among women, men, community members or health workers and program administrators.

For this secondary analysis, apart from the four studies that reported health outcomes in the systematic review, we analysed an additional 18 documents identified through the systematic review as they described interventions promoting rights for maternal health and an additional four that promoted awareness of rights for other health areas [15–18]. Only the studies included in the systematic review [10–13] were assessed for quality using the Effective Public Health Practice Project quality assessment tool [19], designed to assess study quality of quantitative studies across various fields of public health (Table 1).

Data was abstracted and discussed by two persons (AG and CB). Variables included the experiences of key stakeholders, their attitudes and responses to the intervention and contextual factors related to implementation. We conducted a narrative synthesis guided initially by the Supporting the Use of Research Evidence framework (SURE) developed by WHO to highlight relevant implementation and contextual factors [20]. Abstracted findings were reviewed and synthesized by the lead author (AG) following a process of constant comparison. After drafting synthesized findings, authors revisited original articles to check their interpretations.

Results

Study characteristics

The 26 documents that reported interventions that promote awareness of rights for maternal health and other related health areas (Tables 1 and 2) varied widely in nature, methodological orientation, depth and quality. Only four studies included health outcomes, with study quality ranging from strong to weak. Nine were peer reviewed journal articles that were either qualitative [16, 21–23]; used multiple data sources [24–26], or experimental studies [10, 13], with the remaining 17 documents being grey literature.

Across the 26 documents, interventions took place in a broad range of geographical contexts spanning Central Europe, Asia, sub-Saharan Africa and Latin America, with some also in high-income countries [27, 28]. Two initiatives, those supported by SAHAYOG [24, 29–31] and ISOFI India [32, 33] were detailed in more than one document.

Synthesis of study content

Diversity of interventions

Diverse mediums were used to raise awareness of rights through booklets, posters, pamphlets/briefs [10, 12, 16] and in some instances service standards, charters or monitoring tools [11, 13]. In addition, initiatives also raised awareness of rights through mass rallies, campaigns and broader communication efforts [12, 22, 28, 29].

While one intervention focused solely on disseminating information [10], most were embedded within larger efforts to improve the accountability and responsiveness of services through community monitoring and advocacy [11–13, 21, 22, 28, 30, 34]. One also supported women from

Table 1 Studies detailing interventions promoting awareness of women's rights for maternity care services with reported specified health outcomes ($N = 4$)

#	Study	Study type and quality Document type	Setting	Nature of intervention/initiative/project	Reported health outcomes
1	Pandey, Sehfal, Roboud, Levine & Goyal 2007	-Cluster randomized trial -Strong quality Journal article	Uttar Pradesh, India Study in 105 village clusters across 21 districts; Intervention with 22,495 households in 55 village clusters across 11 districts	4–6 public meetings during two visits spaced 2 weeks apart to disseminate information about entitled health and education services and village governance	ANC increase
2	Bjorkman & Svensson 2009	-Cluster randomized trial - Moderate quality Journal article	Uganda Rural Uganda, 4 regions, 9 districts; Study included 50 communities. Intervention with approximately 55,000 households in 25 communities	A community score card process with a week of meetings when communities and health facility staff review local priorities and action plans and agree on contracts monitored by communities, revisited in meetings 6 months later	ANC increase (not statistically significant) Facility delivery increase
3	Ganju, Khanna, Taparia & Hardikar 2014	-Participatory action research -Weak quality Newsletter article	Gujarat, India Intervention with 10,374 people in 12 villages in two districts	Over 2 years local volunteers visit families and prospectively fill a monitoring tool for every woman once during pregnancy and once during post-partum. A report card is developed to dialogue with different stakeholders and support local action.	ANC increase Facility delivery increase
4	Sinha 2008	-Pre- and post-intervention design -Weak quality Working paper	Andhra Pradesh, India Intervention with approximately 40,000 people in 37 villages and poor area of headquarter village in 1 district;	Over 15 months awareness raising and community support for pregnant women through local government and youth committees; involvement of their families through monthly meetings; and home visits by a community organizer who worked with families to create a birth preparedness plan and support access to care.	ANC increase Facility delivery increase

Table 2 Documents detailing interventions promoting awareness of women's rights for maternity care services or rights for other health areas without reported specified health outcomes ($N = 22$)

#	Document	Document type and study type if applicable	Setting	Nature of intervention/ initiative/ project
1	Bajpai 2009	Report	Rajasthan, India 15 villages across 5 districts of Rajasthan, India	The project supported a Maternal Health Right Awareness program. They supported capacity building of community based organizations, women's self- help groups, health committees, observed outreach maternal and child health days, improved linkages with frontline health workers and held public hearings. Booklets on maternal health entitlements were distributed, meetings held and street plays, folk theatre performed.
2	Burket, Hainsworth & Boyce 2008	Report	Angola, Ethiopia, Ghana, Kenya, Nigeria, Mozambique, Tanzania, Uganda	Pathfinder implemented youth friendly post-abortion care across the eight countries tailored to their specific contexts. Across all eight countries the project worked to improve facility level care through facility assessments, action plans, provider training, orientation meetings for the remaining staff, facility renovations and supportive supervision. In addition, community level work supported sensitization meetings and peer educator training. In particular, in Mozambique, youth associations undertook community mobilization and outreach to raise awareness on rights related to accessing post-abortion care.
3	CARE International & ICRW 2010	Report	Uttar Pradesh, India 2 districts in Uttar Pradesh, India	ISOFI (Inner Spaces Outer Faces Initiative) was from 2007 to 2010. Integrated into an existing maternal health program, interventions facilitated dialogues that explored personal values and challenged assumptions related to gender and sexuality. For example, pictorial flash cards that prompted discussion on men's role as supporters for women's rights, the division of household labor, domestic violence, and women's rights to seek care with a skilled provider. The project also brought couples together in a public location to allow them to learn and discuss MNH care in a safe space and carried out media campaigns (e.g., puppet shows, theater, etc.) focused on gender-related discrimination. CARE also worked closely with district health staff to build community-level capacity. Examples include training for CHWs on counseling men on their role in MNH and the integration of iterative and open-ended exercises for discussion on gender and sexuality with district and sub-district health meetings.
4	CARE International 2012	Report	Bangladesh, Bolivia, DRC, India, Peru, Tanzania	The following case studies were documented: Bangladesh-Community Support Systems in two sub-districts from 2006 to 2010 that tracked every pregnant woman, supported community awareness and resources for maternal health, strengthened local governance mechanisms (based on the Dinajpur Safe Mother Initiative); India-Inners Spaces Outer Faces (ISOFI) see above; Bolivia- Participatory Community Management implemented for 1 year in four rural and peri-urban departments that tracked pregnant women and other types of service utilization, raised community awareness, supported community monitoring of services (based on FEMME program in Peru); DRC -Uzazi Bora Project in Kasongo district from 2007 to 2011 supporting local governance mechanisms, raising community awareness; Peru-FEMME program in Ayacucho region from 2000 to 2005, subsequent policy advocacy to scale up through FEMME+ from 2006 onwards; Tanzania - HEqP Initiative – highlighting inequities and rights violations; community scorecard process, community awareness, advocacy and policy work from 2007 to 2011.

Table 2 Documents detailing interventions promoting awareness of women's rights for maternity care services or rights for other health areas without reported specified health outcomes (N = 22) *(Continued)*

5	Crump 2003	Report	Nepal, Mexico	Nepal newborn case study decided against following a rights approach because it brought in too much complexity, though it included Minister of Human Rights into their work. Findings conflict with other case studies on a rights-based approach to maternal health in Nepal; Mexico Safe Motherhood committee worked on a charter for patient's rights and promoted reproductive rights in reviewing policies, working with other stakeholders, but mostly an overview case study; Indonesia Involvement of Minister of Human Rights in maternal health advocacy
6	Das & Dasgupta 2013	Report	Uttar Pradesh, India	Reflects on the experience of the Mahila Swasthya Adhikar Manch (MSAM) or Women's Health Rights Forum in Uttar Pradesh, India, which raised women's awareness of entitlements and supported their role in monitoring service delivery and dialoguing with policy makers to improve access to health services to improve maternal health.
7	Dasgupta 2011	Journal article Descriptive study	Uttar Pradesh, India	Describes the experiences of a NGO, SAHAYOG, developing 'rights based' strategies around maternal health. Uses recent frameworks on accountability and gendered rights to draw out lessons. Multiple initiatives discussed that raised awareness of rights: forums, campaigns, etc.
8	Davis-Floyd, Pascali-Bonaro, Davies & Gomez Ponce de Leon 2010	Newsletter	Includes examples from Bangladesh, Cambodia, Canada, China, Honduras, Ghana, India, Nepal, Romania, Uruguay.	Outlines 10 steps through which IMBCI aims to improve care throughout the childbearing continuum to save lives as well as prevent illness and harm from the overuse of obstetric technologies and promote health for mothers and babies around the world. Cites the approach as a "testament to and an affirmation of women's fundamental rights during childbirth". Cites the launching of a demonstration project in Canada and Uruguay.
9	DFID 2005	Guideline	Includes examples from Bangladesh, Cambodia, China, Ghana, Honduras, India, Nepal, Romania	Provides guidance to program managers specifically on how to put a human rights-based approach into practice and mentions specific case study examples.
10	DFPA 2010	Report	Bangladesh, India, Pakistan, Nepal	Supports civil society engagement for accountability in health governance Women's Health and Rights Advocacy Partnership (WHRAP) with a focus on sexual and reproductive health and rights in India (Sahayog/Chetna), Pakistan (Shirkat Gah), Nepal (Beyond Beijing Committee), Bangladesh (Naripokkho) through ARROW based in Malaysia from 2003 to 2010. Targets vulnerable women in the most remote areas and applies 1) a rights-based approach recognizing that the rights are at all times relational between citizens (rights-holders) and the state (duty-bearers) and between international obligations and local citizens' claims, 2) a policy engagement approach to increase the influence of civil society in political decision making in health. Community mobilization strategy involving community members and organizations in evidence production and in monitoring government accountability; an advocacy strategy to mobilize political will; an alliance strategy to build civil society coalitions; a boomerang strategy to leverage external and national actors.
11	Kayongo, Esquiche, Luna, Frias, Vega-Centeno & Bailey 2006	Journal article Descriptive study	Peru	AMDD and CARE began Femme project in 2000 focusing on 5 facilities improving EmOC and promoting a human rights approach in health care (specific effort to provide non-discriminatory care to local cultures, signs with information on health services, birthing chairs according to women's preference, improved privacy during childbirth, microwave oven for hot

Table 2 Documents detailing interventions promoting awareness of women's rights for maternity care services or rights for other health areas without reported specified health outcomes ($N = 22$) *(Continued)*

				food, name tags to address women by name, community human rights initiatives to demand accountability).
12	Kenney, Siupsinskas, Sharman, Adilbekova & Zues 2005.	Report	Kazakhstan	*ZdravPlus* is a health reform project, supported by USAID, which assists five Central Asian countries in providing effective and efficient health services through technical assistance to improve quality of care, strengthen the financing systems and management of health services, and enhance the population's involvement in health care decisions. Interventions are linked to the context of de-medicalizing and rationalizing care, reducing the number of ANC visits, unnecessary examinations, tests, episiotomies, increasing attendance of partners at birth and empowering women to choose the position they give birth in, more individual vs. shared rooms, use of partograph, changing sterile to clean enough environment so that family members can more readily access laboring woman, increasing skin to skin, breast-feeding on demand, reducing extent of hospitalization.
13	Molina, Michelini, Escobar & Robinson 2010	Report Internal self-evaluation External qualitative study	Argentina	Evaluation of the 'Child Rights Education for Professionals' initiative, including in its annexes references to 'Te Escucho' a project promoting the rights of children and women within health.
14	Natoli, Renzaho & Rinaudo 2008	Journal article Qualitative study	Ethiopia	Lessons learned on reducing harmful traditional practices from the Adjibar Safe Motherhood project.
15	Papp, Gogoi & Campbell 2013.	Journal article Qualitative study	Orissa, India	Case study of efforts to improve accountability focusing on the role of local women, intermediary groups, health providers and politicians. It highlights three drivers of success: [1] generation of demand for rights and better services, [2] leverage of intermediaries to legitimize the demands of poor and marginalized women and [3] the sensitization of leaders and health providers to women's needs.
16	Reis, Deller, Carr & Smith 2012	Report	19 countries	Outlines findings of RMC survey with key stakeholders about their experience implementing interventions to promote respectful maternity care (48 individuals, 19 countries). Discusses how safe motherhood initiatives must beyond the prevention of morbidity or mortality encompass respect for women's basic human rights. Case studies outlining strategies to ensure that women are better informed of their SRHRs and how to exercise them.
17	Schooley, Mundt, Wagner, Fullerton & O'Donnell 2009	Journal article Qualitative study	Guatemala	Qualitative study of women's support groups seeking care at Casa Materna; a maternity waiting home that provides prenatal, postnatal, infant and well women care inclusive of family planning
18	Shepard 2002	Book chapter Qualitative study	Peru	Qualitative case study documenting the experience of *Consorcio Mujer*, an initiative by several feminist NGOs, to work with communities and health providers in six municipalities. The first phase involved sharing the results of an evaluation showcasing violations of women's rights when accessing health centers and initial dialogues about the results. The second phase supported trainings and meetings with both women in communities and providers separately, before bringing them together for dialogues, that would agree on action plans to improve quality of care in facilities in ways that would respect women's rights.
19	SORAK Development Agency 2013	Report	Uganda	Community-based approach that empowers women with relevant knowledge and skills to demand and access care and commodities to exercise their rights. Discussion of SORAK's projects (2011–2012) and key

Table 2 Documents detailing interventions promoting awareness of women's rights for maternity care services or rights for other health areas without reported specified health outcomes ($N = 22$) *(Continued)*

				achievements. Of specific interest is the Women's Maternal Rights Promotion Project, which is only touched upon briefly. The only indicator provided is process-level (number of women trained). Empowers women (particularly members of marginalized groups) to understand and claim their rights through the establishment of a complaint mechanism
20	Stoffregen, Andion, Dasgupta, Frisancho & Mutunga 2010	Report	India, Kenya, Peru	Field projects undertaken 2008–2009 to increase understanding of rights based approaches to maternal mortality reduction efforts by NGOs in three countries: SAHAYOG in India, FCI in Kenya and CARE in Peru. SAHAYOG supported the Mahila Swasthya Adhikar Manch (MSAM) or Women's Health Rights Forum in two districts to document case studies representing women's experiences of facility delivery and to discuss this with national policy makers as part of a 'Voices from the Ground' meeting; briefing kits for elected officials developed and distributed; public hearings with local officials and women facilitated; booklet that supported discussion meetings following Friere methodology with local NGOs and women members. FCI in coordination with government partners implemented the Right to Care project that conducted workshops with community and religious leaders and health providers on maternal health and rights that resulted in action plans to ensure women's rights to maternal health. CARE worked through its DFID funded Participatory Voices Project in Azangaro and Ayaviri provinces of Puno to support capacity building workshops, alliance building among local civil society networks, community monitoring of services, dialogues with community leaders and local authorities responsible for health services.
21	Strecker, Stuttaford & London 2012	Journal article	South Africa	Evaluation of pamphlets developed on the right to health as a part of a broader action research effort supported by a Learning Network for Health and Human Rights between local universities and civil society organisations.
22	Srofenyoh, Ivester T, Engmann, Olufolabi, Bookman & Owen 2012	Journal article Descriptive study	Ghana	Quality improvement in a hospital where "Customer service was addressed including a patient's right to respect, privacy, emotional support, pain relief, communication, and timely access to care. These elements were promoted through lectures, informal discussion, and bedside example. Satisfaction surveys are conducted to monitor progress. Staff members who demonstrate excellent customer care are recognized".

marginalized communities to run for political office [29]. In addition to disseminating information, these broader efforts fostered critical consciousness and attitudinal change across all stakeholders through capacity-building and training; the formation or reformation of community groups; and facilitated dialogue and participatory exercises [3, 12, 21].

While many initiatives focused on women, they were not always the sole target group. Initiatives also engaged with men and other decision makers at the household level, community structures such as health committees, health providers and managers, as well as elected representatives [11, 12, 29].

In the following sections, we seek to better understand these initiatives raising awareness of rights for maternity care by examining the experiences of each key stakeholder, before analyzing cross-cutting implementation factors.

Women's perspectives and experiences

Few documents assessed women's perspectives about the interventions directly, but several did detail women's sense of personal empowerment and increased self-esteem [12, 16, 21–23, 29, 30]. This change was reported not just for women seeking care, but also for female health volunteers from marginalised communities [33]. Valuing themselves and changing their views about their social background entailed revisiting deep- seated social norms, particularly for women from marginalized communities that were marked by gender and other social inequalities [11, 21, 22, 35]. Some women in India were also hard to reach and engage in group processes because they migrated to their natal homes for pregnancy and childbirth [11, 35].

Key implementation factors included supportive friends and family members for sustaining peer-based learning [3, 12, 22, 23, 33]. Support groups were also valued by women [12, 22, 23] as they provided a space for social bonding, changing social norms and building self-esteem. Having safe environments to practice rights through role playing and/or with family members to learn negotiation and two-way communication skills were valued. Women had to strategize to find the right time and way to approach key individuals or groups; sometimes using humor to address issues [22, 23]. Significant time, capacity-building and iterative efforts were needed to overcome barriers such as paternalistic norms and internalized gender bias [20, 22, 23, 29].

Beyond supporting women's awareness and agency in affirming and negotiating health seeking behaviour with family members and providers at an individual level, the promotion of rights awareness also resulted in women's leadership and collectivisation more broadly [29–31]. For example, in Peru, local women replicated trainings on the right to maternal health with their own community as a means of building women's leadership capacity [22]. In Uttar Pradesh, India, women recognized that they needed to organize at various administrative levels if they wanted their voices to be heard [29].

Community perspectives and experiences

Moving beyond the capacity of individuals, communities as a collective entity also provided critical support in promoting awareness of rights and ensuring their translation into action. In Uttar Pradesh, India [29], Peru and Tanzania [32], women's mobilization strategically linked with other community groups to gain further support and foster a broader collective consciousness supportive of women's rights to quality maternity care. Despite these examples of community engagement and mobilization, very few documents examined community perspectives directly. Those that did so reported positive views [12].

Supportive implementation processes included community dialogues combined with participatory social analysis and critical reflection that helped communities clarify the root causes underlying maternal mortality and discuss issues that had previously remained unspoken or unaddressed [28–30, 32]. In Bolivia, health center tours by community representatives also oriented them to the context of health service provision [32]. Before embarking on such community processes, gaining buy-in from community leaders and other influential community representatives was emphasized [3, 12, 17, 30, 32].

Successful projects also drew on community organizers with prior community work experience and who were trusted by community members [11, 12, 18, 22, 23]. Ensuring a gender balance among organizers, volunteers or peer educators was highlighted as critical to reach both female and male members [17, 18]. Strong relationships between volunteers or community organisers and health services, characterised by familiarity, trust and frequent collaboration, helped to ensure that awareness of rights is linked to increases in utilizing services [12, 17, 32].

Several projects supported local health committees and other structures that provide oversight of health centers [3, 10, 12, 13, 28, 30, 32, 35], although functionality was a concern in some cases [10, 32]. In Uganda, community awareness of health committee roles and responsibilities, alongside reconstitution of health committees were linked to increased utilization of maternity care services [13].

Several documents emphasized breadth of participation across social groups [10, 13, 28, 32, 35]. Conversely, disseminating information to key groups, without further community dialogue, facilitation or mobilisation, failed to increase maternity care seeking among low caste community members in Uttar Pradesh, India [10]. Barriers to equitable participation ranged from internalised community biases to pressing livelihood needs [30]. Some of these barriers were overcome by holding separate meetings [13], facilitating individual and group discussions about male resistance [12, 23] or identifying champions from specific groups and providing them with capacity-building [32].

Divisions among communities due to political vested interests, whether by insurgents or by entrenched political parties, also challenged efforts to build critical consciousness with respect to rights [22, 29]. Community members in Uttar Pradesh, India, felt that their elected village leadership were unapproachable and monopolized development work [10].

Health Provider's perspectives and experiences

In general, frontline providers over time saw initiatives that promote awareness of rights as positive, particularly when aligned with generating demand for appropriate services [12, 24, 30]. However, some health providers found it hard to accept challenges to their authority, viewpoints and routines [16, 30, 32]. Others interpreted rights narrowly, without understanding the root causes underpinning the challenges women face in seeking care or conversely felt that social change was a longer term process beyond their influence [21, 22].

Health worker resistance or lack of cooperation was also linked to their difficult work environments, which can be contrary to respecting women's rights [3, 28, 30, 32]. Staffing shortages, limited supplies and inadequate equipment combined with large patient loads inhibited provider ability and motivation to support promotion of rights awareness [22, 28]. In India and Bolivia, advocacy by community representatives to improve local budget allocations and resolve supply chain problems, demonstrated to providers' a mutual commitment to improving health [12, 32].

Some providers, while acknowledging service delivery challenges that are beyond their control, also recognized the need for a change in mindsets on their behalf [18, 21, 22, 28, 30, 32, 33]. Supporting attitudinal changes among providers was aided by reflecting on their own experiences as users [22]. Ongoing refresher trainings for health providers to build solidarity/ motivation, especially when interventions are against the mainstream and challenge discriminatory ideologies, was important [32, 33]. Initiatives also focussed on strengthening interpersonal skills, identifying a group of champions to sustain energy for change and using a team approach so that individual providers are not isolated [15, 17].

In Uganda, provider awareness of patient's rights and of their performance being reviewed in local committee meetings was linked to increased responsiveness and utilization of services [13]. However, measures to work with providers to support women's rights to quality maternity services were short lived if they were not combined with higher-level support and structural changes creating a broader enabling environment [15, 22, 24, 28, 32]. Local providers rarely had the authority to address vacancies or delays in supply chains. In addition, managerial policies in certain contexts pushed service delivery targets that were counterproductive to supporting women's rights to quality maternity care [22].

Health administrators and policy makers perspectives and experiences

Only two documents reported views of government officials, which were positive in nature [21, 30]. In particular, in Orissa, India, government officials reported that public hearings were useful in fostering collective critical consciousness and action. They felt that women from marginalized communities as individuals on their own did not have the confidence to articulate service delivery grievances [21].

Even though health administrator and policy makers viewpoints are not well documented, the importance of involving government counterparts, particularly higher level health administrators, in all steps of the project was stressed [25, 28, 30, 33]. Without efforts to ensure policy maker understanding, decision makers in Peru were found to prioritize purely technical interventions over the capacity building and facilitation required to support awareness of rights [32]. Several projects also found buy-in from senior management to be variable [28] [30, 33, 35], even if health administrators and policy makers were appreciative of women and community members monitoring and highlighting service delivery problems [24]. To overcome such challenges, several initiatives stressed the importance of maintaining relationships with administrators and policy makers at all levels of the health system [11, 12, 28, 30, 33, 34] and across political party affiliation given changes due to turnover and elections [32].

Many initiatives stressed the importance of higher level policies that support community inputs in local health planning and service oversight, whether in terms of broad decentralization measures or specific quality improvement mandates [3, 22, 30]. The lack of policies, guidelines or protocols listing out the obligations of health administrators and providers in supporting awareness and responsiveness to women's rights to quality maternity care was also cited as a challenge [28, 32].

NGO perspectives and contexts

All the initiatives documented were facilitated by NGOs and many reported factors that NGOs perceived as supportive or challenging to their efforts to promote awareness of rights. Apart from a few examples, the majority of the articles did not discuss how NGOs themselves benefited or were at risk from this work, despite being central actors facilitating such initiatives.

In the few documents that discussed NGO experience, the capacity of NGOs to support rights initiatives was reported to have improved overtime [30, 33]. NGO efforts to raise awareness of rights and concomitant advocacy also lead to increased visibility and credibility from state actors, media and community members [12, 24]. At the same time,

NGOs also ran various risks. In India [24] and in Peru [22], feminist organizations found themselves at risk of being co-opted by government, when included in government initiatives over which they had no control and that even at times violated rather than supported rights.

When working on government initiatives to advance rights, NGOs in India, Columbia, Peru and Chile noted that government contracts were underfunded. As a result, unpaid staff time and other administrative resources were often not accounted for, resulting in overworked staff and organizational strain [22, 35]. In India, additional staffing and funding was integrated with existing personnel and program systems so that gender and rights methodologies were not seen as extra work with no corresponding support. Flexibility in funding was also essential in supporting local adaptations [35].

Managing strategic alliances across civil society networks and social movements were critical when negotiating with government counterparts [30, 32, 35]. Doing so was reported to be challenging in Peru, due to the politics of representation. Some NGOs tread a fine line when advocating for the interests of marginalized populations, without coming from such marginalized groups themselves [22].

Cross-cutting implementation considerations

This section reviews implementation factors that were not specific to particular stakeholders.

Characteristics of tools

Posting information on free services and using suggestion boxes [13] was found to be effective, while posters explaining patient rights were not effective on their own in Uganda [13] or seen as empty gestures in other contexts [3]. The visual attractiveness and relevance of print materials was an important part of their use in South Africa and in India [11, 16, 32]. Community monitoring is facilitated if checklists are kept simple with indicators that reflect community priorities and that are observable by them [13, 22]. In India, group exercises facilitating dialogue on gender and rights emphasized fun at appropriate instances [33]. NGO involvement in developing the materials and in subsequent training influenced their use of pamphlets, with those less involved being less likely to use the materials [16]. Most critical was the ability of materials and exercises to act as context specific tools to foster interactive learning and dialogue [16].

Strategic orientation

A process of vernacularisation was cited as being critical for local stakeholders to adopt rights principles [3, 16]. This ensures that rights are articulated in a manner that reflects the local context, enabling their internalisation and ownership by local stakeholders. Authors also stressed that this must not contravene the rights principles they are meant to promote.

Several projects noted the importance of engaging both communities and providers simultaneously to promote awareness of rights [11–13, 30]. Furthermore, some initiatives emphasized a phased approach. Ensuring that services can handle increased demand and offer quality services, where women are treated with dignity and are affirmed/ valued, before promoting rights awareness that directs women to access such services [17, 23]. In addition, efforts that pursued multi-level, stakeholder and sectoral pathways were likely to build synergies that sustain the promotion of rights over the long term [12, 18, 32, 33].

Negotiating strategic dialogues and alliances was not an easy or predictable process. It required preparing groups ahead of time, fostering a common language and clarifying rules to counter power imbalances [11–13, 22, 30, 32]. It was also not a straightforward process. As setbacks and backlash entailed iterative capacity building and restrategizing to emphasize common ground and mutual aims. Expectations needed to be constantly re-aligned for both community members and providers [13, 28, 32]. Frustrations at times undermined women's and community members' confidence in their ability to support change [16, 22].

Strategic planning and sustained concrete operationalization

To overcome such setbacks and to realize the deep social transformation that promoting rights awareness entails, several factors related to strategic planning and operationalization were noted, particularly for initiatives to progress from rhetoric to reality.

At the *community level*, many documents stressed the importance of understanding women's realities and what matters most to communities as a starting point [3, 12, 13, 21, 22, 28, 30, 32]. Involving family and community members in the design of the intervention is one way to ensure that initiatives understand their perspectives. In addition, a careful assessment of the local context and advance preparation between various stakeholders is required prior to events such as public hearings are held, to ensure that grievances aired will be addressed and most importantly that there will be no reprisals [21]. At the level of *health services*, a situation analysis to understand the context in which providers work was essential [3, 17]. Several studies also recommended stakeholder analysis or political mapping to ensure that initiatives secure buy-in from key officials and critical stakeholders [15, 22, 30].

Project experiences also emphasized that rights awareness initiatives be grounded in concrete actions and operational plans, with adequate follow up, monitoring and evaluation to ensure that they do realize their goals and not be only aspirational [22, 28, 30, 32, 35]. Costing studies were found to be particularly helpful in supporting and scaling up initiatives in Tanzania and Peru [32]. In addition, continuity of funding and leadership over several years to achieve change at multiple levels is required [18, 24, 32] to sustain initiatives and continually refresh relationships, as key stakeholders, particularly those within government may change.

Without significant capacity and consensus building among stakeholders, these initiatives can fail and frustrate the participants involved. Time and capacity building through iterative processes that support changed attitudes and norms across all stakeholders was noted as being vital across several contexts [16, 21, 22, 29, 30, 32, 33, 35]. Other elements of success included strong leadership, strategic thinking, political adeptness and management skills to support interventions that entail a mind shift that often runs against prevailing social norms [15].

Discussion

Summary of evidence

Across the various initiatives documented, women reported a sense of empowerment and increased self-esteem. This was supported through group processes that broke down isolation, nurtured social bonding and critical reflection. Women's leadership and collective organizing around health rights were also key. Challenges included low literacy and in India, the mobility of pregnant women to natal homes during the period of pregnancy and childbirth. Significant time and capacity building are required to overcome deep seated gender and other forms of internalized discrimination [36].

Communities play a critical role in supporting women's rights to maternity care services [37, 38]. Community dialogues that supported critical reflection about the root causes undermining women's rights to health were instrumental. Gaining buy-in from community leaders and selecting community volunteers that are trusted, gender balanced, familiar with the local context and have strong relationships linking communities to health care services are important. Working through existing community health and local governance structures, such as health committees was critical if they are functional [39]. In some instances these structures needed to be reconstituted. Throughout efforts need to ensure that community processes reflect marginalized women's perspectives and not further marginalize them [36].

Health providers perceived initiatives to raise awareness of women's rights to quality maternity care services as having instrumental value in increasing utilization of services, but also as an opportunity to receive feedback and improve service provision. Similar to what Filby et al. [40] found, resistance was due to a narrow interpretation of rights or due to poor working conditions that constrained responsive care. Efforts to change provider attitudes included reflecting on their own experiences as patients, trainings focussed on interpersonal skills, identification of champions to model positive behaviour and a team approach to ensure against demoralisation. To be effective such initiatives need support from higher level managers and administrators, who reinforce standards and allocate resources necessary for responsive care.

While close collaboration with government counterparts was emphasized to mainstream interventions within the health sector, understanding and buy-in from senior level administrators and policy makers was not always found. Linkages to decision makers at all levels of the health system and across political party lines was important to ensure continuity of efforts, particularly when considering turnover of administrators and instability of political appointees. Ensuring policy recognition and mandate was also critical in enabling community dialogue and inputs into local service delivery for women's rights, just as it is for community participation more broadly [39].

All initiatives documented were facilitated by NGOs, which in many instances led to increased capacity and visibility for them. At the same time, many NGOs also ran risks as they were under resourced, with insecure or inflexible funding, resulting in teams that were strained or not as well prepared as needed. When integrating such efforts to existing health projects, additional funding and staff may be required. As mentioned by Marston et al. [38], the legitimacy of NGOs also needs to be carefully balanced with representation of marginalized groups they serve. Strategic alliances across civil society and social movements were critical in ensuring broad based support for efforts to raise awareness of and respond to women's rights to quality maternity care services.

Tools and materials used to raise awareness of rights need to be accessible, attractive and relevant to community members and must also foster opportunities for interactive learning and dialogue. Efforts to raise awareness of rights need to be grounded in the contexts of participants and internalised by them, without at the same time contravening their universal core principles. Initiatives in the health sector need to engage at various levels reflecting the multi-dimensional and multi-stakeholder character of women's rights to quality maternity care services. It entails supporting dialogue and balancing power across stakeholders, whether at the individual level among women, at the interpersonal level with families and communities, at the service delivery level with providers and administrators and at the policy level with higher level decision makers. It requires time, capacity building and iterative facilitation to overcome resistance, backlash and setbacks [36]. Careful implementation with sound situational analysis, planning, budgeting, strong leadership, strategic thinking, political adeptness and good management are required.

Table 3 lists the stakeholder experience and implementation factors documented by the four studies that detailed

Table 3 Stakeholder experience and implementation factors in studies detailing interventions promoting awareness of women's rights for maternity care services with reported specified health outcomes ($N = 4$)

Supportive implementation factors	Challenging implementation factors	Studies			
		Pandey et al. 2007	Björkman & Svensson 2007	Ganju et al. 2014	Sinha 2008
Stakeholder Experience And Implementation Factors					
Women					
Increased awareness and self-esteem					X
Supportive friends and family members, peer-based learning					X
Support groups that provide a space for social bonding, discussion, breaking down isolation, building social ties, changing social norms					X
	Low literacy among women, migration of pregnant women			X	
Community					
Support from community leaders					X
Volunteers with prior experience working in intervention communities and trusted by community				X	X
Volunteers with strong relationships with health services enabling better linkages between communities and health services					X
Community awareness and support; participatory analysis and community dialogue combined with critical reflection and social analysis to identify hidden issues and underlying, root causes				X	X
Peer pressure to prevent harmful practices by traditional healers, violence against women, early marriage, dowry					X
Strengthening existing community governance structures related to health and if they are not functional, either dissolving them or creating parallel mechanisms to ensure community voice			X	X	X
Increased frequency of health committee meetings, although community members were not aware of this		X			
Community awareness of health committee roles and responsibilities			X		
Community action to improve inputs for local health care services fostering a sense of mutual commitments to improving health				X	X
Explicit equity considerations: Separate meetings within communities to ensure representation of interests by marginalized groups; Tailored capacity-building and accompaniment processes; Identification of champions from among the most poor and marginalized.	Social inequality, caste hierarchies, gender discrimination	X	X		
	Feeling by community members that sharing information on entitlements was futile, incomprehensible or fearful	X			
		X			

Table 3 Stakeholder experience and implementation factors in studies detailing interventions promoting awareness of women's rights for maternity care services with reported specified health outcomes (*N* = 4) *(Continued)*

	Vested interests from local elected representatives that are unresponsive to community development needs.			
Health Providers				
Health provider knowledge about patients' rights		X		
Health providers awareness that their performance was being discussed at local council meetings		X		X
Health Administrators And Policy Makers				
Relationships between individuals across levels of the health system			X	X
Non Governmental Organisation				
Additional capacity building, credibility and visibility for non-governmental organisation				X
Cross-Cutting Implementation Considerations				
Characteristics of tools				
Posting information on free services and use of suggestion boxes were effective, in contrast to posters on patient's rights and obligations which on their own were not effective		X		
Simple checklists and indicators that reflect community experience and are observable by them		X	X	
Strategic orientation				
Working with communities and health workers to raise awareness of rights, rather than just one side		X		X
Fostering a common language, clarifying rules to counter power imbalances, fostering dialogue and mutual understanding, supporting a constructive rather than confrontational approach		X	X	X
Multi-level and multi-stakeholder initiatives that build synergies from household level interventions, community actions, health facility interventions to broader systems wide initiatives				X
Strategic planning and concrete operationalization				
Situational analysis of community, health care system, local governance and higher level policy and management linkages;		X	X	X
Time and capacity-building of all stakeholders; Iterative processes to support changed attitudes and norms			X	X

interventions promoting awareness of rights and reported increases in antenatal care and facility births. These experiences and factors are only a subset of those elements reported in the larger set of documents examined. While several factors at community level are detailed, information on women, health provider and NGO experiences are notably scarce across these four studies. Few negative experiences or challenges are discussed. Furthermore, in this subset of studies study quality was inversely related to information related to stakeholder experience and implementation factors. This is partly because the high quality studies were published in journals that emphasize succinct reporting and do not emphasize elements related to implementation or stakeholder experiences.

The poor availability and low quality of information in the 26 documents examined indicate that while numerous examples of promoting rights for quality maternity services exists, the capacity, time and resources to support research partnerships to systematically evaluate their processes, learning and effects is lacking.

Strengths and limitations

Strengths of the synthesis include the concerted effort to triangulate multiple potential sources of information, to overcome the challenge of finding quality documentation of interventions that promote awareness of rights for maternity care services, despite consensus of its strategic value. Nonetheless, the variable quality across all documents meant an over-reliance on the few studies and reports that documented stakeholder perspectives and implementation considerations.

Conclusion

Despite the diversity of examples found, initiatives promoting awareness of women's rights to quality maternity care services have a strong commonality. They can have strong positive effects on individual women, nurturing collective dialogue and negotiation skills with other stakeholders to raise awareness of and respond to their rights. While illustrative examples are highlighted in this review, many interventions have yet to be evaluated and several are poorly documented. More investment is required to create and sustain research partnerships that support such initiatives and better elucidate their context specific variations. Rather than being aspirational, promoting awareness of women's rights to quality maternity services is more than just disseminating information about rights. The strongest examples reflected efforts to change mindsets and relationships among varied stakeholders at different levels of the health system through social processes over time to overcome resistance, backlash and setbacks. Promoting and realizing these rights are at the heart of societal and health system transformation. They require sustained investment and are not for the feint hearted or weary.

Abbreviations

ISOFI: Inner spaces outer faces initiatives; NGO: Non governmental organisation; SURE: Supporting the use of research evidence framework; WHO: World Health Organisation

Acknowledgements

The authors would like to thank all the World Health Organization Guidelines Development Group Members involved in the July 2014 consultation to develop guidance on health promotion interventions for maternal and newborn health, as well as all the experts that responded to the emails searching for studies. Lars Åke Persson, Helen Smith, Rajat Khosla and Avni Amin also provided particularly helpful advice. This work would not have been possible without the leadership, guidance and patience provided by Anayda Portela.

Funding

AG's time was supported by the South African Research Chairs Initiative of the Department of Science and Technology and National Research Foundation of South Africa (Grant No 82769). Any opinion, finding, conclusion or recommendation expressed in this material is that of the authors and NRF cannot accept any liability in this regard.

Authors' contributions

AG conceived of the review with inputs from WHO. CB undertook the searches, undertook data extraction and initial analysis. AG drafted the manuscript with CB's inputs. Both authors read and approved the final manuscript.

Competing interests

The authors declare that they have no competing interests.

References

1. United Nations. International conference on population and development program of action. New York: United Nations Population Fund; 1994. p. 296
2. United Nations Secretary General. Global strategy for Women's and Children's health. New York: Partnership for Maternal, Newborn and Child Health; 2010. p. 20.
3. DFID. How to reduce maternal deaths: rights and responsibilities. London: UK Department for International Development (DFID); 2005.
4. World Health Organization. Working with individuals, families and communities to improve maternal and newborn health. Geneva: WHO; 2003. WHO/MPS/09.04
5. World Health Organization. WHO recommendations on health promotion interventions for maternal and newborn health. Geneva: WHO; 2015. p. 94.
6. United Nations Human Rights Council. Resolution of the United Nations human rights council on preventable maternal mortality and morbidity and human rights. New York: United Nations; 2012. p. 3.
7. World Health Organization. State of inequality: reproductive, maternal, newborn and child health. Geneva: WHO; 2015. p. 124.
8. World Health Organization. The prevention and elimination of disrespect and abuse during facility-based childbirth. Geneva: WHO; 2014. WHO/RHR/14.23
9. George AS, Branchini C, Portela A. Do interventions that promote awareness of rights increase use of maternity care services? A systematic review. PLoS One. 2015;10(10):e0138116.
10. Pandey P, Sehgal AR, Riboud M, Levine D, Goyal M. Informing resource-poor populations and the delivery of entitled health and social services in rural India: a cluster randomized controlled trial. JAMA : J Am Med Associat. 2007; 298(16):1867–75.
11. Ganju S, Khanna R, Taparia M, Hardikar N. Promoting accountability for maternal health through report card. COPASAH Communique. 2014;8:3–5,33.
12. Sinha D. Empowering communities to make pregnancy safer an intervention in rural Andhra Pradesh. Population Council: New Delhi; 2008.
13. Björkman M, Svensson J. Power to the people: evidence from a randomized field experiment of a community-based monitoring project in Uganda. Quarterly J Econ. 2009;124(2):735–69.

14. Shakespeare W. The tragedy of hamlet prince of Denmark. Vol. XLVI, part 2. The Harvard classics. New York: P.F. Collier & Son. p. 1909–14.
15. Molina H, Michelini M, Escobar R, Robinson G. Evaluation report for Argentinian child rights education for professionals (CRED PRO). Buenos Aires: Iniciative del Cono Sur (FLACSO-CRED PRO); 2010.
16. Strecker M, Stuttaford M, London L. Health rights pamphlets: critical literacy and inclusive citizenship, South Africa. Health Promot Int. 2012;29(2) doi:10.1093/heapro/das067.
17. Burket M, Hainsworth G, Boyce C. Saving young lives: pathfinder internationals youth-friendly postabortion care project. Pathfinder International: Watertown; 2008.
18. Natoli L, Renzaho AM, Rinaudo T. Reducing harmful traditional practices in Adjibar, Ethiopia: lessons learned from the Adjibar safe motherhood project. Contemp Nurse. 2008;29(1):110–9.
19. EPHPP. Quality assessment tool for quantitative studies. EPHP: Hamilton, Canada; 1988.
20. SURE Collaboration. Identifying and addressing barriers to implementing policy options. Version 2.1 ed. Geneva: WHO; 2011.
21. Papp SA, Gogoi A, Campbell C. Improving maternal health through social accountability: a case study from Orissa. India Global Public Health. 2013; 8(4):449–64.
22. Shepard B. Lets be citizens, not patients!: Womens groups in Peru assert their right to high-quality reproductive health care. Responding to Cairo: case studies of changing practice in reproductive health and family planning. New York: Population Council; 2002. p. 339–54.
23. Schooley J, Mundt C, Wagner P, Fullerton J, O'Donnell M. Factors influencing health care-seeking behaviours among Mayan women in Guatemala. Midwifery. 2009;25(4):411–21.
24. Dasgupta J. Ten years of negotiating rights around maternal health in Uttar Pradesh, India. BMC International Health and Human Rights. 2011;11(Suppl 3):S4.
25. Kayongo M, Esquiche E, Luna MR, Frias G, Vega-Centeno L, Bailey P. Strengthening emergency obstetric care in Ayacucho. Peru International Journal of Gynaecology &Obstetrics. 2006;92(3):299–307.
26. Srofenyoh E, Ivester T, Engmann C, Olufolabi A, Bookman L, Owen M. Advancing obstetric and neonatal care in a regional hospital in Ghana via continuous quality improvement. Int J Gynaecol Obstet. 2012;116(1):17–21.
27. Davis-Floyd R, Pascal-Bonaro, D., Davies, R. and, Ponce de Leon, RG. The international motherbaby childbirth initiative: a human rights approach to optimal maternity care. Midwifery Today. 2010;(94):1–14.
28. Reis V, Deller B, Catherine Carr C, Smith J. Respectful maternity care. Washington DC: USAID; 2012.
29. Das A, Dasgupta J. Claiming entitlements: the story of women leaders' struggle for the right to health in Uttar Pradesh. India: The Center for Health and Social Justice and COPASAH; 2013.
30. Stoffregen M, Andion X, Dasgupta J, Frisanch A, Matunga A. Human rights-based approaches to maternal mortality reduction efforts. India: International Initiative on Maternal Mortality and Human Rights; 2010.
31. Danish Family Planning Association. Promoting women's sexual and reproductive health and rights in South Asia: project document 2011–2014. Denmark: DFPA; 2010.
32. CARE International. Learning, sharing, adapting innovations in maternal health programming. Atlanta: CARE International; 2012. p. 91
33. CARE International, ICW. Inner spaces outer faces initiative (ISOFI) toolkit: tools for learning and action on gender and sexuality. Washington, DC: CARE International, ICRW; 2007.
34. London L, Schneider H. Globalisation and health inequalities: can a human rights paradigm create space for civil society action? Social Science & Medicine(1982). 2012;74(1):6–13.
35. Bajpai S. Enhancing community awareness on maternal health entitlements - a report. Ahmedabad: CHETNA; 2009. p. 21.
36. George AS, Scott K, Mehra V, Sriram V. Synergies, strengths and challenges: findings on community capability from a systematic health systems research literature review. BMC Health Serv Res. 2016;16(Suppl 7):623. doi:10.1186/s12913-016-1860-1.
37. Portela A, Santarelli C. Empowerment of women, men, families and communities: true partners for improving maternal and newborn health. Br Med Bull. 2003;67:59–72.
38. Marston C, Hinton R, Kean S, Baral S, Ahuja A, Costello A, Portela A. Community participation for transformative action on women's, children's and adolescents' health. Bull World Health Organ. 2016 May 1;94(5):376–82.
39. George AS, Mehra V, Scott K, Sriram V. Community participation in health systems research: a systematic review assessing the state of research, the nature of interventions involved and the features of engagement with communities. PLoS One. 2015;10(10):e0141091.
40. Filby A, McConville F, Portela A. What prevents quality midwifery care? A systematic mapping of barriers in low and middle income countries from the provider perspective. PLoS One. 2016 May 2;11(5):e0153391.

4

The role of Community Mobilization in maternal care provision for women in sub-Saharan Africa

Choolwe Muzyamba[1,2*], Wim Groot[3], Sonila M. Tomini[1] and Milena Pavlova[3]

Abstract

Background: While the role of community mobilization in improving maternal health outcomes of HIV positive women in sub-Saharan Africa is continuously emphasized, little is known about how legitimate these claims are. The aim of this study is to systematically review the empirical evidence on this issue.

Methods: A systematic search was conducted in PuBMed, Scopus, Web of Science, MEDLINE, COCHRANE, Allied Health Literature, and Cumulative Index to Nursing.

Results: Our search identified 14 publications on the role of community mobilization in maternal care provision in sub-Saharan Africa, including both HIV negative women and women with HIV, that have used experimental research designs. Regarding HIV negative women, literature has demonstrated that community mobilization is a useful strategy for promoting both positive maternal process results and maternal health outcomes. Most of the literature on women with HIV has focused only on demonstrating the causal link between community mobilization and process results. There has been very little focus on demonstrating the causal link between community mobilization and maternal outcomes for women living with HIV. Overall, the results show that while there is some empirical evidence on a causal link between community mobilization and maternal health outcomes for HIV negative women, this kind of evidence is still missing for HIV positive women. Moreover, as shown by the studies, community mobilization as a maternal health strategy is still in its infancy.

Conclusion: Given the gaps identified in our review, we recommend further research with the aim of providing sound evidence on the role of community mobilization in improving maternal health outcomes of women with HIV in sub-Saharan Africa.

Background

Despite improvements in funding and policy recommendations by international organizations such as World Health Organization (WHO), United Nations (UN), maternal health remains a challenge in low income countries [1–3]. Studies show that on average, in sub-Saharan African countries, 720 women die each day during pregnancy and childbirth from causes which are largely preventable [4]. The worst maternal health outcomes are found in sub-Saharan African countries [1, 5].

* Correspondence: muzyamba@merit.unu.edu
[1]UNU MERIT, Boschstraat, 246211, AX, Maastricht, The Netherlands
[2]A9 Marshlands Village Box 32379, Lusaka, Zambia
Full list of author information is available at the end of the article

A combination of vulnerabilities and health system weaknesses including poor health infrastructure, poverty, inequality, and HIV are seen as the causes of high maternal mortality [5]. Further, women living with HIV are four times more likely to die during pregnancy and childbirth than HIV negative women [6]. HIV positive women suffer intersecting vulnerabilities. The combined burden of pregnancy-related complications and HIV status is intensified by stigma and discrimination, which prevent some women from seeking help [7].

Intersecting vulnerabilities are further compounded by the dominance of the biomedical approach in handling maternal health challenges [8]. This approach undermines the potential benefits of local knowledge and strategies [9]. Some scholars contend that lack of community involvement led to failed maternal health interventions in sub-Saharan Africa, including maternal health of women living with HIV [10]. There is a traditional tendency inherent in dominant maternal health approaches to undermine local competencies. More specifically, as an antidote to deplorable maternal health outcomes in poor sub-Saharan African settings, mainstream researchers have continued to recommend conventional solutions such as infrastructure improvement, construction of more hospitals and roads, and promotion of women's rights [11, 12]. While in theory there is no contention on the usefulness of such conventional solutions, evidence has indicated that in practice, little can be done to operationalize these ideal solutions in a sustainable way in poor settings [10]. This is partly because most of these recommendations are costly and thus the majority of the resource-poor governments have been reluctant to implement them. As a result, these solutions remain largely idealistic, especially when applied while ignoring local experience.

Despite the dominant approach to maternal care, several studies have drawn attention to the role of communities and have reported on how involvement of communities, use of indigenous resources and reliance on peer support help to improve health outcomes [2, 13–16]. This observation has ignited the hypothesis that capitalizing on community competencies can complement conventional maternal health efforts especially in sub-Saharan Africa where health systems are inefficient and sometimes inaccessible to many women living with HIV in the peripherals of the societies [17–19].

This is why community mobilization is increasingly being seen as a useful complement to conventional maternal health initiatives [13, 20]. Some examples of initiatives that rely on community mobilization include: a) the "MaiKhanda programme" in Malawi, which is a comprehensive locally-run maternal care project where Traditional Birth Attendants (TBAs) provide maternal services to communities [21]; b) the "Zambulance project", which connects rural Zambian villages to health centers through a locally manufactured bicycle with an attached trailer used to carry patients and pregnant women to remote health centers [22]; c) the "MaiMwana" project in Malawi, which is an intervention aimed at providing peer support to mothers in rural Malawi [21].

Specific to women living with HIV, Rifkin (2012) also argues that in the absence of an exchange of perspectives and views between professionals and communities, maternal health initiatives for women living with HIV in poor sub-Saharan African communities will continue to meet inaction, mistrust, resistance and failure. It is, however, not known to what extent community mobilization can be a useful strategy for women living with HIV [5, 6]. It is not clear which components of community mobilization actually change conditions among women living with HIV nor how this change is achieved [13, 23].

The aim of this study is to provide an overview of the empirical evidence on the role of community mobilization in maternal care provision to women living with HIV in sub-Saharan Africa. We only include studies with an experimental design in order to identify causal effects. Strong evidence for causal inference is a useful basis for establishing definitive conclusions [24]. The evidence on the role of community mobilization in maternal care provision in general is also reviewed.

Our review is imperative for both policy and research. Researchers have hypothesized that through the generation of locally acceptable, feasible, useful and relevant knowledge and experience, including partnerships with health professionals, community mobilization might be the missing link in the improvement of maternal health [14]. Therefore, our review provides a basis for comparing the role of community mobilization in maternal care provision to HIV negative women and women living with HIV. We also highlight specific areas that need further research. The review can help to guide policy and practice in designing maternal health interventions which are relevant, feasible and accessible to local communities in sub-Saharan Africa [5]. The paper further adds to the gap in literature about how to best operationalize the concept of community mobilization in the context of sub-Saharan Africa.

Definition of Community Mobilization

Although community mobilization is seen as critical in maternal health promotion, there is little agreement on what defines community mobilization. This is partly because of the diversity in theoretical roots in the development of the concept of community mobilization. This includes Coleman's (1988), Bourdieu (1986) and Putnam's (2000) theory of social capital, Michael Foucault's (1977) theory of governmentality, Jovchelovitch's (2008) theory of Cognitive Polyphasia and Paulo Freire's theory of "conscientisation". In general, the theoretical roots of community mobilization suggest that this concept is premised on the principles of equity, empowerment, inclusion in decision-making, social justice, attention to community, respect for diversity and collaboration [20, 23, 25]. These principles work as core-values in different definitions of community mobilization. Different scholars attach different levels of importance to different principles in their definitions. An overview of definitions of community mobilization in maternal health research is provided in Table 1.

Table 1 Summary of community mobilization definitions

Citation	Definition	Central theme
[42]	"A process of creating and harnessing the agency of the marginalized groups most vulnerable to HIV/AIDS, enabling them to build a collective, community response, through their full participation in the design, implementation and leadership of health programmes and by forging supportive partnerships with significant groups both inside and outside of the community"	Campbell et al. (2010) - Community participation - Collaboration between community and professionals - Identity - Indigenous actors
[45]	"Community mobilization is defined as a component of externally-triggered HIV interventions, rather than including indigenous community mobilization initiated by grassroots actors with broader interests than HIV."	Cornish et al (2014). - Collaboration between community and professionals
[46]	"A participatory approach, which involves building on local competences and strategies by ensuring that community members take part in decision- making and bring local knowledge, experiences and problems to the fore."	Tripathy et al (2012) - Use of local knowledge - Community participation - Use of indigenous resources
[25]	A capacity building process through which community members, groups and organizations plan, implement and evaluate on a participatory and sustained basis to improve their health or other conditions either on their own initiative or stimulated by others	Howard- Grabman et al (2007) - Local initiatives - Capacity building - Community participatory
[47]	"Community mobilization constitutes active involvement of the community in information sharing , consultation, collaboration and empowerment strategies aimed at bringing change in communities"	Rifkin (2001) - Use of indigenous strategies - Collaboration - Community involvement - Community mobilization as a process/continuum
[48]	"Community mobilization is seen as health promotion intervention which helps communities to identify and undertake appropriate actions in relation to shared problems. Further, there are two types of community mobilization strategies: community organization and building, and community advocacy. The latter assumes involving citizens in institutions or decision which have an impact on their lives"	McKenzie (2013) - Health promotion intervention - Cooperation for collective action - Involvement of community - Community advocacy - Community support
[49]	"Community mobilization is seen as a process where people come together to take action on an issue by relaying on enhanced social connectedness and efficacy or the ability to have influence and control over their situation"	Watson- Thompson et al (2008) - Peer support - Community cooperation
[50]	"Community mobilization is defined as individuals taking action organized around specific community issues. It involves community empowerment, community participation, capacity- building, community coalitions, community organization and development"	Kim- Ju et al (2008) - Community involvement - empowerment, - Capacity- building - Community coalitions - Use of community resources
[51]	"Low- cost, participatory, community- based approaches involving women's groups aimed at effectively improving home delivery practices and birth outcomes in a range of settings"	Nahar et al (2012) - Participatory low cost - Community based strategies - Use of community resources
[21]	"A health promotion strategy best seen as a continuum of process which include, Community informed of decisions made, Community consultation about decisions tokenistically to gain buy in, Community's views taken into account, Joint decision- making , and Community driven decision- making"	Rosato et al (2006) - Tokenistic - Cooperation - Community consultation - Joint effort - Support
[52]	"Community mobilization is the process of engaging communities to identify community priorities, resources, needs and solutions in such a way as to promote representative participation, good governance, accountability and peaceful change"	Mercy- corps (2009) - Community engagement - Use of Community resources - Community priorities - Community strategies
[19]	"Actions that engage and galvanize community members to take action towards achieving a common goal"	Lippman et al (2013) - Engaging community members - Galvanizing community members

From Table 1, it is clear that any operationalization of the definition of community mobilization should reflect the common principles identified above such as community participation, community empowerment, use of community competence, use of indigenous resources, collaboration, community cooperation, use of peer-support. That notwithstanding, most of these principles are related or just synonyms of each other; thus, in general, they can be grouped into three main ones, namely: (a) *reliance on peer support,* e.g. financial, psychological and social support for pregnant women or new mothers by community members.; (b) *use of indigenous resources in maternal care provision,* e.g. service provision by trained traditional birth attendants (TBA); and/or (c) *collaboration between community and professionals in designing maternal care initiatives,* which is seen through collaborative partnerships between health professionals and communities. Taking this into consideration, for the purpose of our review, we define community mobilization as any initiative that is anchored on at least one of these three principles highlighted above. The central theme among the three principles being community ownership in the form of participation in planning and implementation of the initiative regardless of whether the initiative was externally or locally-initiated.

This operationalization of the concept allows us to capture the community constitutes and health outcomes under investigation. Further, due to the lack of a universally agreed upon definition of the concept of community mobilization, we ensured that we captured as much as possible articles with deeper meaning of community mobilization in which community ownership of an intervention was evident from any of the three principles of community mobilization (reliance on peer support, use of indigenous resources in maternal care provision, collaboration between community and professionals in designing maternal care initiatives).

Methods

To identify studies to include in our review, a search was conducted in PuBMed, Scopus, Web of Science, MEDLINE, COCHRANE, Allied Health Literature, and Cumulative Index to Nursing with the help of a librarian of Maastricht University.. We conducted a search using the following key-words: community mobilization and maternal health. In addition to this, synonyms of the above phrases were added based on our exploration of the definitions of community mobilization highlighted in Table 1. A complete chain of words used in the search process can be found in Table 2. The search was conducted in April 2017.

The procedure included search of articles using different word combinations with the help of a librarian (see Table 2). This was followed by screening of abstracts which lead to exclusion of some papers. Further, thorough reading of retained papers was conducted in order to arrive at the final papers to be included in the study.

Table 2 Search strategy

Community mobilization OR community networks OR community groups OR Community coalitions OR community-based OR participatory OR Traditional birth attendants OR community mobilization OR community OR Community engagement OR indigenous strategies OR Local initiatives OR collective action
AND [postnatal care OR Prenatal OR ANC OR emergency obstetrics care OR maternal mortality OR complications during pregnancy OR duration of postpartum stay at hospital OR duration of postpartum stay at home OR community care OR Transmission of HIV from Mother to Child]

To be included in our study, the publications must have:

- reported studies conducted in sub-Saharan Africa
- reported results in English
- reported on community-based initiatives that engaged one or more community groups in concrete participatory activities in designing maternal care initiatives, or used indigenous resources in maternal care provision, or relied on peer support for pregnant women or new mothers.
- have been peer reviewed
- must have made use of an experimental research design, i.e. a randomized trial or a quasi-experimental design..
- must have also been conducted between 1990 and 2015 reflecting the period when HIV became a serious epidemic in sub-Saharan Africa.
- must have evaluated the initiative in terms of process indicators and quantifiable biomedical maternal health outcome indicators as defined by WHO. These include:
  a) *Process indicators for maternal health,* which capture changes in behavior of pregnant women and new mothers. These changes in behavior are usually a direct result of activities of a given maternal health promotion activity and they may include indicators such as: adoption of maternal health-enhancing behavior, increased access to health facility, adherence to antiretroviral therapy if living with HIV, attendance to antenatal and postnatal care, etc. Although useful, these indicators in themselves do not provide information on the results and impact of the activity [2, 26].
  b) *Quantifiable biomedical maternal health outcome indicators,* which capture the eventual health status of the target population and can be divided into [1, 16, 27]: *primary outcomes* (incl. complications during pregnancy and during childbirth, duration of postpartum stay at

hospital/community care at home and maternal depression, such as antenatal and postpartum depression); *secondary outcomes* (incl. postnatal care and emergency obstetrical care, maternal mortality); *other outcomes* (transmission of HIV from mother to child).

The selected publications were then divided into category one studies, which had looked at HIV negative women living in sub-Saharan Africa, and category two studies for women living with HIV in sub-Saharan Africa. The text of the publications was screened based on the same inclusion criteria presented above, and the final list of publications within each category was defined. In Fig. 1, we provide a diagram showing the summary of the search procedure.

We analyzed the text of the publications using content analysis. Content analysis is an approach that helps to synthesize data around key themes. This helps to systematically and objectively describe the study phenomenon [28]. A coding frame was established illuminating the following themes: community mobilization conceptualization, study designs, generalizability of results, process and outcome maternal health indicators. We also followed PRISMA guidelines to ensure quality of our review, see Fig. 1 [29].

Results

In total, 1334 publications were initially identified, after which 859 publications were excluded because neither the title nor the abstract indicated the use of community mobilization or the reported maternal health outcomes. This left us with 475 publications. After reviewing their abstracts in detail, we excluded another 416 articles leaving us with 59 articles. The full text of the 59 articles were read in detail which led to further exclusion of 46 papers for not meeting the inclusion criteria, thereby leaving us with 14 publications for analysis (Fig. 1). These papers were divided into two categories: those that involved HIV negative women (category one) and those that involved women living with HIV (category two). For category one HIV negative we had nine articles, and for category two women living with HIV, we had five articles. A detailed description of the findings of the publications and their results can be found in Tables 3, 4, 5 and 6.

Overall characteristics of publications

Table 3 presents an overview of the general characteristics of the publications reviewed. The studies were published in peer reviewed journals between 1990 and 2015 and were all based on experimental research designs.

Regarding the definition of community mobilization, overall, the studies operationalized community mobilization

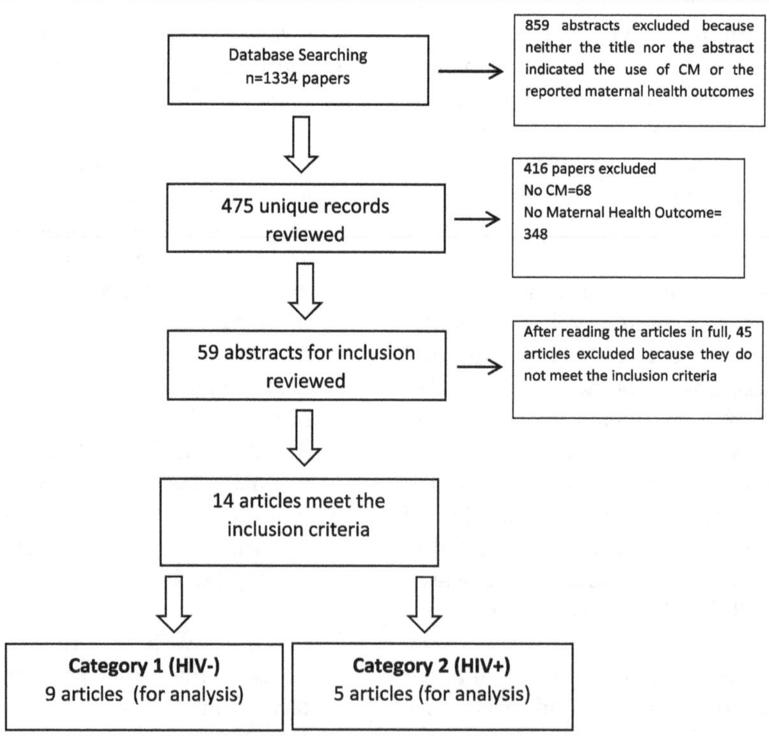

Fig. 1 PRISMA Flow Chat for inclusion and Exclusion of articles

Table 3 Summary of General Characteristics of Result

Characteristic of the publication	Number of publications (%)	Category 1 (HIV-)	Category 2 (HIV+)
Operationalization of Community Mobilization			
-The role of group/peer support for pregnant women or new mothers	5	[8, 17]	[30–32]
-The role of Traditional Birth Attendants (TBA) in maternal care provision	5	[15, 18, 27, 33, 34]	[35]
-The role of partnership between community and professionals in designing initiatives	5	[36–39]	[40]

in accordance with the three main principles namely; *collaboration between community and professionals in designing maternal care initiatives, use of indigenous resources in maternal care provision (e.g. TBA), reliance on peer support for pregnant women and new mothers.* In total, five publications operationalized community mobilization as group/peer support (social, psychological, and financial), another five operationalized community mobilization as the use of indigenous resources in maternal care provision (e.g. TBAs), and another five conceptualized community mobilization as partnership between community and health professionals in the design and implementation of maternal care initiatives.

The role of Community Mobilization among HIV negative women (Category 1) and HIV positive women (Category 2)

Table 4 presents a summary of the indicators used to study the process and outcome of community mobilization among both HIV negative women and women living with HIV.

With regard to HIV negative women, some of the publications reported process indicators which involved adoption of health-enhancing behavior among mothers. The others reported outcome indicators, which included reduction in maternal depression, reduced rates of hemorrhage, reduced neonatal mortality and reduced maternal mortality. On the other hand, the majority of publications on women living with HIV reported process indicators, which included among other things, adoption of maternal health-enhancing behavior among HIV positive mothers. In addition, a few reported outcome indicators such as reduced depression among HIV pregnant women.

Peer support was explicated in the form of regular meetings in women's groups where pregnant women provided each other with emotional, physical, social and psychological support to deal with high levels of psychological

Table 4 Summary of results for HIV Negative (Category 1) and HIV positive women (category 2)

HIV negative (category 1)			
Process outcomes:	Value reported	Number of publications	Publication reference number
Health-enhancing behavioral	Positive change (e.g. increased access to health facility, enhanced the pregnant women's knowledge on how to handle maternal complications)	6	[15, 18, 27, 33, 36, 37]
Outcome indicators			
Depression rate	Reduced depression	3	[8, 17, 38]
Maternal mortality	Reduced maternal mortality	2	[17] [34]
Hemorrhage/sepsis	Reduced hemorrhage	1	[34]
HIV Positive (category 2)			
Process outcomes:	Value reported	Number of publications (%)	Publication reference number
Health-enhancing behavioral	Positive change: increased maternal health knowledge, Increased utilization and access to health-enhancing resources e.g. antenatal & primary healthcare, PMTCT, information on safe delivery services)	5	[30, 31, 32, 35, 40]
Outcome Indicators			
Depression rate	Reduced depression	1	[30]
Maternal mortality	Reduced maternal mortality	0	
Hemorrhage/sepsis	Reduced hemorrhage	0	

Table 5 Category 1: Detailed results for HIV negative women

Citation	Country	Study Design	Community Mobilization Component	Process results	Outcome
1. [36]	Tanzania	Longitudinal	Community Capacity Building & Empowerment support for village health workers; (2) developing community-based plans for transportation to health facilities; & (3) increasing participation by community members in planning;	Significant improvement in access t health facilities due to increased transport options Increased attention to Obstetric complications by 275 Deliveries attended by a relative/community member or no one decreased 4% & 6%, respectively but by a TBA increased 200%	
2. [8]	Malawi	randomized controlled trial	Established participatory women's groups to mobilize communities around maternal and newborn health		A combined community and facility approach using participatory women's groups and quality improvement at health centers reduced newborn mortality in rural Malawi
3. [17]	Malawi	Randomized trial	Established Community women's groups to ensure provision of socioeconomic support	Better health outcomes for infants reduction in disease for both mother and child Better health-seeking behavior Increased Uptake of HIV testing	Reduced MMR, NMR and IMR in treated group, Conclusion: Community mobilisation through women's groups and volunteer peer counsellor health education are methods to improve maternal and child health outcomes in poor rural populations in Africa.
4. [37]	Kenya	Randomized control trials	Involvement of Community Health Workers in provision of maternal health services	Increased visits to health center, increased deliveries by skilled personnel, "Conclusion increase in essential maternal and neonatal care practices	
5. [38]	Ethiopia	randomized controlled trial	Mother to Mother support in recognizing maternal health risks		Reduced MMR, NMR and IMR in treated group
6. [34]	Angola	longitudinal	Involvement of traditional birth attendants (TBAs) prenatal, delivery, and postnatal care		Better MMR, NMR and IMR outcomes
7. [33]	Sahel	Longitudinal	Involving TBAs to promote safe motherhood	- High levels of retained knowledge of risk factors, hygiene and malaria prophylaxis in 2-year followup survey. - Low levels of knowledge of postpartum haemorrhage management, low number of births attended for most"	
8. [27]	Nigeria	Longitudinal	"Involved traditional birth attendants (TBAs) in a rural community maternal health care provision	- Increased referrals to health centers increased use of family planning	Reduced haemorrhage, oedema, extended labour cases
14. [18]	Sudan	Longitudinal	Involvement of Village TBAs to detect high-risk pregnancy and newborns complications	Increased reporting of complications Increased detection of complications	25% reduction in cases of stillbirth and neonatal death

Table 6 Category 2: Detailed results for women living with HIV

Citation	Country of origin	Study Design	Community Mobilization Component	Process results	Outcome
1. [30]	South Africa	Randomized Controlled Trial	Involvement of fellow HIV positive pregnant women to mobilize and provide support to fellow HIV positive mothers.	- Women in Treatment Group (TG) exhibited Increased knowledge on how to improve the health of their children - Increased access to information and resources to improve their health during maternity	- Mothers in Treatment Group (TG) exhibited reduced maternal depression when compared to their counter-parts
2. [31]	Tanzania	Randomized controlled trial	Creation of peer support group that provided a safe space for women with high levels of psychological distress to discuss and share strategies for addressing common concerns related to PMTCT among HIV positive pregnant women.	- Increased disclosure among HIV positive pregnant women in the treatment group as compared to those in the control group. - Women in Treatment Group experienced a significantly higher rate of overall personal satisfaction with response to disclosure,	- a marginally significant reduction in the level of depressive symptoms for HIV-positive pregnant women participating in a group counseling intervention (Treatment Group) 60% of women in the intervention group were depressed post-intervention, versus 73% in the control group [Relative Risk (RR) 0.82, 95% confidence interval (CI): 0.671.01, p0.066]. H
3. [32]	South Africa	cluster randomized controlled	The intervention consisted of four antenatal and four postnatal small group sessions led by Peer Mentors, in addition to Standard Care. HIV positive pregnant Women were recruited during pregnancy and 70 % were reassessed at 1.5 months post-birth.	Compared to Standard Care WLH, EI (treatment Group) were more likely to ask partners to test for HIV (OR = 1.84; two-sided p = 0.014),	Compared to Standard Care WLH, EI (treatment Group) were more likely to have infants with height-for-age z-score ≥ −2 (OR = 3.30; p = 0.006) and were less likely to report depressed mood (OR = 2.55; p = 0.003). - Healthcare utilization was similar across conditions. - Significant improvement in PMTCT
8. [40]	Zambia	(Longitudinal)	Healthcare workers (HCWs) and lay providers conduct rapid HIV testing. support for pregnant women,"	Uptake of services significantly improved HIV testing among pregnant women improved - There was also significant improvement in the percentage of HIV positive pregnant women referred for clinical care	

distress and other practical needs. They also shared strategies for addressing common concerns related to antenatal and primary healthcare, including Prevention of Mother To Child Transmission (PMTCT) among women with HIV. Although there was more emphasis on support for PMTCT for women with HIV, in general, the type of peer support (financial, psychological, and material) given was to a large extent similar for both HIV negative and women positive women [8, 17, 30–32].

For HIV negative women, peer support improved emotional strength and enhanced pregnant women's knowledge on how to handle maternal complications such as antepartum and postpartum hemorrhage, obstructed labor, and sepsis [8]. Further, peer support arising from participation in women's groups in the community significantly reduced the risk of mortality among newly born children [8, 17]. Overall, the majority of publications in this systematic review concluded that peer support in HIV negative women led to improvements in maternal and child health outcomes due to improved access to emotional, psychological, social and physical support, which enabled pregnant women to access information, services and resources that are necessary for improving maternal health outcomes .

Three publications regarding women with HIV reported that peer support among other things, helped to increase access to health-enhancing resources (such as antenatal and primary healthcare, PMTCT, information on safe delivery services) and knowledge, it also increased utilization of health services by providing pregnant women with transport to health centers and safe delivery packages. Women with HIV who had peer support also experienced reduced maternal depression [30–32].

- Use of traditional birth attendants (TBA) in maternal care provision

The studies that reported on TBAs demonstrated how TBAs helped to increase women's knowledge on risk factors during pregnancy, knowledge on hygiene, use of malaria prophylaxis among HIV negative pregnant women who were outside the catchment area of standard health care [18, 27, 33]. One publication highlighted that the use of TBAs helped to reduce maternal depression, hemorrhage, and maternal mortality among HIV negative women [34]. These studies concluded that in general, TBAs contribute positively to maternal health outcomes of HIV negative women in the peripherals of sub-Saharan Africa.

Among women living with HIV, the only publication that was found concluded that using TBAs enhanced the coverage of maternal health care for women living with HIV especially in areas where many pregnant women chose to have home deliveries [35]. TBAs were considered useful because they encouraged women with HIV to take medication (e.g. zidovudine), which helped to prevent mother-to-child transmission of HIV during pregnancy. The evidence examined in this systematic review however does not report exactly on whether and how the TBAs managed to deal with complications such as hemorrhage, sepsis and PMTCT. The only study on women living with HIV was also silent on what mechanisms were available to TBAs for referral purposes in cases of emergency.

- Collaboration between community and professionals in designing and/or implementing initiatives

The role of collaboration in the design and implementation of maternal care initiatives for HIV negative women was studied in four publications [36–39]. Collaboration helped to design initiatives that improved access to professional treatment. Such initiatives included transportation of pregnant women by community members to health centers in case of obstetric emergencies. This sort of collaboration increased the attention to other complications such as sepsis and hemorrhage. This was because the collaboration allowed for easy exchange of knowledge and information regarding these complications between professionals and the community [36–39]. Further, it was deduced from the publications that through the collaboration between the community and professionals, there was an increase in antenatal services and institutional delivery [36, 37]. Other studies showed that through the collaboration between health workers and local community members, there was a significant reduction in child mortality of up to 57% [38]. Another study from Tanzania concluded that through collaboration with community care-givers, health-inhibiting practices during home deliveries were mitigated (e.g. use of unclean thread to tie the umbilical cord, putting "substances" on the cord) [39]. Overall, it is evident from the publications that collaboration between professionals and communities in the design of maternal care initiatives improved access to health information, treatment and services, as well as increased attention to maternal health complications, thereby making this a viable strategy in an attempt to improve maternal health outcomes of HIV negative women.

On the other hand, only one publication evaluated the role of community involvement in promoting maternal health of women living with HIV [40]. This study also only reported positive process results in the form of improved uptake of institutional health services and acceptance of maternal health interventions; both of which are assumed to be important in improving maternal health of women living with HIV. It is therefore clear that the focus of research on community involvement and maternal health outcomes of women with HIV was limited to explication of process results only, without much on outcomes. There is still a gap in linking collaboration in maternal care initiatives to outcome results such as reduced maternal mortality, reductions in complications such as sepsis and hemorrhage in women with HIV.

Discussion

Overall, this systematic review of experimental design studies has produced results which differ somewhat between women living with HIV and HIV negative women. We observe that to date, there is sound causal evidence in support of community mobilization as a useful maternal health care strategy for HIV negative women. On the other hand, strong evidence for women with HIV is still missing. The fact that strong evidence linking community mobilization to maternal health outcomes for women with HIV is still missing confirms Kendall and Langer's (2015) assertion that the intersection of HIV and pregnancy has generally been ignored in social science research [4]. This is despite the fact that women with HIV are more susceptible to morbidity and mortality during pregnancy [5]. Below we demonstrate in detail the differences in empirical evidence between HIV negative women and women living with HIV using the three principles of community mobilization.

Firstly, evidence indicates that for HIV negative women, *peer support* from fellow pregnant women improves maternal health outcomes. Our findings are consistent with a growing body of literature which shows that peer support is necessary in reducing rates of maternal depression, antepartum and postpartum hemorrhage, obstructed labor and sepsis in HIV negative women [41]. This is normally achieved through provision of economic and psychological support to peers, including sharing of different strategies in order to deal with negative maternal outcomes. It is clear from existing literature that peer support is useful for HIV negative women, however, the same cannot be said of women with HIV. Given the relatively high risk associated with HIV/AIDS, and this coupled with the lack of studies focusing on women with HIV, it remains unclear whether peer support can also be useful in reducing maternal complications in women with HIV, and if so, in which ways. This however does not imply that peer support is completely useless for women with HIV. The indication from our results is that peer support is still useful in promoting process results which include enhanced coping, increased access to emotional and economic support, adherence to treatment, utilization of health services [30–32]. While most scholars attach less importance to processes within different maternal health interventions, it should be noted however that these process outcomes are not completely unrewarding. They embody social conditions that are necessary for maternal health improvement [42]. In particular, the processes observed in this review are important for women living with HIV who are usually victims of isolation, stigma and discrimination. Peer support thus gives rise to social spheres which provide opportunities for critical dialogue about maternal health issues among women with HIV [14, 43]. Peer support also necessitates the re-assessment of harmful cultural and social norms affecting women with HIV [41]. While it is true that in general peer support leads to conditions necessary for improving maternal health in women with HIV, this fact alone does not offer any basis for drawing a causal link between peer support and maternal health of women living HIV. Existing evidence does not provide a knock-on effect of peer support on maternal health outcomes such hemorrhage, sepsis, and maternal mortality for women with HIV. Evidence linking peer support to maternal health outcomes of women with HIV is still missing in literature. The evidence provided in support of peer support vis-à-vis women with HIV seems necessary but not sufficient to unequivocally establish peer support as a useful strategy for improvement of maternal outcomes among women with HIV. More research needs to be undertaken to examine this relationship in order to shade light on whether peer support can actually lead to improved maternal health outcomes among women with HIV, and if so, how exactly this change is achieved.

The other important principle of community mobilization is the involvement of TBAs in maternal care provision. Our results in this regard were concomitant with recent studies indicating that TBAs are particularly useful for enhanced maternal care for HIV negative women, especially in areas lacking efficient health systems [18, 27, 33]. TBAs were particularly useful in reducing maternal morbidity and mortality in HIV negative women. However, this evidence only speaks for HIV negative women, whereas no focus has been placed on women living with HIV. The impact of TBAs on maternal health outcomes in women with HIV (who require antiretroviral therapy and cesarean birth in order to promote PMTCT) remains understudied [35, 44]. There is a need for more research to establish the link between use of TBAs and positive maternal health outcomes in women with HIV. Although a stronger case for TBAs is still lacking, it does not automatically mean that TBAs are irrelevant to women with HIV in sub-Saharan Africa. To the contrary, this result only means that to date, there is no study that establishes a significant causal link between TBAs and maternal health outcome of women with HIV. We also note that in sub-Saharan Africa, it is counterproductive to encourage only institutional delivery.

Institutional delivery in poorly equipped, hard-to-reach, remote, and overcrowded health facilities with poor adherence to quality is far from optimal. Given this, TBAs are sometimes the only feasible, cheap, practical and readily available source of maternal care in the peripherals of Africa and as such, it seems more advantageous in the context of sub-Saharan Africa to make use of TBAs and professional midwives complementary to each other [35, 37]. Therefore, a more nuanced understanding of maternal health interventions for women with HIV in sub-Saharan Africa is needed. However, before achieving this, it is vital that we increase our understanding on how exactly TBAs can improve maternal health of women with HIV and what kind of training should be provided to them.

Lastly, collaboration between professionals and the community in the design and implementation of maternal care initiatives, which is another principle of community mobilization, also produced varied results for HIV negative women and for women with HIV. The causal link between collaboration and maternal health outcomes for HIV negative women is established [36–39]. To date, collaboration with regard to women with HIV is only credited for the adoption of health-enhancing behavior. Although not a maternal health outcome in itself, behavioral change is an essential step towards improving maternal health. At the same time, it should be noted that behavioral change does not epitomize improved maternal outcome, it is merely a process through which improvement in maternal health can be achieved. This means that currently, it is less lucid to claim a collaboration-precipitated maternal health improvement in women with HIV on the basis of behavioral change. Therefore, we posit that more evidence is needed to understand how useful collaboration could be for women with HIV. Thus, before advocating for collaboration as a panacea to maternal health challenges among women with HIV in sub-Saharan Africa, there is a need for more research which establishes a causal link beyond behavioral change; one which can clearly show the effect of collaboration on maternal health outcomes in women with HIV.

Our review has several limitations that need to be acknowledged. Key among them is the fact that the search only included publications in English. This may have led to the omission of studies published in other languages within sub-Saharan Africa. The search also just focused on studies published in peer-reviewed journals thereby leaving out any grey literature. Therefore, it is possible that some literature focusing on the role of community mobilization on maternal health outcomes of HIV positive women in sub-Saharan Africa may have been omitted. We also did not find studies reporting undesirable process or outcome results. It should be acknowledged in this regard that positive results are more easily published while negative results tend to remain underreported.

Conclusion

As shown in our systematic review, currently, the evidence on the role of community mobilization on maternal outcomes of HIV negative women in sub-Saharan Africa is more conclusive than for women with HIV. This is embodied in all principles of community mobilization that we analyzed. So far, not much empirical work has been done to provide compelling evidence regarding the impact of community mobilization on maternal outcomes (i.e. sepsis, hemorrhage, and maternal mortality) for women living with HIV. That notwithstanding, there is some evidence suggesting that all three principles of community mobilization provide necessary process results for improving maternal health of women with HIV. It is indeed true that the process results create necessary conditions for improving maternal health. However, evidence on process indicators alone without subsequent causal evidence on the outcomes is not sufficient, and as such, cannot be used as a basis for advocating community mobilization as a useful maternal health care strategy for women with HIV in sub-Saharan Africa. Thus, more research needs to be undertaken to examine whether community mobilization actually leads to better maternal health outcomes in women with HIV and how exactly this change is achieved. Consequently, when it comes to relying on community mobilization for policy recommendation, we observe that there is not enough evidence to recommend community mobilization as a strategy for maternal health care provision for women in sub-Saharan Africa.

Acknowledgements

We like to acknowledge the assistance of some UNU-MERIT staff for assisting with access to publications.

Funding

No funding was obtained for this study.

Authors' contributions

All authors collaborated and contributed in the formulation of objectives of the study and oversaw the development of the study concept and design, data collection and analysis, including the drafting of the manuscript. All authors at every stage contributed in drafting, correcting and perfecting the manuscript. CM was tasked with consolidating all the contributions to the manuscript and taking care of all correspondence. All authors read and approved the final manuscript.

Competing interests
The authors declare that they have no competing interests.

Author details
[1]UNU MERIT, Boschstraat, 246211, AX, Maastricht, The Netherlands. [2]A9 Marshlands Village Box 32379, Lusaka, Zambia. [3]Department of Health Services Research. Room 0.073, Maastricht University, Duboisdomein 30, 6229, GT, Maastricht, The Netherlands.

References
1. WHO. World Health Statistics 2013. Geneva: WHO; 2013.
2. WHO. Child health and development. Geneva; WHO; 2015.
3. UNAIDS. Report on the Global HIV/AIDS Epidemic 2013. Geneva: UNAIDS; 2013.
4. Kendall T, Langer A. Critical maternal health knowledge gaps in low- and middle-income countries for the post-2015 era. Reprod Health. 2015:1-4.
5. Kendall T, Dane I, Cooper D, Dilmitis S, Kaida A. Eliminating Preventable HIV-Related Maternal Mortality in Sub-Saharan Africa: What Do We Need to Know? J Acquir Immune Defic Syndr. 2014;1(64):250–8.
6. Kendall T, Danel I. Research and Evaluation Agenda for HIV and Maternal Health in Sub-Saharan Africa. Women and Health Initiative Working Paper No. 1. Boston: Women and Health Initiative, Harvard School of Public Health; 2004.
7. Lindegren M, Kennedy C, Bain-Brickley D. Cochrane Database Systematic Review. In: Integration of HIV/AIDS services with maternal, neonatal and child health, nutrition, and family planning services; 2012.
8. Colbourn T, Nambiar B, Bondo A, Makwenda C, Tsetekani E. Effects of quality improvement in health facilities and community mobilization through women's groups on maternal, neonatal and perinatal mortality in three districts of Malawi: MaiKhanda, a cluster randomized controlled effectiveness trial. Int Health. 2013;5(3):180–95.
9. Calvert C, Ronsmans C. The contribution of HIV to pregnancy-related mortality: a systematic review and meta-analysis. AIDS. 2013;27:1631–163.
10. Rifkin SB, Pridmore P. Partners in Planning: Information, Participation and Empowerment. New York: Macmillan Education; 2001.
11. Abdool-Karim Q, AbouZhar C, Dehne K. HIV and maternal mortality: turning the tide. Lancet. 2010;375:1948–9.
12. Hanson C. The Epidemiology of Maternal Mortality in Southern Tanzania. London: London School of Hygiene and Tropical Medicine; 2013.
13. Ackerman GL, K Kiragu. Lessons learnt from promising practices in community engagement for the elimination of new HIV infections in children by 2015 and keeping their mothers alive: summary of a desk review. J Int AIDS Soc. 2012;15(12).
14. Campbell C, Cornish F. How can community health programmes build enabling environments for transformative communication? Experiences from India and South Africa. AIDS and Behavior. 2012;16(4):847–57.
15. Lassi ZS, Das JK, Salam RA, Bhutta ZA. Evidence from community level inputs to improve quality of care for maternal and newborn health: interventions and findings. Reprod Health. 2014;11(2).
16. WHO. Declaration-of-Alma-Ata International Conference on Primary Health Care, Alma-Ata, USSR 1978. Alma-Ata: World Health Organization; 1978.
17. Lewycka S, Mwansambo C, Rosato M, Kazembe P, Phiri T, Mganga A, Chapota H. Effect of women's groups and volunteer peer counselling on rates of mortality, morbidity, and health behaviours in mothers and children in rural Malawi (MaiMwana): a factorial, cluster-randomised controlled trial. Lancet. 2013;381:1721–35.
18. Ibrahim S, Omer M, Amin I, Babiker A, Rushwan H. The role of the village midwife in detection of high risk pregnancies and newborns. Int J Gynecol Obstet. 1992;39(2):117–22.
19. Lippman SA, Maman S, MacPhail C, Twine R, Peacock D, Kahn K, Pettifor A. Conceptualizing Community Mobilization for HIV Prevention: Implications for HIV Prevention Programming in the African Context. PLOSE ONE. 2013;8(10):e78208.
20. Campbell C. Community mobilisation in the 21st century: Updating our theory of social change. J Health Psychol. 2014;19(1):46–59.
21. Rosato M, Mwansambo CW, Kazembe PN, Phiri T, Soko QS, Lewycka S, Beata SV, Kunyenge E. Women's groups' perceptions of maternal health issues in rural Malawi. Lancet. 2006;368(9542):1180–8.
22. CHMI. Zambulance. Lusaka: Center for Health Market Innovations; 2015.
23. Altman L, Kuhlmann AKS, Galavotti C. Understanding the black box: A systematic review ofthe measurement of the community mobilization process in evaluations of interventions targeting sexual, reproductive, and maternal health. Eval Program Plann. 2015;49:86–97.
24. Hooijmans CR, Ritskes-Hoitinga M. Progress in Using Systematic Reviews of Animal Studies to Improve Translational Research. PlosOne. 2013;
25. Howard-Grabman L, Storti C, Hummer P, Pooler B. Demystifying community mobilisation: an effective strategy to improve maternal and newborn health. Geneva: USAID; 2007.
26. Mant J. Process versus Outcome indicators in the assesment of quality health care. Int J Qual Health Care. 2001;13(6):475–80.
27. Akpala C. An evaluation of the knowledge and practices of trained traditional birth attendants in Bodinga, Sokoto State, Nigeria. Am J Trop Med Hyg. 1994;97(1):46–50.
28. Hodder I. The contextual analysis of symbolic meanings. In: Pearce SM, editor. Interpreting Objects and Collections. London: Routledge; 1994. p. 12–3.
29. PRISMA. Transparent reporting of systematic reviews and meta analysis. Oxford: Oxford University Press; 2015.
30. Rotheram-Borus M, Richter L, van Heerden A, van Rooyen H, Tomlinson M. A cluster randomized controlled trial evaluating the efficacy of peer mentors to support South African women living with HIV and their infants. PloSe One. 2014;9(1).
31. Kaayaa SF, Blanderb J, Antelmanc G, Cypriana F, Emmonsd KM, Matsumotoe K. Randomized controlled trial evaluating the effect of an interactive group counseling intervention for HIV-positive women on prenatal depression and disclosure of HIV status. AIDS Care. 2013;25(7).
32. Richter L, Rotheram-Borus MJ, Van Heerden A, Stein A, Tomlinson M, Harwood JM, Rochat T, Van-Rooyen H, Comulada W, Tang Z. Pregnant women living with HIV (WLH) supported at clinics by peer WLH: a cluster randomized controlled trial. AIDS Behavior. 2014;18(4):706–15.
33. Dehne K, Wacker J, Cowley J. Training birth attendants in the Sahel. World Health Forum. 1995;16(4):415–9.
34. Schaider J, Ngonyani S, Tomlin S, Rydman R, Roberts R. International maternal mortality reduction: outcome of traditional birth attendant education and intervention in Angola. J Med Syst. 1999;23(2):99–105.
35. Perez F, Aung KD, Ndoro T, Engelsmann B, Dabis F. Participation of traditional birth attendants in prevention of mother-to-child transmission of HIV services in two rural districts in Zimbabwe: a feasibility study. BMC Public Health. 2008;401(8).
36. Schmid T, Kanenda O, Ahluwalia I, Kouletio M. Transportation for Maternal Emergencies in Tanzania: Empowering Communities Through Participatory Problem Solving. American Journal of Public Health. 2001;91(10):1589–90.
37. Wangalwa G, Cudjoe B, Wamalwa D, Machira Y, Ofware P, Ndirangu M, Ilako F. Effectiveness of Kenya's Community Health Strategy in delivering community-based maternal and newborn health care in Busia County, Kenya: non-randomized pre-test post test study. Pan Afr Med J. 2012;13(1).
38. Kidane G, Morrow R. Teaching mothers to provide home treatment of malaria in Tigray, Ethiopia: a randomised trial. Lancet. 2000;356(9229): 550–5.
39. Shamba DD, Schellenberg J, Penfold SC, Mashasi I, Mrisho M, Manzi F, Marchant T, Tanner M, Mshinda H, Schellenberg D, Hill Z. Clean home-delivery in rural Southern Tanzania: barriers, influencers, and facilitators. J Health Popul and Nutr. 2013;31(1):110–7.
40. Torpey K, Kabaso M, Kasonde P, Dirks R, Bweupe M, Thompson C. Increasing the uptake of prevention of mother-to-child transmission of HIV services in a resource-limited setting. BMC Health Serv Res. 2010;10(29).
41. Campbell C, Mzaidume Y. How can HIV be prevented in South Africa? A social perspective. Br Med J. 2002;324:229–32.
42. Campbell C, Cornish F. Towards a "fourth generation" of approaches to HIV/AIDS management: creating contexts for effective community mobilisation. AIDS care. 2010;22(1):569–79.
43. O'Gorman DA, Nyirenda LJ, Theobald SJ. Prevention of mother-to-child transmission of HIV infection: Views and perceptions about swallowing nevirapine in rural Lilongwe, Malaw. BMC Public Health 2. 2010;10(34).
44. Lippmann Q, Mofolo I, Bobrow E, Maida A, Kamanga E. Exploring the feasibility of engaging Traditional Birth Attendants in a prevention of mother to child HIV transmission program in Lilongwe, Malawi. Malawi Med J. 2012;24(4):79–80.

45. Cornish F, Priego-Hernandez J, Campbell C, Mburu G. The impact of Community Mobilisation on HIV Prevention in Middle and Low Income Countries: A Systematic Review and Critique. AIDS Behavior. 2014;18:2110–34.
46. Tripathy P, Nair N, Mahapatra R, Rath S, Gope RK. Community mobilisation with women's groups facilitated by Accredited Social Health Activists (ASHAs) to improve maternal and newborn health in underserved areas of Jharkhand and Orissa: study protocol for a cluster-randomised controlled trial. Trials. 2011;12(182):2–12.
47. Rifkin S, Pridmore P. Partners in Planning. Oxford: Macmillan; 2001.
48. McKenzie J, Neiger B, Thackeray R. Planning, Implementing & Evaluationg Health Promotion Program. 6th ed. Boston: Pearson Education; 2013.
49. Watson-Thompson J, Fawcett SB, Schultz JA. A Framework for Community Mobilization to Promote Healthy Youth Development. Am J Prev Med. 2008; 34(3):S72–81.
50. Kim-Ju G, Mark GY, Cohen DR, Garcia-Santiago O, Nguyen P. Community Mobilization and Its Application to Youth Violence Prevention. Am J Prev Med. 2008;34(3):S5–S12.
51. Nahar T, Azad K, Aumon BH, Younes L, Shaha S, Kuddus A. Scaling up community mobilisation through women's groups for maternal and neonatal health: experiences from rural Bangladesh. BMC Pregnancy Childbirth. 2012;12(5).
52. MERCY-CORPS. COMMUNITY MOBILIZATION Approach. Portland: MERCY-CORPS; 2009.

5

Improving quality of care for maternal and newborn health: a pre-post evaluation of the Safe Childbirth Checklist at a hospital in Bangladesh

Herfina Y. Nababan[1,2*], Rubana Islam[1,3], Shabnam Mostari[4], Md Tariqujjaman[1], Malabika Sarker[4], Mohammad Tajul Islam[5] and Corrina Moucheraud[6]

Abstract

Background: Bangladesh has achieved major gains in maternal and newborn survival, facility childbirth and skilled birth attendance between 1991 and 2010, but excess maternal mortality persists. High-quality maternal health care is necessary to address this burden. Implementation of WHO Safe Childbirth Checklist (SCC), whose items address the major causes of maternal deaths, is hypothesized to improve adherence of providers to essential childbirth practices.

Method: The SCC was adapted for the local context through expert consultation meetings, creating a total of 27 checklist items. This study was a pre-post evaluation of SCC implementation. Data were collected over 8 months at Magura District Hospital. We analysed 468 direct observations of birth (main analysis using 310 complete observations and sensitivity analysis with the additional 158 incomplete observations) from admission to discharge. The primary outcome of interest was the number of essential childbirth practices performed before compared to after SCC implementation. The change was assessed using adjusted Poisson regression models accounting for clustering by nurse-midwives.

Result: After checklist introduction, significant improvements were observed: on average, around 70% more of these safe childbirth practices were performed in the follow-up period compared to baseline (from 11 to 19 out of 27 practices). Substantial increases were seen in communication between nurse-midwives and mothers (counselling), and in management of complications (including rational use of medicines). In multivariable models that included characteristics of the mothers and of the nurse-midwives, the rate of delivering the essential childbirth practices was 1.71 times greater in the follow-up compared to baseline (95% CI 1.61–1.81).

Conclusion: Implementation of SCC has the potential to improve essential childbirth practice in resource-poor settings like Bangladesh. This study emphasizes the need for health system strengthening in order to achieve the full advantages of SCC implementation.

Keywords: Maternal and newborn health, Safe Childbirth Checklist, Quality of care, Health worker performance, Health service delivery, Bangladesh

* Correspondence: herfina.nababan@gmail.com
[1]Centre for Universal Health Coverage, Health Systems and Population Studies Division, International Centre for Diarrhoeal Disease Research, 68 Shahid Tajuddin Ahmed Sharani, Mohakhali, Dhaka 1212, Bangladesh
[2]Nossal Institute for Global Health, Melbourne School of Population and Global Health, the University of Melbourne, 333 Exhibition Street, Melbourne, Victoria 3004, Australia
Full list of author information is available at the end of the article

Background

The end of the Millennium Development Goals (MDGs) era offers an opportunity to examine successes and failures in global health and development, and to identify priorities for the future [1]. Overall, the world achieved major gains in maternal and child survival and in coverage of facility-based childbirth and skilled birth attendance [2, 3]. Many women and newborns, however, continue to die during and shortly after childbirth, and disparities persist across countries as well as across groups within countries [1, 2]. This suggests that the global strategy, which has focused on increasing coverage of skilled birth attendance, did not eliminate all excess burden [4]. Utilization alone is not sufficient; high-quality maternal health care is essential for reducing excess mortality [5, 6].

Mirroring global trends, Bangladesh made great progress towards MDG 4 and 5 targets [1]. While the current neonatal mortality rate of 28 per 1000 live births has been lower than the target of 48 deaths per 1000 live births, its maternal mortality ratio (MMR) decreased from 574 maternal deaths per 100,000 live births in 1991 to 176 deaths per 100,000 live births in 2015 [7, 8]; and use of facility delivery increased over this period [9]. However, there is an unfinished agenda for improving childbirth outcomes in Bangladesh. Still only 37% of births occur at health facilities, with much lower rates among poorer women, and provision of quality care during childbirth remains a particular challenge [9–11].

High-quality childbirth care requires facility readiness (physical infrastructure, equipment, medicines and supplies) and availability of human resources with the knowledge, skills, and capacity to effectively manage uncomplicated and complicated childbirth events [12]. In 2008, World Health Organization (WHO) designed the Safe Childbirth Checklist (SCC), a 29-item quality improvement tool to help reduce adverse childbirth events by facilitating frontline health workers' adherence to evidence-based essential childbirth practices [13]. The items on the SCC address the major causes of maternal deaths, intrapartum-related stillbirths and early neonatal deaths [13].

In the current study, we examined the effectiveness of the SCC in improving childbirth practices at a district hospital in Bangladesh. The use of SCC is hypothesized to facilitate adherence to essential childbirth practices demonstrated to be effective in reducing maternal and newborn deaths, by reminding nurse-midwives to perform the practices and in the proper sequence [13]. The results from this study were expected to expand the emerging body of empirical evidence about the SCC – including evaluation results from India and Sri Lanka [14, 15].

Methods

Study setting

This study was conducted at a 100-bedded district level secondary care hospital (Magura District Hospital (DH)) in Khulna division in Southwestern Bangladesh, around 260 km from the capital Dhaka. This hospital was purposively selected because it sees a high annual volume of births (on average more than 1200 uncomplicated vaginal deliveries per year) and was implementing no other safe childbirth interventions during this evaluation period [16]. It also had all requisite supplies and materials to perform the SCC activities, except the partograph and disposable surgical gloves which were provided for the purposes of this study for the entire study period.

Adaptation of the SCC

There was a series of consultative meetings between study investigators and external experts (obstetricians and neonatologists from Bangabandhu Sheikh Mujib Medical University, Shaheed Suhrawardy Medical College Hospital; and public health scientists and researchers affiliated with BRAC, the International Center for Diarrhoeal Disease Research, Bangladesh (icddr,b), Japan International Cooperation Agency (JICA), and James P. Grant School of Public Health – BRAC University) to reach consensus on how to adapt the SCC for the local context. This is a recommended first step by WHO for each instance of local implementation [17]. These proposed adaptations were shared with WHO for their review and feedback, and a revised checklist version was pre-tested in February 2014 at the Narsingdi district hospital (Dhaka division), which has characteristics similar to the study hospital. The key differences between the final checklist used in this study and WHO SCC are: removal of HIV-related items (due to low prevalence in Bangladesh); and addition of a question to identify women who had already received oxytocin outside of the hospital. The later was added to prevent double dose in women who were sent to Magura DH by traditional birth attendants or village doctors, given the wide practice of oxytocin at the community level by these providers [18]. In total, there are 27 checklist items adopted in the current study, consisting of practices such as partograph use, checking the need for antibiotics or magnesium sulfate and ensuring the availability of bedside supplies. These practices were organized into four pause points: on admission, just before pushing, soon after birth, and before discharge (See Additional file 1: Table S1 for the full checklist items).

Study design and data collection

A pre-post study design was used to measure the association between SCC implementation and changes in safe childbirth care. Baseline (pre) data were collected at the obstetric unit of Magura DH between April and June 2014. Then the SCC was introduced: eight nurse-midwives (all with more than 10 years of working experience) responsible for care in delivery ward were trained to use SCC, with special focus on the partograph because this was not routine in Magura DH. They were subsequently requested to use the SCC during all childbirth practices. There were additional orientation sessions on the SCC for obstetricians, health care managers and medical officers working in the obstetric unit. The follow-up (post) phase began in July 2014, with 5 months of data collection (ending in November 2014).

The sample size for the active intervention phase was calculated at a power of 80% and significance level of 5%. The formula was used assuming a 150% increase in partograph use, given the extremely low rate of current practice (5%) [19]. The total sample size calculated was 440 i.e. 220 deliveries for each phase of the study. Only uncomplicated vaginal deliveries admitted before the active stage of labor was observed. Pregnant women who required Caesarean birth were excluded from the study, as well as pregnant women who were HIV positive.

Data at baseline and follow-up were collected by three research assistants who were nursing school graduates with working experience in obstetric care, with supervision on-site provided by a retired senior nurse. The data collectors received extensive preparatory training on the study objectives, data collection procedure and skill, informed consent, as well as on the SCC and evidence-based essential practices incorporated in the SCC. To ensure that observation was done in a similar manner, a pilot data collection was conducted in a different district hospital. Data were collected via direct observation of birth events to record providers' behavior. All births were observed for 24 h per day for 6 days each week except during official holidays, for all the eight nurse-midwives at Magura DH. Research assistants worked an eight-hour shift (including the night shift) and then handing the observation over to the next research assistant in duty when required.

Data analysis

The primary outcome of interest was the number of essential childbirth practices—operationalized as items on the SCC—performed per childbirth event. We tested how this was associated with the SCC intervention by performing statistical tests of difference (Wald test) between births occurring during baseline and follow-up periods. Additionally, we examined whether other factors were related to childbirth practices, comprising of mothers' characteristics (age, parity, and number of antenatal care (ANC) visits completed which were treated as continuous variables, and educational attainment which was categorized into no education/primary, secondary and higher) and nurse-midwives' characteristics (age, years of experience in healthcare, and months after the last refresher training; all treated as continuous variables). This was tested using multivariable Poisson regression models with reported Incidence Rate Ratios (IRR), accounting for clustering by nurse-midwives. The first multivariate model was unadjusted, the second model included covariates for mothers, and the third model included covariates for mothers and nurse-midwives. The main analysis was done using complete observations i.e. childbirth events whose all 100% of pause points were observed. However, the incomplete observations were incorporated for the sensitivity analysis. Data were entered and verified with SPSS version 20. Analyses were performed with Stata version 13 (Stata Corp.).

Results

The analysis included 310 complete observations of childbirth events from Magura DH, comprising of 153 and 157 observations at baseline and endline respectively. Characteristics of the mothers represented in this sample are presented in Table 1. The majority of the women were between 20 and 29 years old and had given birth to their first child. There were no statistically significant differences between characteristics of women examined at baseline and endline.

Table 1 Demographic characteristics of mothers at baseline and endline

Characteristics	Baseline ($N = 153$) n (%)	Endline ($N = 157$) n (%)	*P*-Value
Age (years)			
< 20	19 (12)	17(11)	0.156
20–24	66 (43)	73(47)	
25–29	48 (31)	35(22)	
≥ 30	20 (13)	32 (20)	
Median age (IQR) (years)	23 (20, 25)	23 (20, 28)	0.52
Education			
Primary or no education	45 (29)	57 (36)	0.122
Secondary	85 (56)	69 (44)	
Higher	23 (15)	31 (20)	
Parity			
0	84 (55)	84 (54)	0.941
1	44 (29)	48 (31)	
≥ 2	25 (16)	25 (16)	
Number of ANC visit			
0	25 (16)	17 (11)	0.27
1	82 (54)	96 (61)	
≥ 2	46 (30)	44 (28)	

Additional file 2 Table S2 includes information about the eight nurse-midwives from Magura DH who provided care for the births in this sample. All nurse-midwives had at least 10 years of experience, and three had recently received refresher training on childbirth care. The numbers of childbirth observation of each nurse-midwife varied (See Additional file 2: Table S2), likewise the numbers of observation completed by each observer also varied (See Additional file 3: Table S3).

Following implementation of the SCC, the average number of safe childbirth practices performed per childbirth increased by approximately 70%, from 11 out of 27 practices in baseline to 19 out of 27 practices in endline (See Table 2). This was a statistically significant increase according to a series of multivariable Poisson regression models that included covariates for mothers' and nurse-midwives' characteristics (See Table 3). The result was robust for all specifications, with the rate of delivering the essential childbirth practices being 1.71 times greater in the follow-up compared to baseline (95% CI 1·61–1·82), and no covariates were found significant.

Some checklist items related to appropriate management of maternal infection and of eclampsia as well as appropriate newborn infection management were composite measures representing a series of sub-actions, consisting of checking for symptoms and giving the medicine when needed (See Additional file 1: Table S1 for the full checklist items). In the absence of any symptom, it was expected that the nurse-midwives would not give the medicine. Following SCC implementation, the largest improvement for these items for mothers was in the first component i.e. checking for symptoms (Table 4). Provision of antibiotics and of magnesium sulfate at endline was more likely to occur after symptoms were checked, although at endline 89% of the mothers who were prescribed antibiotics at discharge had been checked for symptoms and no symptoms were present.

When examining the improvements seen on specific activities (See Table 2), maternal counseling on admission, soon after birth, and before discharge improved considerably, from near-zero rates to near-universal coverage by endline. Statistically significant improvements were also seen in the active management of the third stage of labor (AMTSL) (from 88% to 99%) and the bedside availability of supplies for mothers and babies such as oxytocin 10 IU in syringe and sterile blade to cut the cord (from 0% to 11%). Only two women received oxytocin at the community level prior to admission (results not shown).

Some safe childbirth practices were already commonly performed at baseline, such as hand hygiene (99%), encouraging the presence of a birth companion (97%), assessing and treating postpartum maternal blood loss (99%), breastfeeding and skin-to-skin contact soon after birth (99%), newborn feeding assessment (99%), and counseling for family planning and for a follow-up visit (99% each). Other behaviors were not performed at baseline and did not improve with introduction of the SCC: partograph use (0% at baseline and endline), appropriate management of newborn infection (1% at baseline and endline), and checking the need for newborn special care (0% at baseline and endline). Appropriate newborn thermal and resuscitation practices (special care) declined between baseline and endline (from 11% to 0%).

As a sensitivity analysis, we reran the analysis on a dataset that also included incomplete observations (In total 468 observations, with additional 76 and 82 incomplete observations at baseline and endline respectively) (See Additional file 4: Table S4), and all results remained the same.

Discussion

Main findings and interpretation

We observed a significant and substantial increase in the number of evidence-based safe childbirth practices following the introduction of the SCC. The magnitude of this improvement is similar to results from a previous evaluation of the SCC in India [14], and the endline results from Sri Lanka [15]. This result is also consistent with previous studies showing that health worker reminders and prompts were associated with improvements in quality care for maternal and child health care in low and middle income countries (LMICs) [20].

Maternal counselling on admission, soon after birth, and before discharge saw considerable improvement in this study. Such counselling is important to ensure that women are treated with respect and are empowered to participate in decisions about their own care [21], which may encourage health service utilization [22, 23]. It has previously been reported that poor provider-patient communication can discourage health service use [24] – so the SCC offers a model for how to improve such exchanges. The improvement in bedside availability of birth supplies is likewise noteworthy, as it is important that medicine and supplies are readily available to providers to encourage the performance of childbirth practices [14]. An important practice that relies upon the availability of supplies was among others the AMTSL.

Some other childbirth practices were already commonly performed at baseline in this study – including breastfeeding and handwashing. A 2014 health facility survey in Bangladesh found that 79% of district hospitals had the requisite supplies for hand hygiene (i.e. soap and running water) [25], which suggests that, where infrastructure and supplies were available, they were being used for safe childbirth care. In line with the current findings, the results from previous study assessing essential newborn practices in Bangladesh also demonstrated

Table 2 Number of essential childbirth practices (SCC items) performed at baseline and endline (complete observations)

Childbirth practices	Baseline (*N* = 153) n (%)	End line (*N* = 157) n (%)	*P*-value
On admission			
Partograph use	0 (0)	0 (0)	–
Appropriate maternal infection management	1 (0.65)	149 (95)	<0.001
Appropriate eclampsia management	6 (4)	129 (82)	<0.001
Hand hygiene	152 (99)	157 (100)	0.318
Birth companion present	148 (97)	157 (100)	0.024
Intrapartum counseling	3 (2)	121 (77)	<0.001
Just before pushing			
Emergency birth helper was identified	152 (99)	156 (99)	0.99
Appropriate maternal infection management	1 (0.65)	147 (94)	<0.001
Appropriate eclampsia management	4 (3)	125 (80)	<0.001
Supplies for mothers and babies	0 (0)	18 (11)	<0.001
Soon after birth (within 1 h)			
AMTSL	134 (88)	156 (99)	<0.001
Appropriate newborn thermal and resuscitation	17 (11)	0 (0)	<0.001
Maternal blood loss assessment and treatment	152 (99)	157 (100)	0.318
Appropriate maternal infection management	3 (2)	148 (94)	<0.001
Appropriate eclampsia management	3 (2)	119 (76)	<0.001
Newborn referral	149 (97)	157 (100)	0.044
Appropriate newborn infection management	0 (0)	0 (0)	–
Newborn special care	0 (0)	0 (0)	–
Breastfeeding and skin to skin contact	152 (99)	157 (100)	0.318
Postpartum counseling	3 (2)	133 (85)	<0.001
Before discharge			
Maternal blood loss assessment	152 (99)	157 (100)	0.318
Appropriate maternal infection management	0 (0)	35 (22)	<0.001
Appropriate newborn infection management	1 (0.65)	1 (0.64)	0.985
Newborn feeding assessment	152 (99)	157 (100)	0.318
Family planning counseling	152 (99)	157 (100)	0.318
Discharge counseling	1 (0.65)	108 (69)	<0.001
Follow-up visit counseling	151 (99)	157 (100)	0.156
Median total practices performed	11 (41)	19 (70)	<0.000

The *P*-values were generated from Wald tests

that the coverage of practices such as handwashing and breastfeeding were high [26].

Some practices including partograph, appropriate management of newborn infection and checking the need for newborn special care were not performed in the baseline and did not see any improvement after SCC introduction. At the same time, newborn thermal and resuscitation practices declined in the endline. Other than inappropriate attitude, inadequate knowledge and skills can deter good health care [27]. Nonetheless, today it is widely recognized that health workers' performance is not only a function of these individual characteristics [28]. An enabling environment, managerial culture and organizational context as well as the overall health system also play interrelated crucial roles [28, 29]. Factors including absence of teamwork, high workload, shortage of drugs, unavailability of equipment and supplies, and the lack of supervision and training opportunities can demotivate health workers [27]. Furthermore, factors such as resources allocation, planning and deployment of health workers, policy and regulatory framework, communication and decision-making processes, and

Table 3 Multivariable Poisson regression models assessing factors associated with improvement in essential childbirth practices

Variable	Model (1) IRR (95%CI)	Model (2) IRR (95%CI)	Model (3) IRR (95%CI)
WHO SCC use			
Yes (endline)	1.71[a] (1.68-1.73)	1.70[a] (1.68–1.73)	1.71[a] (1.61–1.82)
Nurse-midwives' age[b]			1 (1.00-1.03)
Nurse-midwives' year of experience[b]			0.96 (0.94–0.98)
Months since nurse-midwives' last refresher training[b]			1 (0.98-1.02)
Mothers' age[b]		1 (1.00-1.03)	1 (1.00–1.03)
Mothers' education background			
Primary or no education		(ref)	(ref)
Secondary		0.99 (0.97–1.01)	0.99 (0.97–1.01)
Higher		1 (0.96–1.03)	1 (0.96–1.03)
Parity[b]		1 (0.98-1.02)	1 (0.98–1.02)
Number of ANC visit[b]		1 (0.99-1.02)	1 (0.99–1.02)
Constant	11.04 (10.92–11.16)	11.2 (10.18–12.32)	11.33 (9.98–12.86)
Number of observations	310	310	310

Outcome variable is number of SCC practices performed per childbirth
Model (1) includes no covariates; Model (2) includes covariates for the mothers; Model (3) includes these plus covariates for the nurse-midwives
[a]denotes significance at the 1% level
[b]indicates a continuous variable

accountability mechanisms also influence performance from the broader health system perspective [28].

The non-use of partograph found in this study is disheartening, given its importance in preventing prolonged labor and subsequent possible events such as postpartum haemorrhage, maternal or newborn infection, as well as birth asphyxia [30]. Partograph is a low technology tool that graphically represents key events during labor and is recommended by WHO for routine monitoring of labor to provide an early warning system and take action according to a clinical management protocol [29]. Its underuse is unfortunately often found in LMICs, including Bangladesh [19, 29, 31]. In accordance with health workers' performance in general, the barrier of its use also ranges from individual, social and organizational contexts [29]. It is perceived as time-consuming [32], especially in the settings with high workload and/or understaffed [33]. Some organizational barriers include shortage of clinical equipment, medicine and supply [32, 34], including unavailability of partograph itself. These underlying issues are often problematic in LMICs, including Magura DH [30]. Training was deemed important to improve the ability of midwives to use partographs [35]. Nevertheless, with training and constant supply, partograph use didn't improve in the current study. Since partograph was not available and its correct use was not a norm prior to the study, it was probable that no proper enforcement i.e. supervision and monitoring was in place to maintain its use [36]. Consequently, although it was made available for this study and training was provided to the nurse-midwives, a lack of experience and/or low confidence may have limited its uptake [29]. Recognizing the fundamental role of policy and leadership, it is suggested that an implementation strategy should also include policy level interventions to ensure quality assurance and improvement activities including rigorous implementation of management protocols [30, 37].

Other practices that did not improve in the current study were related to newborn care. Twenty-four hours period immediately after birth holds the highest risk of neonatal deaths resulting from conditions such as birth asphyxia, pre-term birth related problems, and neonatal infection, suggesting the need for high quality newborn care [38]. Acknowledging this risk, WHO developed a course to strengthen the capacity of health workers to deliver a set of minimum evidence-based newborn care called the Essential Newborn Care (ENC) that has been proven to improve care for newborns and lead to a decrease in neonatal death [39]. The practices within ENC that address the major causes of neonatal death were also incorporated into SCC [13]. The finding from this study therefore suggest the need to strengthen care in this area if a decline in neonatal death is to be achieved. Improving the competence of nurse-midwives is important given the low numbers of staff in district hospitals in Bangladesh who had ever received training in newborn care and resuscitation. However, improvement in organizational and structural context including adequacy of health workforce, supportive supervision and availability of necessary supply is also necessary [25, 26]. In addition. The decline in newborn thermal and resuscitation practice found in this study following SCC implementation was likely prompted by SCC, showing that these practices should be performed only when the need for these practices were confirmed.

An encouraging finding from this study was the increase in checking for symptoms to ensure appropriate use of medicines to manage maternal infection and

Table 4 Appropriate use of medicines at baseline and endline

	Received medicine, n		Had any symptoms checked, n		Had any symptoms present, n	
	Baseline (n = 153)	Endline (n = 157)	(as % of those who received medicine)		(as % of those who had symptoms checked)	
Maternal antibiotics						
On admission	0	1	0	1 (100%)	0	1 (100%)
Just before/after birth	0	1	0	1 (100%)	0	1 (100%)
One hour postpartum	4	3	0 (0%)	3 (100%)	0	1 (33%)
Before discharge	90	111	2 (2.2%)	99 (89%)	0 (0%)	0 (0%)
Magnesium sulfate						
On admission	2	2	0 (0%)	2 (100%)	0	1 (50%)
Just before/after birth	2	2	0 (0%)	1 (50%)	0	1 (100%)
One hour postpartum	2	2	0 (0%)	2 (100%)	0	2 (100%)

eclampsia after implementation of the SCC – especially at discharge, although 89% of women at endline were still given antibiotics despite having no infection symptoms. WHO has found widespread substandard medicine use worldwide [40], which may be due to misinformation, provider and/or patient bias and preference, prescribing habits, peer pressure, system constraints including lack of diagnostics, or economic incentives from the pharmaceutical industry that may promote overuse [41–43]. This study did not explore these hypothesized mechanisms, but other studies from Bangladesh have identified these as salient factors for misuse of medicines locally [44]. It can be difficult to identify women at risk of developing infections during childbirth – which may be more prevalent among women who deliver at health facilities due to unhygienic conditions, poor water and sanitation systems, overcrowding and poor quality care [45] – since symptoms (such as fever and abnormal vaginal discharge) can be non-specific and may manifest only after childbirth [46]. Therefore providers may be overly cautious, and as a result prescribe broad-spectrum antibiotics during childbirth [42]. This may be one reason for the persisting use of antibiotics at discharge in this study; these reasons were echoed in informal discussions with providers at Magura DH about this finding. Irrational medicine use has serious public health and clinical consequences, including increased adverse drug events and accelerating rates of antimicrobial resistance [40]. This study suggests that there is a need for tools to address the issue of dispensing even in the absence of symptoms, for example via continuous quality improvement to encourage rational use [42].

Finally, the result of the Poisson model that included nurse-midwives' characteristics showed that the number of years of experience was associated with worse childbirth practices, even though this result was not significant. Previous studies have found both positive and negative correlations between experience and health workers' performance [47–49]. The association could likely be explained by better self-confidence of more experienced nurse-midwives of their clinical experience and intuition which made them less willing to follow a new tool or guideline or less open to new ideas [47]. In line with this, different studies revealed that higher-level cadres of health workers who are usually also more experienced tend to perform less well at following new guidelines compared to their lower level counterparts [50, 51].

Strength and limitation

A key advantage of this study over previous evaluations was its continuous measurement of SCC activities for each observed childbirth – from admission to discharge. But several limitations should also be noted. First, a randomized trial design – including a control arm (with no SCC implementation) – would have allowed for stronger causal inference in this evaluation, but such an evaluation was beyond the resources available for this study. The current study was also not designed to detect any change in outcome of maternal and neonatal morbidity and mortality. Second, some supplies (i.e. gloves and partograph) were provided by the investigators, to enable the assessment of SCC' use without supply constraints. These results may therefore not be generalizable to other settings where such supplies are unavailable. Third, the 310 complete observations analyzed in this study were falling short of the sample size calculated of 440 observations. Nonetheless, the sensitivity analysis incorporating incomplete observations didn't alter the results. Fourth, direct observation of nurse-midwives' practices could introduce bias, such as a Hawthorne effect whereby performance is improved due to the act of observation. However, the same groups of nurse-midwives were observed pre- and post- intervention, therefore cancelling this effect. Fifth, the findings from the current study may not be generalizable to providers with less than 10 years of experience, providers other than nurse-midwives, or providers working in different settings. Lastly, it was difficult to measure certain SCC items, such as blood loss and management of newborn infection, which involved subjective or otherwise challenging observation. This may have caused some under-reporting, so more detailed measurement guidelines and instructions (as part of WHO SCC program) might be useful for future studies.

Conclusion

The overall improvement in nurse-midwives' practices was significant and strong. It suggests that implementing the SCC may facilitate health worker' compliance to essential childbirth practices. The study has identified areas of practice that should be strengthened in Bangladesh, such as prevention of prolonged labor using partograph as well as essential newborn care. It also pointed out the importance of available workforce, infrastructure and supplies, of strengthening the role of leadership and continuous quality assurance and improvement, as well as of strengthening the overall health system to achieve the full advantages of SCC implementation. The results of SCC implementation evaluation in Bangladesh presented in this paper offers new evidence and insights for expanding use of the SCC in low-income settings.

Additional files

Additional file 1: Table S1. Final SCC used in the current study.

Additional file 2: Table S2. Characteristics of nurse-midwives.

Additional file 3: Table S3. Distribution of observation completion.

Additional file 4: Table S4. Number of essential childbirth practices (SCC items) performed at baseline and endline (including incomplete observations).

Abbreviation

AMTSL: Active management of the third stage of labor; ANC: Antenatal care; DGHS: Directorate General of Health Services; DH: District hospital; icddr,b: International Center for Diarrhoeal Disease Research, Bangladesh; JICA: Japan International Cooperation Agency; MDGs: Millennium development goals; MMR: Maternal mortality ratio; SCC: Safe Childbirth Checklist; WHO: World Health Organization

Acknowledgments

We would like to thank Magura District Hospital authorities, physicians, nurse-midwives, and patients who supported and participated in this study. We would also like to extend our deep appreciation to the field research team for their dedication. We are grateful for Dr. Iqbal Anwar who encouraged us to initiate the study and provided invaluable support throughout the study period. We are thankful for Dr. Alayne Adams who supported us with tangible and non-tangible support. We would also like to thank Maternal Health Task Force and icddr,b who funded the study and James P. Grant School of Public Health through which the study made possible.

Funding

This study is supported by Maternal Health Task Force (MHTF) through icddr,b. The funding source had no role in the design of the study, data collection, data analysis, interpretation of the data, decision to publish, or preparation of the manuscript.

Authors' contributions

HYN, RI, and SM conceived the study. MS and MTI contributed in the study design. HYN, RI and CM conceptualized the paper, designed the analysis, and interpreted the results. MT performed the statistical analysis and contributed to the interpretation. HYN drafted the manuscript. CM edited the manuscript. RI, SM, MS, MTI, and CM provided critical review of the manuscript. All authors read and approved the final manuscript.

Competing interests

Dr. Moucheraud reports grants from Maternal Health Task Force, outside the submitted work. Other co-authors declare no competing interests.

Author details

[1]Centre for Universal Health Coverage, Health Systems and Population Studies Division, International Centre for Diarrhoeal Disease Research, 68 Shahid Tajuddin Ahmed Sharani, Mohakhali, Dhaka 1212, Bangladesh. [2]Nossal Institute for Global Health, Melbourne School of Population and Global Health, the University of Melbourne, 333 Exhibition Street, Melbourne, Victoria 3004, Australia. [3]School of Public Health & Community Medicine, Faculty of Medicine, University of New South Wales, Sydney, Australia. [4]James P. Grant School of Public Health, BRAC University, 68 Shahid Tajuddin Ahmed Sharani, Mohakhali, Dhaka 1212, Bangladesh. [5]Japan International Cooperation Agency (JICA), 3rd Floor, Bay's Galleria, 57 Gulshan Avenue (CWS-A19), Gulshan-1, Dhaka 1212, Bangladesh. [6]Department of Health Policy and Management, UCLA Fielding School of Public Health, 650 Charles E Young Dr S, Los Angeles, CA 90095, USA.

References

1. Victora CG, Requejo JH, Barros AJ, Berman P, Bhutta Z, Boerma T, Chopra M, de Francisco A, Daelmans B, Hazel E, et al. Countdown to 2015: a decade of tracking progress for maternal, newborn, and child survival. Lancet. 2015; 387(10032):2049–59.
2. Souza JP, Gülmezoglu AM, Vogel J, Carroli G, Lumbiganon P, Qureshi Z, Costa MJ, Fawole B, Mugerwa Y, Nafiou I. Moving beyond essential interventions for reduction of maternal mortality (the WHO multicountry survey on maternal and newborn health): a cross-sectional study. Lancet. 2013;381(9879):1747–55.
3. PMNCH WHO, World Bank. AHPSR: success factors for Women's and Children's health: policy and programme highlights from 10 fast-track countries. Geneva: WHO; 2014.
4. Moyer CA, Adanu RM, Engmann CM. The relationship between facility-based delivery and maternal and neonatal mortality in sub-Saharan Africa. Int J Gynaecol Obstet. 2013;122(3):263–5.
5. Kruk ME, Larson E, Twum-Danso NA. Time for a quality revolution in global health. Lancet Glob Health. 2016;4(9):e594–6.
6. Koblinsky M, Moyer CA, Calvert C, Campbell J, Campbell OM, Feigl AB, Graham WJ, Hatt L, Hodgins S, Matthews Z, et al. Quality maternity care for every woman, everywhere: a call to action. Lancet. 2016;388(10057):2307–20.
7. WHO, UNICEF, UNFPA, World Bank Group, the United Nations Population Division. Trends in maternal mortality 1990 to 2015: Estimates by WHO, UNICEF, UNFPA, World Bank Group and the United Nations population division. Geneva: WHO; 2015.
8. UNICEF, WHO, the United Nations Population Division, World Bank Group. Levels and trends in child mortality Estimates Developed by UN Inter-agency Group for Child Mortality Estimation. New York: UNICEF; 2015.
9. Arifeen S, Hill K, Ahsan KZ, Jamil K, Nahar Q, Streatfield PK. Maternal mortality in Bangladesh: a countdown to 2015 country case study. Lancet. 2014;384(9951):1366–74.
10. Islam F, Rahman A, Halim A, Eriksson C, Rahman F, Dalal K. Perceptions of health care providers and patients on quality of care in maternal and neonatal health in fourteen Bangladesh government healthcare facilities: a mixed-method study. BMC Health Serv Res. 2015;15(1):237.
11. NIPORT, Mitra and Associates, ICF International. Bangladesh Demographic and Health Survey 2014. Dhaka, Bangladesh and Rockville, Maryland:

National Institute of Population Research and Training, Mitra and Associates, and ICF International; 2015.
12. Tuncalp, Were WM, MacLennan C, Oladapo OT, Gulmezoglu AM, Bahl R, Daelmans B, Mathai M, Say L, Kristensen F et al. Quality of care for pregnant women and newborns-the WHO vision. BJOG. 2015;122(8):1045–9.
13. WHO. Safe Childbirth Checklist programme: An overview. Geneva: WHO; 2013.
14. Spector JM, Agrawal P, Kodkany B, Lipsitz S, Lashoher A, Dziekan G, Bahl R, Merialdi M, Mathai M, Lemer C. Improving quality of care for maternal and newborn health: prospective pilot study of the WHO Safe Childbirth Checklist program. PLoS One. 2012;7(5):e35151.
15. Patabendige M, Senanayake H. Implementation of the WHO Safe Childbirth Checklist program at a tertiary care setting in Sri Lanka: a developing country experience. BMC Pregnancy Childbirth. 2015;15(1):12.
16. Management Information System, DGHS, Government of Bangladesh and UNICEF. Emergency Obstetric Care (EmOC) Performance Report. In: Voice of MIS-Health, vol. 11. Dhaka: Directorate General of Health Service, Government of Bangladesh and UNICEF; 2013.
17. WHO, WHO Safe Childbirth Checklist Implementation Guide. Improving the quality of facility-based delivery for mothers and newborns. Geneva: WHO; 2015.
18. Moran A, Wahed T, Afsana K. Oxytocin to augment labour during home births: an exploratory study in the urban slums of Dhaka, Bangladesh. BJOG. 2010;117(13):1608–15.
19. Anwar I, Kalim N, Koblinsky M. Quality of obstetric care in public-sector facilities and constraints to implementing emergency obstetric care services: evidence from high-and low-performing districts of Bangladesh. J Health Popul Nutr. 2009;27(2):139.
20. Althabe F, Bergel E, Cafferata ML, Gibbons L, Ciapponi A, Alemán A, Colantonio L, Palacios AR. Strategies for improving the quality of health care in maternal and child health in low-and middle-income countries: an overview of systematic reviews. Paediatr Perinat Epidemiol. 2008;22(s1):42–60.
21. WHO. Counselling for Maternal and Newborn Health. A Handbook for Building Skill. Geneva: WHO; 2014.
22. Osamor PE, Grady C. Women's autonomy in health care decision-making in developing countries: a synthesis of the literature. Int J Womens Health. 2016;8:191.
23. Upadhyay UD, Hindin MJ. Do higher status and more autonomous women have longer birth intervals? Results from Cebu, Philippines. Soc Sci Med. 2005;60(11):2641–55.
24. Callaghan-Koru JA, McMahon SA, Chebet JJ, Kilewo C, Frumence G, Gupta S, Stevenson R, Lipingu C, Baqui AH, Winch PJ. A qualitative exploration of health workers' and clients' perceptions of barriers to completing four antenatal care visits in Morogoro Region, Tanzania. Health Policy Plan. 2016; 31(8):1039-49.
25. NIPORT, ACPR, ICF International. Bangladesh Health Facility Survey 2014. Dhaka: National Institute of Population Research and Training (NIPORT), Associates for Community and Population Research (ACPR), and ICF International; 2016.
26. Pagel C, Prost A, Hossen M, Azad K, Kuddus A, Roy SS, Nair N, Tripathy P, Saville N, Sen AI. Essential newborn care provided by institutions and after home births? Analysis of prospective data from community trials in rural South Asia. BMC Pregnancy Childbirth. 2014;14(1):99.
27. Dieleman M, Harnmeijer JW. Improving health worker performance: in search of promising practices. Geneva: WHO; 2006. p. 5–34.
28. WHO. The World Health Report 2006: Working together for health. Geneva: WHO; 2006.
29. Ollerhead E, Osrin D. Barriers to and incentives for achieving partograph use in obstetric practice in low- and middle-income countries: a systematic review. BMC Pregnancy Childbirth. 2014;14(1):1–7.
30. Mathai M. The partograph for the prevention of obstructed labor. Clin Obstet Gynecol. 2009;52(2):256–69.
31. Landry E, Pett C, Fiorentino R, Ruminjo J, Mattison C. Assessing the quality of record keeping for cesarean deliveries: results from a multicenter retrospective record review in five low-income countries. BMC Pregnancy Childbirth. 2014;14(1):1–11.
32. Fatusi AO, Makinde ON, Adeyemi AB, Orji EO, Onwudiegwu U. Evaluation of health workers' training in use of the partogram. Int J Gynaecol Obstet. 2008;100(1):41-4.
33. Opiah MM, Ofi AB, Essien EJ, Monjok E. Knowledge and utilization of the partograph among midwives in the Niger Delta Region of Nigeria. Afr J Reprod Health. 2012;16(1):125-32.
34. Dietsch E, Mulimbalimba-Masururu L. The experience of being a traditional midwife: living and working in relationship with women. J Midwifery Womens Health. 2011;56(2):161-6.
35. Theron GB. Effect of the maternal care manual of the perinatal education programme on the ability of midwives to interpret antenatal cards and partograms. J Perinatol. 1999;19(6 Pt 1):432-5.
36. Asp G, Sandberg J, Ezechi O, Odberg PK. Challenges of immediate newborn care in maternity units in Lagos, Nigeria: An observational study. J Obstet Gynaecol. 2011;31(7):612-6.
37. Kwast B, Lennox C, Farley T, Olayinka I. World health organization partograph in management of labour. Lancet. 1994;343(8910):1399.
38. Kanté AM, Chung CE, Larsen AM, Exavery A, Tani K, Phillips JF. Factors associated with compliance with the recommended frequency of postnatal care services in three rural districts of Tanzania. BMC Pregnancy Childbirth. 2015;15(1):341.
39. Carlo WA, McClure EM, Chomba E, Chakraborty H, Hartwell T, Harris H, Lincetto O, Wright LL. Newborn care training of midwives and neonatal and perinatal mortality rates in a developing country. Pediatrics. 2010; 126(5):e1064–71.
40. WHO. Medicine use in primary health care in developing and transitional countries: Fact book summarising results from studies reported between 1990 and 2006. Geneva: WHO. p. 2009.
41. Holloway KA. Combating inappropriate use of medicines. Expert Rev Clin Pharmacol. 2011;4(3):335–48.
42. Radyowijati A, Haak H. Improving antibiotic use in low-income countries: an overview of evidence on determinants. Soc Sci Med. 2003;57(4):733–44.
43. Hulscher ME, Grol RP, van der Meer JW. Antibiotic prescribing in hospitals: a social and behavioural scientific approach. Lancet Infect Dis. 2010;10(3):167–75.
44. Sultana F, Rahman A, Paul TR, Sarwar MS, Islam MAU, Rashid M. Prescribing pattern and prescription errors: a study at a tertiary care hospital of Bangladesh. Bangladesh Pharmaceutical Journal. 2015;18(1):20–4.
45. Hussein J, Walker L. Puerperal sepsis in low and middle income settings: past, present and future. In: Maternal and infant deaths: chasing millennium development goals. Volume 4. Edited by Sean Kehoe JN, Jane Norman; 2010. p. 131–47.
46. Bonet M, Ota E, Chibueze CE, Oladapo OT. Routine antibiotic prophylaxis after normal vaginal birth for reducing maternal infectious morbidity: Cochrane. 2016. http://onlinelibrary.wiley.com.ezp.lib.unimelb.edu.au/doi/10.1002/14651858.CD012137.pub2/full.
47. Steinhardt LC, Onikpo F, Kouamé J, Piercefield E, Lama M, Deming MS, Rowe AK. Predictors of health worker performance after integrated Management of Childhood Illness training in Benin: a cohort study. BMC Health Serv Res. 2015;15(1):276.
48. Rowe AK, Onikpo F, Lama M, Cokou F, Deming MS. Management of childhood illness at health facilities in Benin: problems and their causes. Am J Public Health. 2001;91(10):1625–35.
49. Selemani M, Masanja IM, Kajungu D, Amuri M, Njozi M, Khatib RA, Abdulla S, de Savigny D. Health worker factors associated with prescribing of artemisinin combination therapy for uncomplicated malaria in rural Tanzania. Malar J. 2013;12(1):334.
50. Baiden F, Owusu-Agyei S, Bawah J, Bruce J, Tivura M, Delmini R, Gyaase S, Amenga-Etego S, Chandramohan D, Webster J. An evaluation of the clinical assessments of under-five febrile children presenting to primary health facilities in rural Ghana. PLoS One. 2011; 6(12):e28944.
51. Zurovac D, Tibenderana JK, Nankabirwa J, Ssekitooleko J, Njogu JN, Rwakimari JB, Meek S, Talisuna A, Snow RW. Malaria case-management under artemether-lumefantrine treatment policy in Uganda. Malaria J. 2008;7(1):181.

6

Correlation between maternal and umbilical cord blood in pregnant women of Pokhara Valley

Sameer Timilsina[1*], Sirisa Karki[2], Aajeevan Gautam[3], Pujan Bhusal[1], Gita Paudel[2] and Deepak Sharma[1]

Abstract

Background: Complete blood count is one of the routinely advised blood investigation during pregnancy. It is also utilized as a diagnostic tool for neonatal anemia, sepsis and determining hemostatic status of the newborn. The present study aims at estimating the complete blood count of maternal and umbilical cord blood at the time of delivery and to establish its correlation.

Method: This cross sectional study included 114 mothers and their healthy neonates born through normal vaginal delivery. Complete blood count of umbilical cord blood and maternal blood was estimated using automatic hematology analyzer.

Results: The mean maternal and neonatal hemoglobin concentration was 11.14 ± 1.39 g/dL and 16.34 ± 2.01 g/dL respectively. A significant positive correlation was found between maternal and fetal hemoglobin concentration ($p < 0.001$ and Pearson $R = 0.496$). The correlation between maternal and fetal WBC, RBC and Platelet count was not statistically significant. A significant positive correlation was found between maternal and fetal MCV and MCH while PCV showed a non-significant positive correlation.

Conclusion: There was moderately positive correlation between maternal and fetal hemoglobin, MCV and MCH. The cord blood hemoglobin was lower in babies born to anemic mothers. The decrease in hemoglobin followed the severity of anemia, however, the correlation did not exist in anemic mothers. It suggested that fetal hematological parameters are not reflective of maternal hemogram.

Keywords: Hematology, Umbilical cord blood, Hemoglobin, Mother

Background

Maternal physiology endures several alterations in hematological parameters with an average rise of 40–50% in blood and plasma volume during pregnancy [1]. This hemodilution produces pronounced effect in hematocrit values. Complete blood count is the most commonly advised blood investigation. It is often the first step in evaluating hematologic function and diagnosis of related diseases [2]. During embryonic period, hematopoiesis occurs in different parts of the developing fetus. It starts initially in the embryonic yolk sack migrating to the fetal liver and preterm marrow. However, hematopoiesis is primarily restricted to the bone marrow in adults [3].

Anemia is a clinical condition in which the number of circulating red blood cells is insufficient to meet the body's physiologic demands. WHO classifies anemia [4] in pregnancy as non-anemic (> 11 g/dL), mild anemia (10–10.9 g/dL), moderate anemia (7–9.9 g/dL) and severe anemia (< 7 g/dL).

Umbilical cord blood hemoglobin is a dominant hematologic parameter of newborns at birth. Hemoglobin along with hematocrit values together have been customarily used in the diagnosis and follow-up of the neonatal anemia [5]. Besides this, other hematologic parameters like white blood cell count and platelet count are worthwhile in assessing neonatal sepsis and hemostatic status of infant [5]. Studies have shown some relationships between

* Correspondence: timilsina.sameer@cmc.edu.np; sawmer@gmail.com
[1]Department of Physiology, Chitwan Medical College, Tribhuwan University, Post Box No, Bharatpur-13, Chitwan 42, Nepal
Full list of author information is available at the end of the article

maternal and fetal hemogram but the extent of effect on maternal and neonatal health is still uncertain. This study was conducted to assess the effect of maternal hematologic profile during normal pregnancy on cord blood hematology.

In an attempt to achieving Millennium Development Goals (MDG) 4 and 5 Nepal has made noteworthy progress in the field of maternal, newborn and child health. Nepal Government has implemented certain health related policies like free ion supplementation and ANC visits even in the remote parts of the country. The policy also includes rewards for delivering babies in health care facilities. As a result, substantial improvement has been observed in maternal mortality rate plummeting from 450 in 2004 to 260 in 2014 [6]. As of yet, no studies have been conducted in Pokhara Valley of Nepal on maternal and neonatal hemogram. The present study aims at obtaining a complete picture of maternal and fetal hemogram thereby enabling to maintain referencing in the general population of this region. The anticipated advantage of this study was to determine the fetal outcomes beforehand and building up a strategy in order to prevent adverse outcomes.

Methods

This was a hospital based cross-sectional study conducted from April 2014 to March 2015 at Manipal Teaching Hospital, Pokhara (827 m above sea level), Nepal. A total of 114 normal singleton pregnant mothers and their healthy newborn babies were included in the study. All pregnant women were residents of Pokhara Valley. They all have had 4 routine antenatal checkups during the course of pregnancy and all of them were supplemented with iron and folic acid. A written consent was obtained from the mother for participation in the study for both the mother and their newborn child. A brief history of the mother was taken during presentation for delivery. 3 ml of blood was collected in a sterile syringe from ante cubital vein and stored in an EDTA containing vial. After 2 min of delivery of the baby, 3 ml of umbilical cord blood was collected and was stored in an EDTA containing vial. Upon collection of the sample, it was analyzed within 3–6 h using an automatic hematology analyzer (Diagnova RFCL lablife h3d premier). Appropriate internal quality controls were run before assay of samples. Statistical analysis was performed by using the program Statistical Packages of Social Sciences (SPSS) version 20.0. The results were evaluated by using Pearson correlation test and Independent sample 't' test. Shapiro Wilk test was done to check the normality of distribution of different variables. Multiple regression analysis was performed for multivariate analysis. Statistical significance was considered at $p < 0.05$.

Results

The study included a total of 114 pregnant women and their newborns (86 males and 28 females). Of the total participants, 68(59.64%) were multi gravida and 46 (40.36%) were primigravida. The mean age of pregnancy was 26.04 ± 3.47 years with 86% (98/114) between the age of 21–30 years. The result presented here affirms the existence of variations in red cell indices of umbilical cord blood reported for Pokhara

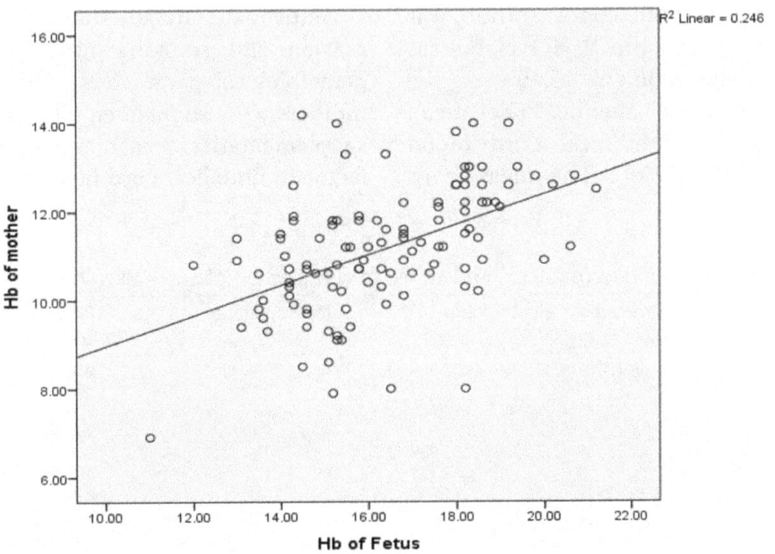

Fig. 1 Scatter plot showing mean hemoglobin concentration of maternal and umbilical cord blood

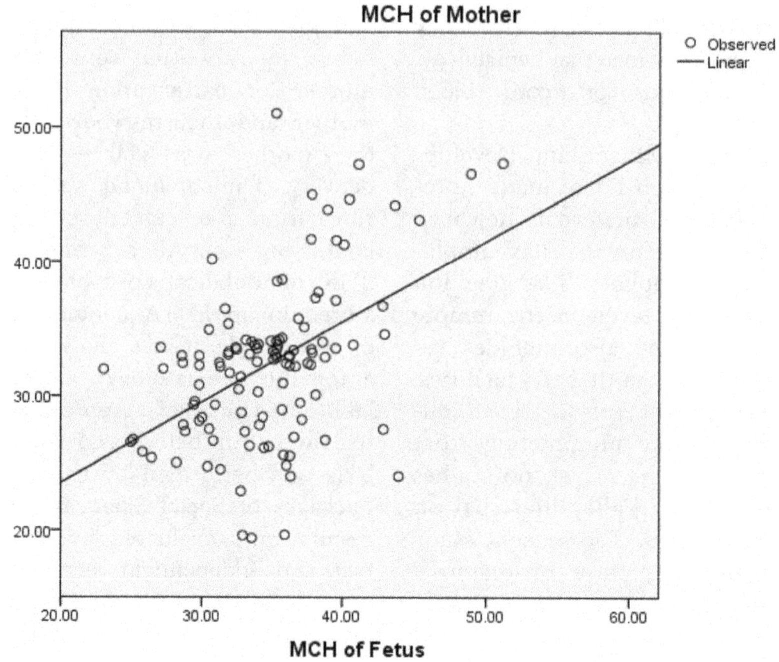

Fig. 2 Scatter plot showing mean MCH concentration of maternal blood and umbilical cord blood

valley of Nepal. These results could be helpful in providing a baseline data for further studies as to establish a reference value for maternal and umbilical cord hemogram in the locality.

The result showed no significant correlation between total white blood cell count of mother with that of the fetus ($p > 0.01$). The normally distributed variables were hemoglobin, RBC count, hematocrit, MCV and platelets while the remaining variables were non-normally distributed.

The mean maternal hemoglobin concentration was 11.14 ± 1.39 g/dL. According to the WHO classification of anemia in pregnant women, 46.49% of the participants were found to be anemic. The mean hemoglobin concentration of umbilical cord blood was found to be 16.34 ± 2.01 g/dL. The mean cord blood hemoglobin concentration in anemic and non-anemic mothers was 15.38 ± 1.7 g/dL and 17.21 ± 1.87 g/dL respectively. Figure 1 represents the scatter plot of mean hemoglobin of mother with that of the umbilical cord blood showing a linear correlation which was found to be statistically significant ($p < 0.05$). Likewise, Fig. 2 shows the scatter plot of mean MCH of mother with that of the umbilical cord blood indicating a linear correlation and was also found to be statistically significant (Tables 1 and 2).

Multivariate analysis showed maternal factors like age, gravida and smoking history did not influence the hematological parameters of the fetus. As all pregnant mothers were supplemented with iron and folic acid, ion supplementation was not considered as a confounding factor to umbilical cord hemogram.

Table 1 Mean Hemoglobin concentration of mothers in reference to classification of anemia by WHO.

Maternal Hemoglobin g/dL (WHO Classification)	Mean maternal Hemoglobin g/dL	No of patients	Pearson's correlation coefficient R	*p* value
Non anemic Hb > 11 g/dL	12.17 ± 0.81	60	0.460	$p < 0.05$
Mild anemia Hb = 10–10.9 g/dL	10.57 ± 0.27	33	0.456	$p < 0.05$
Moderate Anemia Hb = 7–9.9 g/dL	9.18 ± 0.65	20	0.499	$p < 0.05$
Severe anemia Hb < 7 g/dL	....	1	....	....

Table 2 Correlation between maternal and fetal hemogram

Parameters	Mother	Fetal	Pearson's correlation coefficient R	*p*-value
WBC (X 10^3/mm3)	10.20 ± 3.36	15.52 ± 5.60	−0.040	NS
Hb (g/dL)	11.14 ± 1.39	16.34 ± 2.01	0.496	$p < 0.001$
RBC X 10^6/mm^3)	4.04 ± 0.46	4.72 ± 0.59	0.083	NS
Hematocrit (%)	33.29 ± 4.02	48.79 ± 6.88	0.109	NS
MCV (fL)	82.33 ± 6.46	102.85 ± 8.58	0.058	NS
MCH (pg)	33.34 ± 5.94	34.70 ± 4.73	0.478	$p < 0.001$
MCHC (g/dL)	33.40 ± 1.25	33.26 ± 1.09	−0.069	NS
Platelets (X 10^4/mm3)	22.29 ± 6.61	229.20 ± 73.39	0.005	NS

Discussion

The mean age of pregnancy was found to be 26.04 ± 3.47 years and the median age was 26 years which was slightly above the national data of census of Nepal 2011. WHO's [4] report of 44% prevalence of anemia in Nepal was consistent with the present study. The result of the present study was homogenous to WHO survey for mean hemoglobin concentration of average Nepali pregnant women estimated at 11.1 g/dL (10.8–11.5 g/dL with 95% credibility interval) [4]. Similar to studies in other parts of the country, [7–10] 45.61% of pregnant women were found to have hemoglobin concentrations less than 10 g/dL and 0.8% with hemoglobin concentration less than 7 g/dL. This finding was far from similar to the 2016 Nepal DHS Key indicators [11] which reported anemia in this part of Nepal to be around 28%. The prevalence of anemia throughout the country is however similar to the present study (46%). [10].

The present study showed significant positive correlation between maternal and fetal hemoglobin concentrations like Dapper DV et al. [12] in Nigeria, McElroy PD et al. [13] in Kenya, and Alizadeh L et al. [14] in Iran. No significant correlation was observed between maternal and fetal white cell count and MCHC [12–14]. A positive linear Pearson correlation was observed between mean hemoglobin and PCV of cord blood and maternal blood. All these results were similar to the ones observed by Nneli R et al. [15] Singla PN et al. [16] and Al-hilli NM et al. [17]. In contrast to the present study, some previous investigators including Qaiser DH et al., [18] Kilbride J et al., [19] and Mamoury GH et al. [20] have failed to find a relationship between the maternal and cord blood hemoglobin.

The present study showed 5.7% of the fetuses had low hemoglobin concentration, 23.94% had low MCV, 18.24% had low MCH and none of the fetuses had low MCHC which was a constant finding with Abdelgader EA et al. [21] and Steer PJ [22]. The cord blood hemoglobin (16.8 g/dL) of healthy term neonates in this study was uniform with those reported from studies in the west [23, 24].

Qaiser DH et al. [25] measured the mean of all CBC parameters aiming to maintain refrencing, and found the mean hemoglobin = 14.99 ± 1.47 g/dL, RBC = 4.29 ± 0.44, PCV = 45.65 ± 4.83, MCV = 105.81 ± 6.24, MCH = 34.96 ± 2.11, MCHC = 32.47 ± 2.12, TC = 13.61 ± 4.23 and platelet count = 256.25 ± 76.54 in the umbilical cord blood. The result showed similar findings with the present study but with a slightly higher total WBC count.

As the study was conducted in only one tertiary care center and that too with a limited number of patients, the result does not represent the pregnant women in Western Development Region of Nepal. Also, the study only included the patients attending hospital for delivery so the results cannot be generalized as it may not be a true reflection of the general population. However researchers have found the increasing trend of hospital based deliveries in urban population and Pokhara being an urban city, the data and results presented could actually represent the urban population of Pokhara valley. Socioeconomic status of the pregnant women was also not considered in the study. Moreover, further studies are to be conducted in the field to achieve complete results.

Conclusions

There was moderately positive correlation between maternal and fetal hemoglobin, MCV and MCH. There was a decrease in the cord blood hemoglobin in different severities of anemia, however, the correlation between maternal and fetal hemoglobin did not exist. It suggested that the fetal hematological parameters are not reflective of maternal hemogram.

Anemia in pregnancy should be properly evaluated and treated accordingly in order to avoid unwanted fetal and maternal outcomes.

Abbreviations

ANC: Ante-natal Checkup; CBC: Complete Blood Count; EDTA: Ethylene Diamine Tetra Acetic acid; Hb: Hemoglobin; MCH: Mean Corpuscular Hemoglobin; MCHC: Mean Corpuscular Hemoglobin Concentration; MCV: Mean Corpuscular Volume; MDG: Millennium Development Goals; PCV: Packed Cell Volume; RBC: Red Blood Cells; SPSS: Statistical Package for Social Sciences; TC: Total Count; WBC: White Blood Cells; WHO: World Health Organization

Acknowledgements

We would like to thank the ethical committee of Manipal College of Medical Sciences for providing us the consent to conduct this study at this esteemed institute. We would also like to whole heartedly thank the participants of the study without whom the study would not have been possible. We are highly indebted to Prof Dr. C G Saha, HOD and all faculties of Department of Physiology, Manipal College of Medical Sciences for their continuous encouragement and support in the field of research. We would also like to thank Dr. Indu Tiwari, Mr. Bhuwan Baskota and Mr. Madhav Poudel for their help and support. Our sincere gratitude to Dr. Santosh Timalsina for his untiring and ever encouraging words during data analysis. Also, we would like to thank Dr. Nikki Shrestha for her English language assistance.

Funding

No funding of any sort was received for the study.

Authors' contributions

ST wrote the proposal, participated in data collection, analyzed the data and drafted the paper. SK assisted in data collection, laboratory procedures and helped in revising the draft. AG and PB helped in the analysis of the data and writing manuscript. GP and DS participated in manuscript editing and final writing. All authors read and approved the final manuscript.

Competing interests

The authors declare that they have no competing interests.

Author details

[1]Department of Physiology, Chitwan Medical College, Tribhuwan University, Post Box No, Bharatpur-13, Chitwan 42, Nepal. [2]Department of Pharmacology, Chitwan Medical College, Tribhuwan University, Bharatpur-13, Chitwan, Nepal. [3]Department of Anatomy, Chitwan Medical College, Tribhuwan University, Bharatpur-13, Chitwan, Nepal.

References

1. Pritchard JA. Changes in blood volume during pregnancy and delivery. Anesthesiology. 1965;26:393.
2. eMedicine Health [Internet]. Nabili SM.: ©2015 Web MD. Complete blood count (online). 2017 Feb 21 Available from URL: http://www.emedicinehealth.com/complete_blood_count_cbc/article_em.htm
3. Fristma GA, Keohane E. Hematology: Clinical principles and applications. 4th ed. New York: Elsevier Health Sciences; 2012.
4. WHO. The global prevalence of anaemia in, vol. 2011. Geneva: World Health Organization; 2015.
5. Paiva AD, Rondo PH, Pagliuisi RA, Latorre MR, Cardoso MA, Gondium SS. Relationship between the iron status of pregnant women and their newborns. Rev Saude Publica. 2007;41:321–7.
6. Ministry of Health and Population Nepal. Partnership for Maternal, Newborn & Child Health, WHO, World Bank and Alliance for Health Policy and Systems Research. Success factors for women's and children's health: Nepal. Geneva: World Health Organisation; 2014.
7. Bhandary S, Shrestha A. Prevalence of anemia among non-pregnant and pregnant women of reproductive age in Nepal. JGPEMN. 2011 Jan-June;2: 21–6.
8. Rana SS, Sharma S, Chand A, Malla R. Relationship between maternal Haemoglobin and fetal weight. NJOG. 2013 Jan-Jun;8(1):37–40.
9. Raut BK, Jha MK, Shrestha A, Sah A, Sapkota A, Byanju S, et al. Prevalence of iron deficiency anemia among pregnant women before iron supplementation in Kathmandu University/ Dhulikhel hospital. Journal of Gynecology and obstetrics. 2014;2(4):54–8.
10. Tuladhar H. Anaemia in adolescent pregnancy. JNMC. 2000 Jan;2(1):19–21.
11. Ministry of Health, Nepal; New ERA; and ICF. Nepal demographic and health survey 2016: key indicators. Kathmandu, Nepal: Ministry of Health, Nepal; 2017.
12. Dapper DV, Didia BC. Haemorheological parameters of umbilical cord blood of Nigerian newborns: correlations with maternal parameters. WAJM Jan-Mar. 2006;25(1):226–30.
13. McElroy PD, Lal AA, Hawley WA, Bloland PB, Kuile OAJ, et al. Analysis of repeated hemoglobin measures in full-term, normal birth weight Kenyan children between birth and four years of age. The ASEMBO Bay cohort project. Am J Trop Med Hyg. 1999;61(6):932–40.
14. Alizadeh L, Raoofi A, Salehi L, Ramzi M. Impact of maternal hemoglobin concentration on fetal outcomes in adolescent pregnant women. Iran Red Crescent Med J. 2014 Aug 1;16(8):e19670.
15. Nneli R, Amadi S, Nwafia W. Certain red blood cell indices of maternal and umbilical cord blood in Owerri, Nigeria: a preliminary report. Ann Med Health Sci Res 2011 Jan;1(1):1–8.
16. Singla PN, Chand S. Effect of maternal anaemia on the placenta and the newborn infant. Acta Paediatr. 2008 June;67(5):645–8.
17. Al-hilli NM. The Effect of Maternal Anaemia on Cord Blood Haemoglobin & Newborn Birth Weigh Karbala. J Med. 2010;2:8–9.
18. Qaiser DH, Sandhila MP, Omair A, Ghori GM. Correlation of routine Haematological parameters between normal maternal blood and the cord blood of healthy newborns in selected hospitals of Karachi. J Coll Physicians Surg Pak. 2013 Feb;23(2):128–31.
19. Kilbride J, Baker TG, Parapia LA, Khoury SA, Shuqaidefd SW, Jerwoode D. Anaemia during pregnancy as a risk factor for iron-deficiency anaemia in infancy: a case-control study in Jordan. Int J Epidemiol. 1999 June;28:461–8.
20. Mamoury GH, Hamedy AB, Alkhlaghi F. Cord haemoglobin in newborn in correlation with maternal haemoglobin in northeastern Iran. Iran J Med Sci. 2003;28:166–8.
21. Abdelgader EA, Sana E, Abdalla SE, Kordofani AA, Omer IM. Haematological pictures in full term new born children in Sudan. Basic research journal of medicine and clinical. Sciences. 2013 Oct;2(9):88–93.
22. Steer PJ. Maternal hemoglobin concentration and birth weight. Am J Clin Nutr 2000 May;71(5 Suppl):1285S–1287S.
23. Doyle JJ, Schmitdt B, Avery GB, Fletcher MA, Macdonald MG. Neonatology, pathophysiology management of the newborns. 5th ed. Philadelphia: Lippincott; 1999.
24. Chirstenson RD. Expected hematologic values for term and preterm neonates. In: Cristensen P, editor. Hematologic problems of the neonatel. 11th ed. Philadelphia: Saunders; 2005. p. 118–22.
25. Qaiser DH, Ahmed ST, Sandila MP, Kazmi T. Hematological reference values for full term, healthy, newborns of Karachi. Pakistan JPMA. 2009;59:618.

7

The effect of Kenya's free maternal health care policy on the utilization of health facility delivery services and maternal and neonatal mortality in public health facilities

C. M. Gitobu[1*], P. B. Gichangi[2,3†] and W. O. Mwanda[4†]

Abstract

Background: Kenya abolished delivery fees in all public health facilities through a presidential directive effective on June 1, 2013 with an aim of promoting health facility delivery service utilization and reducing pregnancy-related mortality in the country. This paper aims to provide a brief overview of this policy's effect on health facility delivery service utilization and maternal mortality ratio and neonatal mortality rate in Kenyan public health facilities.

Methods: A time series analysis was conducted on health facility delivery services utilization, maternal and neonatal mortality 2 years before and after the policy intervention in 77 health facilities across 14 counties in Kenya.

Results: A statistically significant increase in the number of facility-based deliveries was identified with no significant changes in the ratio of maternal mortality and the rate of neonatal mortality.

Conclusion: The findings suggest that cost is a deterrent to health facility delivery service utilization in Kenya and thus free delivery services are an important strategy to promote utilization of health facility delivery services; however, there is a need to simultaneously address other factors that contribute to pregnancy-related and neonatal deaths.

Keywords: Free maternal health care policy, Maternal mortality ratio, Neonatal mortality rate and health facility delivery services utilization

Background

The reduction and elimination of pregnancy-related mortality remain a challenge in most low income countries [1]. The maternal mortality ratio and the neonatal mortality rate in Kenya have been found to be 362/100,000 live births and 22/1000 live births, respectively [2]. Given that only 61.2% of deliveries in the country are conducted in health facilities, pregnancy-related deaths have been attributed to delivery without skilled birth attendance [2]. Globally, high quality health facility delivery services have been recommended as a solution to preventable maternal and neonatal deaths [3]. For this reason, many African countries have either reduced or eliminated delivery fees to promote health facility delivery service utilization [4].

Kenya joined other African countries in the abolishment of delivery fees in all public health facilities through a presidential directive signed into effect on June 1, 2013 [5]. Through this policy, public health facilities are reimbursed for costs incurred while providing delivery services through a capitation fund provided by the Ministry of Health. This policy provides equal reimbursement for both spontaneous vaginal deliveries and caesarean sections. The amounts reimbursed to health facilities are based on their capacity to manage pregnancy and delivery complications. As such, 2500 Kenya shillings (25 US dollars) are reimbursed for every delivery conducted in level 2 facilities (health centers) and level 3 health facilities (sub district hospitals); 5000 Kenya shillings (50 US dollars) are reimbursed for every delivery carried out in level 4 health facilities (district hospitals) and level 5 health facilities

* Correspondence: cosmgambi@gmail.com
†Equal contributors
[1]Institute of Tropical and Infectious Diseases (UNITID), University of Nairobi, Nairobi, Kenya
Full list of author information is available at the end of the article

(provincial hospitals); and 17,500 Kenya shillings (175 US dollars) are reimbursed for every delivery performed in national referral health facilities [6].

While eliminating delivery fees is a commendable intervention, pregnancy-related mortality due to the following "three delays" remains a concern: delays in deciding to seek skilled delivery services, delays in arriving at health facilities and delays in receiving adequate treatment and referral [7]. Cost is not the only factor hindering the utilization of health facility delivery services. In Kenya, maternal and neonatal deaths have been attributed to other factors, including lack of transport, long distances to health centers, poorly equipped health facilities, low quality of care in health facilities and traditional and cultural practices [8, 9]. Therefore, while elimination of delivery fees in Kenyan public health facilities partially addresses economic barriers to maternal health care utilization, other economic barriers, health system gaps, quality of health facility delivery services and political, social, environmental and religious factors that may influence the utilization and outcomes of maternal health care in the country have not been addressed [10–15].

In addition, initial assessments of the implementation of this policy have identified various gaps, such as drug and supply shortages, insufficient funding, skilled health care worker shortages, lack of skills among health workers, stakeholder non-involvement in the policy design, delayed reimbursement of costs incurred while providing free maternal health care, heavy workloads, health worker demotivation, healthcare worker attitudes, low privacy levels in public health facilities and unavailability of ambulances for emergencies occurring at community level [16, 17]. In light of these contextual gaps, this study aimed to investigate the effects of the free maternal health care policy in Kenya on health facility delivery service utilization and maternal mortality ratio and neonatal mortality rate in public health facilities.

Methods

A time series analysis was performed with the period of interest being 24 months before policy implementation (June 1, 2011, to May 31, 2013) and 24 months after policy implementation (June 1, 2013, to May 31, 2015).

The study was conducted in 77 public health facilities selected from 14 counties in the Republic of Kenya. At the time of data collection, Kenya's public health care facilities were organized in a hierarchical pyramidal structure comprising six levels, namely, level 1 health facilities (health centers), level 2 health facilities (dispensaries), level 3 health facilities (sub district hospitals), level 4 health facilities (district hospitals), level 5 health facilities (provincial hospitals) and level 6 health facilities, which were national referral hospitals [18]. Caesarean sections are carried out in level 4, 5 and 6 health facilities and therefore, health facilities in these three levels were the study sites. This hierarchical pyramidal structure is expected to change from six to four tiers once relevant legislation is passed by the national parliament [19–22].

Deceased mothers and deceased neonates from the selected health facilities were included in the assessment of maternal and neonatal mortality. Mothers who had delivered in the selected health facilities during the 4 years under consideration were included in the assessment of health service utilization.

Fourteen of the forty-seven counties in the Republic of Kenya were selected for inclusion in the study after single-stage cluster sampling and subsequent simple random sampling procedures were applied [23]. The 47 counties were classified into high risk, medium risk and low risk maternal mortality categories based on their perennial maternal mortality ratios. Of these counties, five with a high risk (maternal death to females population ratio above 0.00018), five with a medium risk (maternal death to females population ratio between 0. 00012 and 0.000183) and four with a low of risk maternal mortality (maternal death to females population ratio below 0.00012) were included in the study; these studies were selected via simple random sampling. Of the 97 health facilities eligible for inclusion in the study, 77 in 14 counties were selected through stratified multi-stage sampling with the maternal mortality risk, counties, status of health facilities and location being the strata [18]. These health facilities were one maternity nursing home (equivalent of a level 5 health facility in terms of infrastructure and human resource), 58 level 4 health facilities, 17 level 5 health facilities and one level 6 public health facility.

Written consent was obtained from heads of health facilities included in the study as well as from the Director of medical services, Ministry of Health Kenya. Health facilities were assigned unique identification codes which are only known to the authors.

The authors relied on primary data sources in every health facility (maternity ward registers, audited records of maternal deaths, neonatal ward registers and death registers) as opposed to DHIS records to ensure data accuracy in the study. The instruments for data collection in this study were tabulated questionnaire to capture monthly figures on neonatal mortality rate, maternal mortality ratio and health facility delivery services utilization in each of the 77 health facilities. The data collection instruments were pre tested at a level 4 health facility. Four research assistants, we recruited, trained and used in data collection.

The instrument used for data collection was a tabulated questionnaire designed to capture monthly neonatal mortality rates, maternal mortality ratios and health facility delivery service utilization data for each of the 77 health facilities. SPSS (IBM version 23) was used for data analysis, and the results were stratified by geographical location and health facility level. Interrupted time series analyses of quarterly (3-month) maternal mortality ratios, neonatal mortality rates and health facility delivery service numbers were performed using autoregressive integrated moving average (ARIMA) models, and the level of significance was set at $p < 0.05$. Diagnostic tests were performed to assess the general fit of the model, and stationary R-squared and traditional R-squared (R^2) values were calculated. Root Mean Square Error (RMSE) which is the standard deviation of the residuals (prediction errors) was used to measure the spread out of residuals. Lastly, Ljung-Box statistic, which is a function of the accumulated sample autocorrelations, was used as a diagnostic tool to test the lack of fit of a time series model through autocorrelations of the residuals.

Results

Health facility delivery service utilization

A statistically significant increase in the number of deliveries in the health facilities was identified; this number increased from 234,601 before policy implementation to 303,705 after policy implementation, representing a 29.5% increase ($p < 0.05$; Table 1).

The results of the analysis of quarterly deliveries in the 77 health facilities indicated a decreasing trend in deliveries (slope = – 13.131, $p = 0.00$) during the 24 months preceding implementation of the policy. Thus during the 24 months before the intervention, no significant change was identified in the number of facility-based deliveries. A significant increase, however, in the quarterly number of facility-based deliveries (slope = 124.90, $p < 0.01$) in the 77 health facilities was identified after policy implementation (Table 2).

Table 1 Total Deliveries in the different levels of health facilities

Variable	Variable Description	Total Deliveries Pre- Policy	Total Deliveries Post-Policy	*P* Value
Location	Rural-Based facilities	88,153.00	112,321.00	< 0.001
	Urban-Based facilities	146,448.00	191,384.00	< 0.01
Facility Level	Maternity Nursing Home	39,729.00	43,411.00	< 0.05
	Level 4 facilities	113,950.00	159,956.00	< 0.001
	Level 5 facilities	60,303.00	74,646.00	0.06
	Level 6 facility	20,619.00	25,692.00	0.10
All 77 facilities		234,601.00	303,705.00	< 0.001

A closer look at the delivery service utilization trends identified during the 6 months before policy implementation indicates the presence of a decreasing trend in the utilization of facility-based delivery services (slope = – 124.90, $p = 0.02$). During the 6 months after policy implementation, this trend reversed, and a significant increase in the number of deliveries in health facilities was observed (slope = 111.77, $p < 0.001$).

Both the stationary and the traditional R^2 tests yielded a value of 0.73, implying that 73% of the model was explained by the policy intervention. In addition, a root mean square error (RSME) value of 384.22 was identified, suggesting that a large portion of the variability observed in the number of deliveries could be explained by the predictive model. The mean absolute percentage error (MAPE) value of 7.25 indicated that the values predicted using the policy implementation model were, on average, within 7.25% of the actual values (Additional file 1).

Both the stationary R-squared and traditional R-squared values for all 77 health facilities were 81.5% ($P = 0.15$; Additional file 2). The stationary R-squared and traditional R-squared values varied from 73.1% to 43.7% across various categories of health facilities. This finding indicated that although policy implementation resulted in a remarkably higher number of facility-based deliveries, this intervention had a non-uniform effect on delivery service utilization across the 77 health facilities ($p = 0.15$).

Maternal mortality ratio

A nonsignificant decrease in the ratio of maternal mortality in the 77 health facilities was identified, with the mortality ratio decreasing from 258.3/100,000 live births to 237.1/100,000 live births ($p = 0.07$) following policy implementation (Table 3). It is only in the rural areas that a significant decline in maternal mortality ratio was recorded.

The ARIMA model parameters for the pre-intervention slope that was calculated using data from the 77 health facilities showed a nonsignificant decrease in the rate of quarterly maternal mortality (slope = – 1.64, $p = 0.20$) during the 24 months preceding user fee removal. During the 24 months after free maternity health care services were first offered, a significant increase in the rate of quarterly maternal mortality was observed in the health facilities under consideration (slope = 3.49, $p = 0.01$). This finding indicated that the free maternal health care policy did not have a significant effect on facility-based maternal mortality ratios (Table 4).

Both the stationery R-squared and traditional R-squared (R^2) values for the model were 0.126, implying that only 12.6% of the variance observed in maternal mortality ratio could be explained by the free maternal health care policy intervention. The RSME value of 112.67 indicated that the interrupted time series model was

Table 2 Quarterly Patterns in Health Facility Delivery Service Utilization

	Slope 24 months pre-policy	Slope 12 months pre-policy	Slope 6 months pre-policy	Slope 3 months pre-policy	Slope 3 months post-policy	Slope 6 months post- policy	Slope 12 months post-policy	Slope 24 months post-policy
All 77 facilities	−13.13 ($p = 0.63$)	−13.13 ($p = 0.63$)	− 124.90 ($p < 0.05$)	− 13.13 ($p = 0.063$)	111.77 ($p < 0.05$)	111.77 ($p < 0.05$)	− 26.65 ($p = 0.18$)	124.90 ($p < 0.05$)
Urban-based facilities	− 17.37 ($p = 0.46$)	− 17.37 ($p = 0.46$)	−77.10 ($p < 0.05$)	−17.37 ($p = 0.46$)	59.74 ($p < 0.05$)	59.74 ($p < 0.05$)	111.77 ($p < 0.05$)	77.10 ($p < 0.05$)
Rural-based facilities	4.65 ($p = 0.44$)	4.65 ($p = 0.44$)	−47.34 ($p < 0.05$)	4.65 ($p = 0.44$)	51.99 ($p < 0.05$)	51.99 ($p < 0.05$)	59.74 ($p < 0.05$)	47.34 ($p < 0.05$)
Maternity hospital	−3.12 ($p = 0.87$)	−3.12 ($p = 0.85$)	23.54 (0.45)	−3.12 ($p = 0.87$)	−26.66 ($p < 0.052$)	− 26.66 ($p < 0.05$)	51.99 ($p = 0.0$)	− 23.54 ($p = 0.45$)
Level 4 facilities	18.79 ($p = 0.15$)	18.79 ($p = 0.15$)	−68.00 ($p < 0.05$)	18.79 ($p = 0.15$)	86.79 ($p < 0.05$)	86.789 ($p < 0.05$)	86.98 ($p < 0.05$)	68.00 ($p < 0.05$)
Level 5 facilities	−19.59 (0.13)	19.59 ($p = 0.13$)	−53.63 ($p < 0.05$)	− 19.59 ($p = 0.13$)	34.04 ($p < 0.05$)	34.04 ($p < 0.05$)	34.04 ($p < 0.05$)	53.63 ($p < 0.05$)
Level 6 facility	−0.75 ($p = 0.87$)	− 0.76 ($p = 0.09$)	− 0.76 ($p < 0.05$)	16.26 ($p < 0.05$)	16.26 ($p < 0.05$)	16.26 ($p < 0.05$)	16.26 ($p < 0.05$)	17.01 ($p < 0.05$)

Table 3 Maternal Mortality Ratios

Variable	Variable Description	MMR Pre-Policy	MMR Post-Policy	*P* Value
Location	Rural-Based facilities	158.20	116.70	0.02
	Urban-Based facilities	326.00	324.40	0.83
Facility Level	Maternity Home	44.80	43.10	0.52
	Level 4 facilities	181.50	182.60	0.19
	Level 5 facilities	254.10	196.70	0.11
	Level 6 facility	1125.80	983.30	0.48
All 77 facilities		258.30	237.10	0.07

reliable in predicting maternal mortality trends. The calculated MAPE indicated a 33.77% variation from the model prediction following the policy intervention (Additional file 3).

Overall, the Ljung-Box test statistics were not significant for the 77 health facilities ($p = 0.54$). Significant Ljung-Box test statistics were identified for level 5 health facilities only (30.64, $p < 0.05$). The stationary R-squared and traditional R-squared values indicated that only a minimal decline in maternal mortality ratio occurred in the 77 health facilities (0.19), with the greatest decline in maternal mortality ratio identified in the level 6 health facility (0.56; Additional file 4). The maternal mortality ratios demonstrated a decreasing trend in the health facilities but exhibited marked although not consistently uniform seasonality. Thus, the free maternal health care policy intervention had a random and nonsignificant effect on maternal mortality ratios across all health facilities.

Neonatal mortality rate

A nonsignificant decline in neonatal mortality rates was identified, with rates decreasing from 23.3/1000 live births to 22.9/1000 live births ($p = 0.14$) following policy implementation (Table 5).

The pre-intervention slope indicated a nonsignificant decreasing trend in the quarterly neonatal mortality rates across all health facilities over the course of the 24 months preceding policy implementation (slope = – 0.09, $p = 0.24$). Implementation of the policy did not significantly affect neonatal mortality rates during the first 24 months following policy implementation (slope = 0.12, $p = 0.10$; Table 6).

Only 32.90% of the minimal and nonsignificant change observed in the neonatal mortality rates could be attributed to policy implementation. The RSME and MAPE values for this model were 688.10 and 17.96, respectively (Additional file 5).

The general fit of the model for all 77 health facilities was not significant ($p = 0.06$). Both the stationary R-squared and traditional R-squared values indicated that only 10.5% of the variation could be explained by the model, implying that policy implementation was associated with only a minimal difference in neonatal mortality rates when compared with baseline figures (Additional file 6).

Discussion

A statistically significant increase in facility deliveries was observed in Kenya following the implementation of the free maternal health care policy in 2013. This result is similar to observations of the implementation of free maternal health care policies in other African countries [24–27]. Applying user fees for delivery services in health facilities may limit the demand, and thus elimination of user fees may improve access to health facility delivery services. The increase in facility-based deliveries remained consistently high over the 2 years post-policy implementation. This finding is in contrast with other regional studies, in which increased utilization of delivery care services was documented during the initial 3 months following user fee removal [27, 28]. The high utilization of free delivery services over a long period of time in this study creates an opportunity to reduce maternal and neonatal mortality.

Implementation of the free maternal health care policy in Kenyan public health facilities did not have a significant effect on maternal and neonatal mortality. This observation is consistent with results of other local and international studies, which have shown user free health policies to have limited or no effect on maternal and neonatal mortality [28–32].

A significant decline in maternal mortality ratio was noted in the rural based health facilities; the Kenya household health expenditure and utilization survey shows that 66% of the country's population lives in rural areas and the rural population is more likely to use public health services than the urban residents [33]. The Kenya household health expenditure and utilization survey also showed that those in the poorest quintile were more likely to use public health facilities than those in the richest quintile. Although only 12% of the change in maternal mortality ratio is attributed to the free maternal health care policy in Kenya, the reduction in maternal mortality ratio in rural based health facilities may be attributed to a high utilization of free delivery services in rural areas where the largest population and poorer population reside.

As pregnancy-related deaths may be attributed to delays in deciding to seek health facility delivery services, delays in arriving at health facilities and delays in receiving adequate treatment and referral, the findings of this study emphasize the fact that other factors may contribute to pregnancy-related deaths in Kenyan public health facilities [34]. The service readiness availability mapping in 2013 when the free maternal health care policy was

Table 4 Quarterly Trends in Maternal Mortality Ratio

Facility	Slope 24 months pre-policy	Slope 12 months pre- policy	Slope 6 months pre-policy	Slope 3 months pre-policy	Slope 3 months post-policy	Slope 6 months post-policy	Slope 12 months post-policy	Slope 24 months post-policy
All 77 health facilities	−1.64 ($p = 0.20$)	−1.64 ($p = 0.20$)	−5.12 ($p < 0.05$)	− 1.64 ($p = 0.20$)	3.486 ($p < 0.05$)	3.49 ($p < 0.05$)	3.48 ($p < 0.05$)	3.47 ($p < 0.05$)
Urban-based facilities	− 1.92 ($p = 0.51$)	− 1.92 ($p = 0.51$)	−7.00 ($p = 0.09$)	− 1.92 ($p = 0.51$)	5.09 ($p = 0.08$)	5.09 ($p = 0.08$)	5.09 ($p = 0.08$)	5.09 ($p = 0.08$)
Rural-based facilities	− 1.38 ($p = 0.40$)	− 1.38 ($p = 0.40$)	− 2.37 ($p = 0.31$)	− 1.38 ($p = 0.40$)	0.99 ($p = 0.54$)	0.99 ($p = 0.54$)	0.99 ($p = 0.54$)	0.99 ($p = 0.54$)
Maternity hospital	− 0.08 ($p = 0.94$)	− 0.08 ($p = 0.94$)	− 2.25 ($p = 0.17$)	− 0.08 ($p = 0.94$)	2.17 ($p = 0.06$)	2.17 ($p = 0.06$)	2.17 ($p = 0.06$)	2.17 ($p = 0.06$)
Level 4 facilities	−2.61 ($p = 0.20$)	− 2.61 ($p = 0.20$)	−6.85 ($p < 0.05$)	− 2.61 ($p = 0.20$)	4.24 ($p < 0.05$)	4.24 ($p < 0.05$)	4.24 ($p < 0.05$)	4.24 ($p < 0.05$)
Level 5 facilities	−4.51 ($p = 0.06$)	− 4.51 ($p = 0.06$)	− 6.70 ($p = 0.05$)	− 4.51 ($p = 0.06$)	2.19 ($p = 0.36$)	2.19 ($p = 0.36$)	2.19 ($p = 0.36$)	2.19 ($p = 0.36$)
Level 6 facility	8.50 ($p = 0.42$)	8.50 ($p = 0.42$)	11.05 ($p = 0.46$)	8.50 ($p = 0.42$)	− 2.55 ($p = 0.81$)	− 2.55 ($p = 0.81$)	− 2.55 ($p = 0.81$)	− 2.55 ($p = 0.81$)

Table 5 Neonatal Mortality Rates

Variable	Variable Description	NMR Before Policy Implementation	NMR After Policy Implementation	*P* Value
Location	Rural-Based facilities	10.30	9.90	0.21
	Urban-Based facilities	35.10	34.20	0.45
Facility Level	Maternity Hospital	24.20	24.90	0.51
	Level 4 facilities	7.30	6.60	0.17
	Level 5 facilities	26.90	26.40	0.81
	Level 6 facility	102.30	104.40	0.54
All 77 facilities		23.30	22.90	0.14

implemented in the country shows that only about 28% of health facilities in the country had essential medicines for handling pregnancy related emergencies with 51% having Oxytocin injectables, 26% having magnesium sulphate injectables and 53% having gentamicin injectables [35]. The unavailability of these essential drugs points to the inability of health facilities to handle pregnancy and child birth related complicates hence no changes in maternal and neonatal mortality.

The adequacy of pre-existing healthcare infrastructure, human resources for health, and supply of medical commodities ought to be addressed before waiver of delivery fees given the high demand of services that comes with fees abolishment [36]. As a signatory to the Abuja Declaration, Kenya committed itself to allocating at least 15% of the national budget to the health sector. However, close to two decades after signing the declaration, government funding for health care has remained consistently below 8% of the national annual budget [37]. The national reproductive health strategy in Kenya notes that there are gaps in funding reproductive health services in Kenya (MOH, 2016) [38]. Loss of revenue due to abolishment of delivery fees may lead to poor quality of services despite the increase in health facility delivery services utilization, this would in turn result in shortages of inputs like drugs and other supplies necessary to avert pregnancy related mortalities and demotivation of health care workers [31].

Delays in utilizing free delivery services may occur because of low levels of autonomy, low awareness of the availability and importance of health facility delivery services and low perception of pregnancy risk factors in pregnant women. In addition, the long distances from health facilities, unavailability and high costs of transport services, poor roads and rugged geography may also hinder accessibility of free delivery services [34]. Previous assessments in Kenyan public health facilities have reported health systems gaps in service delivery [37, 38]. These gaps include drug and supply shortages, inadequate health staff to provide care to a high number of mothers seeking delivery services, health worker demotivation, delayed reimbursement of costs incurred when providing free maternal health care services, apathy related to free delivery services due to privacy concerns, poor referral channels and poor quality of care in general. The interplay between these challenges and pregnancy-related mortality needs to be further analyzed and addressed.

User fees have traditionally been seen as a major source of income for health facilities [39]. Given that the free maternal health care policy reimbursements are provided by the National Hospital Insurance Fund (NHIF) which also reimburses health facilities for providing general health services to NHIF members, this double payment is not only duplicative but also inefficient and poorly understood by county health managers who report that they do not know exactly how the funds from the free maternal health care policy should be utilized [40]. With devolution, several changes have occurred regarding health care financing protocols in the counties [39]. Before devolution of health services, facilities kept user fee revenue in their own bank accounts, but these funds are now deposited at the county bank accounts, as such not all health facilities keep the regular NHIF reimbursements and the free maternal health care policy reimbursements. In view of this, concerns have been raised over diversion of the free maternal health care funds by county governments and this too has a negative implication on the quality of delivery services offered by the counties [41]. It is for this reason that stakeholders in health are advising that reimbursement for offering free maternal health care services should be done through the Health Sector Services Fund (HSSF) channel. They also note that the current level of compensating health facilities for delivering free maternal health care services is challenging given that it favours facilities with richer catchment areas thus reducing the facility revenues in areas serving smaller population groups hence compromised quality of services. Similarly, despite all health facilities conducting deliveries, the amounts reimbursed varies per facility level.

Limitations

Data used in the analyses presented in this manuscript have several notable limitations:

- Given that reimbursement of costs incurred in delivery services is based on the number of deliveries conducted in each health facility, the accuracy of data prior to the policy may have been

Table 6 Quarterly Trends in Neonatal Mortality Rate

Facility	Slope 24 months pre-policy	Slope 12 months pre-policy	Slope 6 months pre-policy	Slope 3 months pre-policy	Slope 3 months post-policy	Slope 6 months post- policy	Slope 12 months post- policy	Slope 24 months post-policy
All 77 health facilities	−0.09 ($p = 0.24$)	−0.09 ($p = 0.24$)	−0.21 ($p = 0.05$)	−0.09 ($p = 0.24$)	0.12 ($p = 0.10$)	0.12 ($p = 0.10$)	0.12 ($p = 0.10$)	0.12 ($p = 0.10$)
Urban-based facilities	−0.10 ($p = 0.48$)	−0.10 ($p = 0.48$)	−0.41 ($p < 0.05$)	−0.10 ($p = 0.10$)	0.32 ($p < 0.05$)	0.32 ($p < 0.05$)	0.32 ($p < 0.05$)	0.32 ($p < 0.05$)
Rural-based facilities	−0.08 ($p = 0.10$)	−0.08 ($p = 0.10$)	−0.05 ($p = 0.49$)	−0.08 ($p < 0.05$)	−0.04 ($p = 0.48$)	−0.04 ($p = 0.48$)	−0.04 ($p = 0.48$)	−0.04 ($p = 0.48$)
Maternity hospital	−0.16 ($p = 0.24$)	−0.16 ($p = 0.24$)	−0.53 ($p < 0.05$)	−0.161 ($p = 0.24$)	0.37 ($p < 0.05$)	0.37 ($p < 0.05$)	0.37 ($p < 0.05$)	0.37 ($p < 0.05$)
Level 4 facilities	−0.09 ($p = 0.06$)	−0.09 ($p = 0.06$)	−0.12 ($p < 0.05$)	−0.09 ($p = 0.06$)	0.09 ($p = 0.05$)	0.09 ($p = 0.05$)	0.09 ($p = 0.05$)	0.09 ($p = 0.05$)
Level 5 facilities	0.17 ($p = 0.27$)	0.17 ($p = 0.27$)	0.39 ($p = 0.07$)	0.17 ($p = 0.27$)	−0.22 ($p = 0.14$)	−0.22 ($p = 0.14$)	−0.22 ($p = 0.14$)	−0.22 ($p = 0.14$)
Level 6 facility	−0.15 ($p = 0.83$)	−0.15 ($p = 0.83$)	−0.64 ($p = 0.52$)	−0.15 ($p = 0.83$)	0.50 ($p = 0.48$)	0.50 ($p = 0.48$)	0.50 ($p = 0.48$)	0.505 ($p = 0.48$)

poor when compared to the post policy implementation data.

- Although most of the findings from this study are consistent with other local and international studies, generalization of findings to depict the national picture in the implementation of the free maternal health care policy may be questioned given the shortcomings in equal sampling of the various facility levels, religious dynamics, geographical dynamics and other contextual factors affecting health facility delivery services utilization in the country.
- The free maternal health care policy has been implemented in all public health facilities in Kenya. This provided limitations in getting control groups (public health facilities where the policy was not implemented) for comparisons.
- The study has focused on the outcomes of the policy implementation during the first 2 years of the policy intervention. The trends before 2011 and the trajectory of the outcomes after the 2 years of consideration are unknown, and it is impossible to know whether the observed trends continues after the 2 years of policy implementation under consideration.
- This study was based on retrospective data based on maternal death audits over a period of 4 years. They may have been confounded by population dynamics and context-specific factors in maternal audits. Data on the exact timing of seeking medical help by mothers was not available as such some of the maternal deaths may have been as a result of late presentation in health facilities.

Conclusion

The elimination of user fees for delivery services in Kenya resulted in a significant increase in the number of deliveries conducted in Kenyan public health facilities; this result indicates that cost may be a key deterrent to delivery service utilization. This finding implies that removal of user fees for delivery services may serve as an important strategy to increase health facility delivery service utilization. However, this policy intervention appeared to have no significant effect on maternal and neonatal mortality. This lack of effect indicates that low utilization of health facility delivery services may not be the only factor contributing to pregnancy-related deaths in low income countries such as Kenya; low quality of delivery services in health facilities could be a contributing factor. In addition to eliminating fees to improve health service access, there is a need to simultaneously address other social, economic, political and contextual factors that are known to contribute to pregnancy-related deaths.

Additional files

Additional file 1: Fitness of health facility delivery services Model. This additional file is derived from an analysis of the mean absolute percentage error (MAPE) on all health facilities' deliveries.

Additional file 2: Model statistics of health facility delivery services generated through Ljung. Box analysis of all health facilities' deliveries.

Additional file 3: Fitness of maternal mortality ratio model. This additional file is derived from an analysis of the mean absolute percentage error (MAPE) of maternal mortality ratio in all the 77 health facilities.

Additional file 4: Model statistics of maternal mortality ratio generated through Ljung. Box analysis of maternal mortality ratio in the 77 health deliveries.

Additional file 5: Fitness of maternal mortality ratio model. This additional file is derived from an analysis of the mean absolute percentage error (MAPE) of neonatal mortality rate in all the 77 health facilities.

Additional file 6: Model statistics of neonatal mortality rate generated through Ljung. Box analysis of neonatal mortality rate in the 77 health deliveries.

Abbreviations

APHRC: Africa Population and Health Research Center; ARIMA: Autoregressive Moving Averages; CS: Caesarean Section; DF: Degrees of Freedom; HSSF: Health Sector Services Fund; IBM: International Business Machines; IDRC: International Development Research Centre; MAPE: Mean Absolute Percentage Error; MBChB: Bachelor of Medicine and Surgery; MD: Doctor of Medicine; MMED: Master of Medicine in Obstetrics and Gynecology; MMR: Maternal Mortality Ratio; NHIF: National Hospital Insurance Fund; NMR: Neonatal Mortality Rate; PhD: Doctor of Philosophy; PMRCPath: Masters in Human Pathology; RMSE: Root-Mean-Square Error; SE: Standard Error; SPSS: Statistical Package for Social Sciences; UNITID: Institute of Tropical and Infectious Diseases; US: United States; WHO: World Health Organization

Acknowledgements

Not applicable.

Funding

Partially funded by an African Doctoral Dissertation Research Fellowship (ADDRF) award offered by the African Population and Health Research Center (APHRC) in partnership with the International Development Research Centre (IDRC). APHRC reviewed the study protocol, trained Gitobu CM on protocol development, data analysis and manuscript writing.

Authors' contributions

All the three authors (GCM, GPB, MWO) made substantial contributions to conception and design of the study, acquisition of data, analysis and interpretation of data; and they have been involved in drafting the manuscript or revising it critically for important intellectual content; and they have given final approval of the version to be published; and they have agreed to be accountable for all aspects of the work in ensuring that questions related to the accuracy or integrity of any part of the work are appropriately investigated and resolved.

Competing interests

The authors declare that they have no competing interests.

Author details

[1]Institute of Tropical and Infectious Diseases (UNITID), University of Nairobi, Nairobi, Kenya. [2]Department of Human Anatomy, University of Nairobi, Nairobi, Kenya. [3]Department of Obstetrics and Gynecology, University of

Ghent, Ghent, Belgium. [4]Department of Human Pathology, University of Nairobi, Nairobi, Kenya.

References

1. Campbell OM, Graham WJ. Strategies for reducing maternal mortality: getting on with what works. Lancet. 2006;368(9543):1284–99.
2. Kenya National Bureau of Statistics and ICF Macro. Kenya demographic and health survey report, 2013–2014. Kenya: Ministry of Health; 2015. https://dhsprogram.com/pubs/pdf/fr308/fr308.pdf.
3. McKinnon B, Harper S, Kaufman JS, Bergevin Y. Removing user fees for facility-based delivery services: a difference-in-differences evaluation from ten sub-Saharan African countries. Health Policy Plan. 2015;30(4):432–41.
4. De-Allegri M, Tiendrebéogo J, Müller O, Yé M, Jahn A, Ridde V. Understanding home delivery in a context of user fee reduction: a cross-sectional mixed methods study in rural Burkina Faso. BMC Pregnancy Childbirth. 2015;15:330.
5. Ministry of Health Kenya: "Speech by H.E. Hon. Uhuru Kenyatta, C.G.H., President and Commander-in-Chief of the Defence Forces of the Republic of Kenya During the Madaraka Day Celebrations" (Nyayo National Stadium, June 1, 2013). 2013. www.nation.co.ke/blob/view/-/1869340/data/521193/-/ttjgrk/-/speech.pdf. Accessed 24 Mar 2014.
6. Ministry of Health, Kenya: Free maternal health care policy launch.2013. http://www.knchr.org/Portals/0/EcosocReports/Implementing%20Free%20Maternal%20Health%20Care%20in%20Kenya.pdf. Accessed 13 May 2015.
7. McCarthy J, Maine D. A framework for analyzing determinants of maternal mortality. Stud Fam Plan. 1992;23:23–33.
8. Kenya National Bureau of Statistics and ICF Macro. Kenya demographic and health survey report. Kenya: Ministry of Health; 2010. http://apps.who.int/medicinedocs/documents/s17116e/s17116e.pdf. Accessed 12 June 2014.
9. Wubs E, Brals D, Van der List M, Elbers C: Lessons learned from a maternal health study in Nandi County, Kenya. Learning & analysis brief. Amsterdam Institute for Global Health and Development, Pharm Access Foundation. Healthcare quality. 2016; No 5 April 2016.
10. Watt S, Sword W, Krueger P. Implementation of a health care policy: an analysis of barriers and facilitators to practice change. BMC Health Serv Res. 2005;5:53.
11. Simkhada B, Porter M, Teijlingen E. The role of mothers-in-law in antenatal care decision making in Nepal: a qualitative study. BMC Pregnancy Childbirth. 2010;10(34). https://doi.org/10.1186/1471-2393-10-34.
12. Cheptum J, Gitonga M, Mutua E, Mukui S, Ndambuki J, Koima W: Barriers to Access and Utilization of Maternal and Infant Health Services in Migori, Kenya. Dev Countr Stud. 2014; ISSN 2225–0565, Vol.4, No.15.
13. Cairney P. Understanding public policy – theories and issues. New York: Palgrave Mcmillan; 2012. https://onlinelibrary.wiley.com/doi/pdf/10.1111/padm.12008. Accessed 9 Mar 2016.
14. Nawaz F. Exploring the actors and factors involved in public policy implementation in Bangladesh: a case study of reproductive health policy. Soc Sci Res Network. 2013; https://doi.org/10.2139/ssrn.2228582. Accessed 10 Oct 2016.
15. Sanneving L, Kulane A, Ahgren B. Health system capacity, maternal health policy implementation in the state of Gujarat, India. Glob Health Action. 2013;6:1–8.
16. Lang'at E, Mwanri L. Healthcare service providers' and facility administrators' perspectives of the free maternal healthcare services policy in Malindi District, Kenya: a qualitative study. Reprod Health. 2015;12:59. https://doi.org/10.1186/s12978-015-0048-1.
17. Wamalwa EW. Implementation challenges of free maternity services policy in Kenya: the health workers' perspective. Pan Afr Med J. 2015;22:1–5://doi.org/10.11604/pamj.2015.22.375.6708
18. Bill-Godden W: Sample size determination for finite populations. 2004. http://www.williamgodden.com/samplesizeformula.pdf. Accessed 27 Mar 2015.
19. Government of Kenya: The Kenya constitution, 2010. 2010. http://www.kenyalaw.org/lex/actview.xql?actid=Const2010. Accessed 1 July 2016.
20. Wamai RW. The Kenya health system—analysis of the situation and enduring challenges. Jpn Med J. 2009;52(2):134–40.
21. Government of Kenya: The Health Bill 2014. http://kenyalaw.org/kl/fileadmin/pdfdownloads/bills/2015/HealthBill2015.pdf. Accessed 1 July 2016.
22. Ministry of Health, Kenya: Kenya health policy 2014–2030. 2017. https://www.google.com/url?sa=t&rct=j&q=&esrc=s&source=web&cd=4&cad=rja&uact=8&ved=0ahUKEwj90lzt56XSAhWjJcAKHeLFDaoQFggvMAM&url=http%3A%2F%2Fwww.health.go.ke%2F%3Fwpdmdl%3D272%26ind%3D1&usg=AFQjCNF6HA2Ew0Vwi1TZqAm7RLBl8t__Xg&sig2=gTpLg9r1ppg6mXtrX2JoCA&bvm=bv.147448319,d.d24>. Accessed 1 Feb 2017.
23. Kombo DK, Tromp DL. Proposal and thesis writing: an introduction. Nairobi: Pauline Publications Africa; 2006. http://jaysean.com/index.php?option=com_k2&view=itemlist&task=user&id=11072. Accessed 13 June 2014
24. McPake B. User charges for health services in developing countries: a review of the economic literature. Soc Sci Med. 1993;36:1397–405.
25. Penfold S, Harrison E, Bell J, Fitzmaurice A. Evaluation of the delivery fee exemption policy in Ghana: population estimates of changes in delivery service utilization in two regions. Ghana Med J. 2007;41(3):100.
26. Witter S, Dieng T, Mbengue D, Moreira I, De Brouwere V. The national free delivery and caesarean policy in Senegal: evaluating process and outcomes. Health Policy Plan. 2010;25:384–92.
27. Witter S, Khadka S, Nath H, Tiwari S. The national free delivery policy in Nepal: early evidence of its effects on health facilities. Health Policy Plan. 2011;26(Suppl 2):84–91.
28. Xu K, Evans DB, Kadama P, Nabyonga J, Ogwang-Ogwal P, Nabukhonzo P, Mylena-Aguilar A. Understanding the impact of eliminating user fees: utilization and catastrophic health expenditures in Uganda. Soc Sci Med. 2006;62:866–76.
29. Burgert CR, Bigogo G, Adazu K, Odhiambo F, Buehler J, Breiman RF, Laserson K, Hamel JM, Feikin DR. Impact of implementation of free high-quality health care on health facility attendance by sick children in rural western Kenya. Trop Med Int Health. 2011;16(6):711–20.
30. Lagarde M, Palmer N. The impact of user fees on health service utilization in low- and middle-income countries: how strong is the evidence? Bull World Health Organ. 2016; http://www.who.int/bulletin/volumes/86/11/07-049197.pdf. Accessed 11 Sept 2016.
31. Hatt LE, Makinen M, Madhavan S, Conlon CM. Effects of user fee exemptions on the provision and use of maternal health services: a review of literature. J Health Populnutr. 2013;31(4 Suppl 2):S67–80.
32. Chuma J, Musimbi V, Okungu C, Goodman C, Molyneux C. Reducing user fees for primary health care in Kenya: policy on paper or policy in practice? Int J Equity Health. 2009;8:15.
33. Ministry of Health. The 2013 Kenya household health expenditure and utilization survey. Available at :< https://www.healthpolicyproject.com/pubs/745_KHHUESReportJanuary.pdf >. Accessed 20 July 2017.
34. Thaddeus S, Maine D. Too far to walk: maternal mortality in context. Soc Sci Med. 1994;38(8):1091–10.
35. Ministry of Health Kenya and WHO. Kenya Service Availability and Readiness Assessment Mapping, A Comprehensive mapping of health services, capacity for service provision, sector investments and readiness to provide services by County (SARAM) report 2013. Available online :< apps.who.int/healthinfo/systems/datacatalog/index.php/catalog/42/download/145>. Accessed 8 July 2017.
36. Meessen B, Hercot D, Noirhomme M, Ridde V, Tibouti A, Bicaba A, Kirunga-Tashobya C, Gilson L. Removing user fees in the health sector in low-income countries – a multi-country review. New York: UNICEF; 2009.
37. Ministry of Finance, Kenya. Health sector budget 2017. http://www.healthpolicyplus.com/ns/pubs/6138-6239_FINALNationalandCountyHealthBudgetAnalysis.pdf. Accessed 11 Aug 2017.
38. Ministry of Health. Kenya reproductive, maternal, newborn, child and adolescent health (RMNCAH) investment framework, Government of Kenya, 2016, January 31, 2016. Available at :< http://globalfinancingfacility.org/sites/gff_new/files/documents/Kenya%20RMNCAH%20Investment%20Framework_March%202016.pdf>. Accessed 8 Aug 2017.

39. Ministry of Health, University of Nairobi and KEMRI-Wellcome Trust. Time for comprehensive healthcare costing in Kenya, a report on the feasibility to develop, pilot & implement a unit cost system for key health interventions, 2015. http://publications.universalhealth2030.org/uploads/kenya_healthcare_costing_feasibility_report_moh_version_2015.pdf. Accessed 18 Aug 2017.
40. Ministry of Health. Status of implementation of free maternity services (FMS) program in the devolved health system in Kenya. Nairobi; 2015. [Online]. Available at: http://publications.universalhealth2030.org/uploads/free_maternal_health_services_report_feb_2015_final1_doc_.pdf.
41. Waweru E., Nyikuri M., Tsofa B., Sarah Kedenge S., Goodman C., Molyneux S. Review of health sector services fund implementation and experience, 2013. http://researchonline.lshtm.ac.uk/2869479/1/Review%20of%20Health%20Sector%20Services%20Fund%20implementation%20and%20experience.pdf. Accessed 18 Aug 2017.

8

Exploring barriers to the use of formal maternal health services and priority areas for action in Sidama zone, southern Ethiopia

Aschenaki Z. Kea[1*], Olivia Tulloch[2], Daniel G. Datiko[1,2], Sally Theobald[2] and Maryse C. Kok[3]

Abstract

Background: In 2015 the maternal mortality ratio for Ethiopia was 353 per 100,000 live births. Large numbers of women do not use maternal health services. This study aimed to identify factors influencing the use of maternal health services at the primary health care unit (PHCU) level in rural communities in Sidama zone, south Ethiopia in order to design quality improvement interventions.

Methods: We conducted a qualitative study in six *woredas* in 2013: 14 focus group discussions (FGDs) and 44 in-depth interviews with purposefully selected community members (women, male, traditional birth attendants, local *kebele* administrators), health professionals and health extension workers (HEWs) at PHCUs. We digitally recorded, transcribed and thematically analysed the interviews and FGDs using Nvivo. The 'three delay model' informed the analytical process and discussion of barriers to the use of maternal health services.

Results: Lack of knowledge on danger signs and benefits of maternal health services; cultural and traditional beliefs; trust in TBAs; lack of decision making power of women, previous negative experiences with health facilities; fear of going to an unfamiliar setting; lack of privacy and perceived costs of maternal health services were the main factors causing the first delay in deciding to seek care. Transport problems in inaccessible areas were the main contributing factor for the second delay on reaching care facilities. Lack of logistic supplies and equipment, insufficient knowledge and skills and unprofessional behaviour of health workers were key factors for the third delay in accessing quality care.

Conclusions: Use of maternal health services at the PHCU level in Sidama zone is influenced by complex factors within the community and health system. PHCUs should continue to implement awareness creation activities to improve knowledge of the community on complications of pregnancy and benefits of maternal health services. The health system has to be responsive to community's cultural norms and practices. The mangers of the woreda health office and health centres should take into account the available budgets; work on ensuring the necessary logistics and supplies to be in place at PHCU.

Keywords: Maternal health, Three delays, Service utilization, Health extension workers, Ethiopia, Quality improvement

* Correspondence: aschenakizer@yahoo.com
[1]REACH Ethiopia, P.O. Box 303, Hawassa, Ethiopia
Full list of author information is available at the end of the article

Background

Globally, about 3 million maternal deaths occurred in 2015. The estimated maternal mortality ratio (MMR) for high income regions was 12/100,000 live births and, for low income regions was 239/100,000. The estimated MMR for Ethiopia is 353 /100,000 live births. The sustainable development goals (SDGs) call for an accelerated reduction in maternal deaths, so that the global MMR falls to 70 or below by 2030, working towards a vision of ending all preventable maternal mortality [1].

Use of maternal health services is instrumental for preventing maternal mortality and morbidity. Factors influencing the use of maternal health services have been the subject of research worldwide. In 1994, Thaddeus and Maine devised a model to categorize the main factors shaping three phases of delay in accessing services. Phase I presents the delay in the decision to seek medical care, including a range of factors at the individual level, driven by culture, illness characteristics, costs and previous experiences with the health care system. Phase II includes physical accessibility factors, such as the distribution of facilities, travel time to the facility, availability, and costs of transport and the condition of roads. Phase III is the provision of quality care: factors here include adequacy of the referral system; supplies and equipment and the availability and competence of health workers [2].

Studies, such as those carried out in Uganda, Pakistan, Myanmar, Egypt, and Ethiopia, have applied the model to examine and describe the three delays leading to maternal mortality [3–8]. These studies identified that factors which interplay at the first delay level contributed to maternal mortality, followed by the third delay factors which are associated with lack of adequate and quality care. Other research conducted in Brazil, Tanzania and Ethiopia used the model to assess the three delays in the provision of emergency obstetric care [9–11]. Studies done in Nicaragua and Ethiopia used the model to assess factors that affect women's health seeking behaviour during pregnancy and delivery [12–15]. Also in Tanzania a study has been done using the three delays in relation to perinatal mortality [16]. In Ethiopia, two studies used the three delays framework to investigate the reasons for high perinatal deaths among newborns delivered in health facilities [8, 17]. These studies demonstrate that socio-demographic and cultural factors, perceived quality of care and previous maternal health care experiences affect health seeking behaviour of pregnant women.

In recent years, Ethiopia has invested in the expansion of health facilities as well as the training and deploying of community and mid-level health workers such as health extension workers (HEWs), public health officers, midwives and nurses, to improve access to health care. Primary health care is delivered through the *woreda* (district) health system comprising a primary hospital, 6–10 health centres and satellite health posts which together form a primary health care unit (PHCU). Maternal health services provided by a PHCU; range from simple preventive services at health posts to comprehensive maternal health services and emergency obstetric care at primary hospitals. Health centres provide comprehensive maternal health services and basic emergency obstetric services [18]. Health posts are staffed with two HEWs, who are female community health workers recruited from the community (*kebele*)'[1] delivering 16 primary health care packages at the community level. HEWs are trained for 1 year and provide maternal health services like antenatal care (ANC), "safe and clean"[2] delivery services and postnatal care (PNC) [19]. Health centres provide technical and administrative supervision to HEWs and the *woreda* health office has the general oversight of the health centres and health posts.

The government of Ethiopia promotes skilled birth attendance; HEWs should refer pregnant women to the health centre or primary hospital, especially in cases where there is a high risk or complications [19]. HEWs generally have good connections in their communities and work together with volunteers who are part of the health development army (HDA). The HDA is a formal system of community-based model families trained by the HEWs to deliver health extension packages independently [20], they are also referred to as the "1 to 5 network".

Despite the expansion of primary health care delivery through PHCUs, the use of maternal health services remains low, which contributes to the country's high MMR. In 2014, 41% of mothers made one ANC visit during pregnancy, 16% gave birth by a skilled provider and 13% received PNC within the first 2 days of delivery [21]. Official data suggest that, of the total women receiving ANC, 41% received ANC from nurses or doctors and 18% from a HEW. Over three quarters of all births were assisted by a relative, a traditional birth attendant (TBA) or another non-skilled person. About 2% of births were assisted by a HEW [21].

In Ethiopia, studies have identified factors that influence the use of maternal health services. Pregnant women who lived in urban areas, were literate, had approval from their husbands and families and had good knowledge of the danger signs of pregnancy were more likely to use maternal health services [22–26]. These studies were primarily quantitative and did not capture in-depth perspectives of mothers and other key stakeholders or focus on the PHCU. Given the rich cultural and linguistic diversity within Ethiopia [27, 28], there is need to understand the factors influencing use of maternal health services at community level within very specific cultural contexts, in order to develop locally appropriate interventions. This in-depth qualitative study explored, from multiple perspectives, factors affecting maternal health service use in rural Sidama, to provide context-specific information on experiences and delays in seeking care and to support the design of interventions focused on improving maternal health outcomes.

Methods

Study setting

The study was conducted in Sidama zone of the South Nation Nationalities and Peoples Region of Ethiopia in 2013. The capital of the zone is Hawassa. The zone comprises 19 rural *woredas* with a total population of 3.4 million. In Sidama, 12% of pregnant women gave birth assisted by a skilled birth attendant, 88% made one ANC visit, 48% made four ANC visits and 58% received PNC in 2013. Around 14% of births were assisted by HEWs [29].

Study design, population, and sampling

This explorative qualitative study involved focus group discussion (FGDs) and in-depth interviews (IDIs). FGDs were held to understand the views and norms of different groups regarding factors influencing use of maternal health services. Interviews were carried out with community members and health professionals who were expected to be knowledgeable, have experience or were directly involved in services delivery at the primary health care unit.

A total of 14 FGDs were conducted: 6 FGDs with HEWs (one in each *woreda*), 6 FGDs with women (one in each *woreda*) and two FGDs with male (in two purposively selected *woreda* amongst the six).

We conducted a total of 44 IDIs: 12 IDIs with pregnant women or women who delivered recently (two in each *woreda*), 12 IDIs with HEWs (two in each *woreda*), 6 IDIs with TBAs (one in each *woreda*), 3 IDIs with *Kebele* administrators (in three purposively selected *woredas*), 6 IDIs with persons in charge of the health centre or leaders of the labour room workers (one in each *woreda*), 3 IDIs with *woreda* health extension program coordinators (in three purposively selected *woredas*), 1 IDI with the zonal health department health extension program (HEP) coordinator and 1 IDI with the regional health bureau HEP coordinator (Table 1).

We focused on the first two levels (health post and health centres) of the PHCU, as they are the first point of contact for the rural community to access maternal health services. Participants were purposefully selected eligible women comprised of those who had given birth in the previous 2 years or were pregnant at the time of data collection. Male participants for the FGDs were selected on the basis of having an influential position in the community: husbands (of women with babies), influential elders, religious leaders and other influential male in the community were included. HEWs and health professionals were those who served for three or more years so they had sufficient experience to share.

The study took place in six purposively selected *woredas*, taking into account the rate of skilled delivery in 2012 and the distance from the zonal capital. We took 12% skilled delivery, which was the average coverage of the zone in the year, as a cut off point to categorize the *woredas'* performance. The *woredas* achieving 12% or more were classified as "relatively well performing" and those below 12% were considered "poor performing". We included three *woredas* which were performing relatively well and three *woredas* which were performing poorly, and ensured that half were close to the regional capital Hawassa, and half further away to explore differences in level settings.

Table 1 An overview of participants in IDIs and FGDs

Level	Type of participants	Method	Number	Total
Community	Women	FGD	1 per woreda	6
	Male	FGD	In 2 woredas	2
	Women	Interview	2 per woreda	12
	TBA	Interview	1 per woreda	6
	Kebele administrator/Chair person	Interview	In 3 woredas	3
Health Workers	HEW	Interview	2 per woreda	12
	HEW	FGD	1 per woreda	6
	Person in charge of health centre / leader of labor room health workers	Interview	1 per woreda	6
HEP Coordinators	HEP Coordinator at woreda level	Interview	In 3 woredas	3
	HEP Coordinator at zonal health department	Interview	1 from zonal health department	1
	HEP Coordinator at regional health bureau	Interview	1 from regional health bureau	1
Total				58

To identify and recruit participants for the study at *woreda* level, the research team approached the *woreda* health office, discussed the objectives of the study, the sampling approach and strategies to be used for identification of participants. *Woreda* health office, HEWs and *kebele* administration supported the identification and recruitment of women for the study. Health centre and *woreda* health office staff assisted in the identification of HEWs and health professionals for inclusion in the study, and HEWs were involved in the recruitment of TBAs and community representatives.

Data collection

Data were collected by four Ethiopian researchers who had experience in conducting qualitative studies and were trained for 1 week. Semi-structured interview guides were developed in English, translated to *Sidamigna* and *Amharic* (Additional file 1), and back translated and checked for consistency by an independent person from Ethiopia, who was able to speak both languages.

The interview guides contained questions eliciting factors that facilitate or hinder the use of maternal health services at different levels. During the interview and FGDs, participants were asked about their knowledge on maternal health services, health seeking behaviour, the factors influencing decision-making process, experience with pregnancy, use of services, possible barriers to use of the services and perceptions of service quality. Background information of participants such as age, education level, roles and responsibilities, services years (for health workers) were gathered and queries were run to see their effect on responses of respondents.

The interview guides were piloted in one *woreda,* were not included in the analysis and the questions were modified where needed. Debriefing sessions were held daily to discuss key findings, identify saturation of themes, refine questions and support the quality of the research process.

The interviews were carried out in the usual work settings of participants: health posts, health centres, offices and homes (TBAs only). The FGDs were conducted at schools and *kebele* administration offices. The duration of the IDIs was 60–90 min and for the FGDs 90–130 min. The FGDs were conducted by two facilitators: one recorder and one discussion facilitator, whereas the IDIs were conducted by one interviewer.

Data analysis

All interviews and FGDs were digitally recorded, transcribed and translated into English. A sample of transcripts was randomly checked against the recordings to support quality assurance. Key themes were identified and a coding frame was developed after reading the transcripts in two pairs of two researchers. The coding frame and analytical process was informed by the three delays model to enable demarcation of experiences and challenges at different levels [2]. Transcripts were coded using Nvivo (v.10) software. The coded transcripts were further analyzed and summarized in narratives for each theme and sub-theme. The three delays model was used to frame our findings, as the model supports critical and integrated analyses exploring how individual, community and health system related factors hinder the use of maternal health services. Study findings were presented, discussed and validated in stakeholders meetings at the *woreda* and zonal level.

Results

The results are presented according to the different levels of the three delays model which informed our analytical process (Fig. 1) and supported by direct quotations from study participants.

Delay I: Delay in recognizing the need for maternal health services and deciding to seek treatment or advice.

Lack of knowledge, perception of risks and previous childbirth and health facility experience

HEWs and male FGD participants described how some women chose not to use maternal health services because they are neither aware of danger signs during pregnancy and childbirth nor the benefits of obtaining maternal health services.

> *"...lack of knowledge about the use and benefit of delivering at the health centre is the main reason; if she had the knowledge and awareness about the importance [of skilled delivery] she wouldn't have given birth at home."* (HEW, interview).

Most of the HEWs and some *kebele* administrators supported the opinion that women had low perceptions of risks in pregnancy and therefore do not seek any maternal health services if they feel well during their pregnancy. Some women who participated in the study confirmed that they did not seek care unless they were sick and recognized there were complications; this was also confirmed by some male participants.

> *"If there is no clear sickness, they [women] don't come to visit health institutions." (Male, FGD).*

Some women who had complications during previous pregnancies mentioned they had chosen to use routine maternal health services, while women who had experience with safe home delivery in the past seemed more

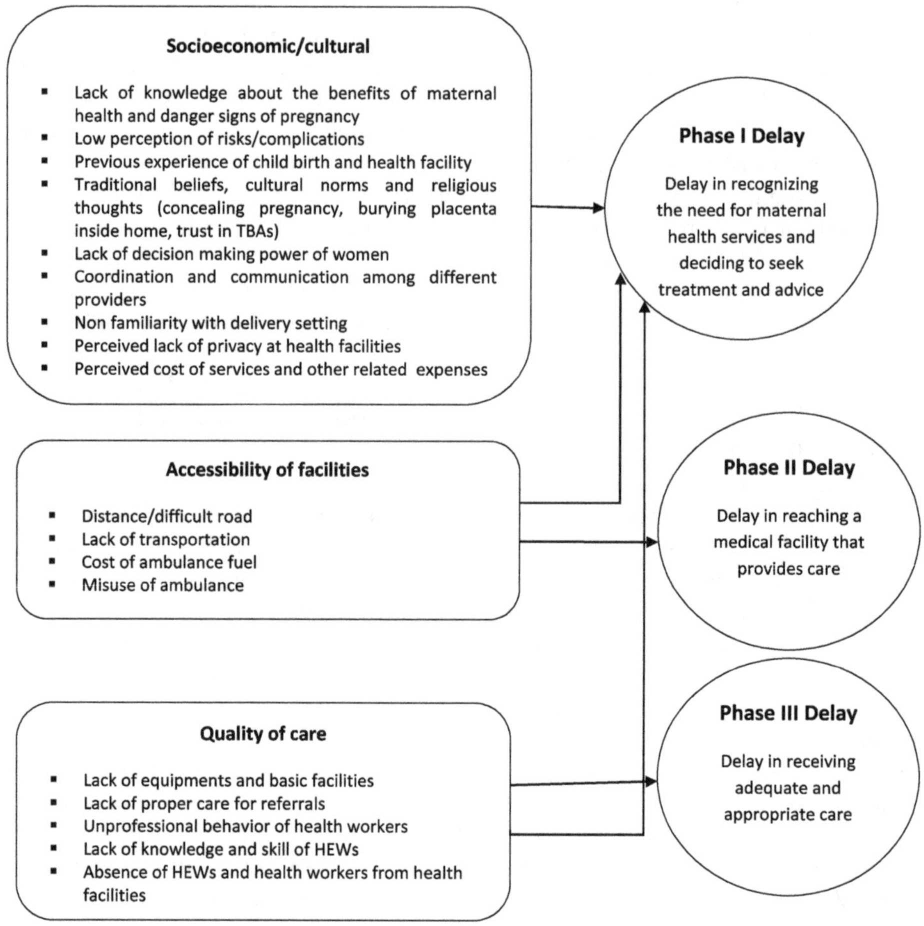

Fig. 1 Applying the three delay model to understand factors limiting utilization of maternal health services in Sidama zone, Southern Ethiopia

likely to choose giving birth at home for subsequent deliveries.

> *"They [women] want to give birth at their home. Especially those who experienced their previous labor at home say, 'we were safe while we gave birth at home, so we don't want to come here (health post)'"* *(HEW, FGD).*

Some pregnant women reported that they did not plan to visit health facilities for their current pregnancy and would not recommend others to use maternal health services, as they felt they had not received proper care during their previous visit.

> *"One time I (HEW) sent a pregnant woman who had some problems to the health centre. They sent her back without giving her any help. Another time I met this woman while I was telling another woman to go to the health centre to give birth. She said 'I will never go there and don't recommend others to go.'" (HEW, FGD).*

Traditional beliefs, religious practices, and cultural norms

There is a range of local behaviours that influence uptake of maternal health services. The tradition of concealing pregnancy during the early stages prevented some women from timely booking for ANC.

> *"In our culture, we don't want to talk to people [about pregnancy]. People should know after the birth of the baby or when our abdomen becomes big. It is shameful and secret because we are not sure about the continuation of the pregnancy. There may be a miscarriage."* (Woman, interview).

In the community, giving birth at home was customary and women who gave birth at health facilities were considered weak. This may be related to the perception that health facilities are a place for managing severe illnesses rather than normal conditions like pregnancy and the fear that those women who visited health facilities were sometimes assumed to end up with surgical procedures or death.

The first and the big challenge is traditional belief, they (women) say "my mum gave birth to eight of us at home, what happened to her? Even our grandma was delivering at home..." (Interview, *woreda* HEP coordinator)

The culture of burying the placenta inside the home was reported as an important practice after the birth, and the worry that this may not be possible was an important deterrent factor against institutional delivery.

"In the culture of this community they don't want to throw the placenta outside their home. Because of this, they don't want to go outside [to health facility] and lose the placenta. If the placenta is not buried inside the home it is considered as bad fortune for the baby. In the health facility, they don't get the placenta to take back to their home and consider it as a big loss, similar as if they lost the delivered baby." (HEW, FGD).

Christian beliefs, for example, that God will help pregnant women during labour, were mentioned by the HEWs, male and female community members and influence health-seeking behaviour. It appeared to encourage women to deliver at home

"The problem is, even though some people have awareness, they don't want to show this in practice. They say 'God will help a mother'" (Interview, HEW)

The decision-making process of when and where a woman should get maternal health services was also influenced by family members, notably husbands and mother-in-laws. Women were expected to follow the same practice as their mothers and ancestors even if that was sometimes against their own preference.

"...some women after being identified by voluntary community health workers [HDAs] don't want to come to the health post for ANC. They complain about their husband and mother-in-law: 'My husband and mother-in-law don't allow me to go for ANC.'" (HEW, interview).

Coordination of maternal health services with community-based providers

Most HEWs reported there was good coordination of maternal health services with HDA leaders, which increased use of services. HDAs are volunteers organized in a 1 to 5 group, with one leader. The role of HDAs is to support HEWs to perform health promotion activities and coordination of referral in the community. HEWs described how HDAs were involved in the identification of new pregnancies, counselling of mothers for ANC and health facility delivery and facilitation of referral of pregnant and laboring women.

"We [HDAs] taught women in our community... the leaders of 1 to 5 networks give us the advice to convince pregnant mothers. When their labor starts we call to the health extension worker...." (Woman, FGD).

Some HEWs mentioned that not all the HDA leaders were active in performing their tasks; this was partly due to the burden of housework, but also because they expected incentives from the government which they did not receive. In the past, some members of the HDAs had received incentives from government and non-governmental organizations during training and campaigns. Currently the government advocates not providing financial incentives for HDAs, given the large number of HDAs nationwide, for whom payment would be difficult to sustain.

Many participants reported that the role of TBAs has shifted. They are no longer formally supported by the government to provide delivery services; rather they are expected to support the referral of pregnant women to health facilities. Many community members supported the new roles of TBAs, however; the change in policy was said not to have been properly communicated to, nor acknowledged by the TBAs. Demand for TBA services persisted and some TBAs continued to provide delivery services in the community, as they were perceived to be more skilled and experienced than the HEWs and health professionals. There were different opinions from community members regarding HEWs' skills: some described them as young and inexperienced, whilst others believed them to be better skilled than TBAs.

"...TBAs receive only a little information [training] from the government but they are famous in the kebeles so the people say 'the known devil is better than unknown God' and the people believe in them [TBAs]." (HEW, FGD).

"...I never attended a mother after I got the order of the government. The health centre head warned us not to attend delivery. He said that you are not allowed to attend birth of any women, only to refer women to the health post and health centre." (Interview, TBA).

"...but after we were told to stop conducting delivery, I got disappointed, because we were not told what problems were created by us, they directly announced to stop our activities." (Interview, TBA).

Non-familiarity with delivery setting, health professionals, and privacy

For some women, visiting unfamiliar settings and not wanting to expose their bodies to unknown health professionals was a hindrance to their giving birth at health facilities. Women indicated that they would prefer their husband and relatives to be present at delivery rather than health workers. Another concern was that women would be expected to use the delivery bed, to lie down and stretch their legs, which differs from the customary squat position taken during birth at home. They believed it would expose them and make them vulnerable to illness. Some HEWs also mentioned women prefer female over male health professionals.

"...the women hang their legs on the bed, which exposes them to "Qilleessa" bad wind which makes the women get sick and be in pain." (HEW, interview)

Perceived costs

Several types of cost had an impact on the decision of where to give birth. Anticipating costs or confusion about which services should be free at the primary hospital was a cause for concern. Indirect costs for food, transport and accommodation associated with a facility delivery also influenced the willingness of women and their families to accept referrals made by HEWs.

".... I paid in the hospital for the medical card and operation service. I paid around 350 birr in the hospital for all the services (drugs, bed and operation) for my first pregnancy." (Woman, interview).

Some participants complained that payment was required by the hospital and this is against the rule of free maternal health service provision.

"...the government stated [has a policy] maternal health services are to be provided free of charge, but women pay at hospital for delivery services, so I [HEW] stopped referring mothers to this hospital." (HEW, FGD).

Ambulances were available and are, in theory, free, but some participants had payment requested for ambulance fuel. This was a hindrance to some taking up referral and is closely linked to the second delay.

Delay II: Delay in reaching a health facility.

Distance and transport problems

Accessibility of maternal health services at distant health facilities was problematic for some communities, this was characterised by the difficult terrain and large size of the geographical area served by a health facility. In the absence of transport, the community sometimes resorted to using locally made stretchers, "*kareza*", to carry pregnant women.

"...there is a place where it's hard to go even by motorbike. There are occasions where pregnant women have to walk 2 to 3 days to reach here. I met a mother who took three days... the biggest problem in this area is the problem of road and transport, while she was travelling here she gave birth on the road..." (Delivery case team leader, interview).

Some areas reported poor availability of the *woreda* ambulance; this was due to an array of reasons, for example, appropriation of the ambulance by officials, drivers being uncooperative, or lack of fuel. Ambulance services were more likely to be impeded when called to areas where the topography and roads were difficult.

"... We observe that mothers who live in a challenging geographical area don't come for institutional delivery. If mothers who live in a good geographical area call for an ambulance, they will benefit from the service..." (HCH, interview).

Delay III: Delay in receiving adequate care.

Availability of logistics, equipment, and basic facilities

Most participants felt that the local health posts and some health centres did not have the necessary medical equipment and basic facilities needed for provision of maternal health services. Lack of supplies appeared to affect motivation and performance of health professionals and HEWs as well as women's willingness to seek services from these facilities.

"We have a newly built health centre but nothing is supported there [no medical equipment], there are not even enough health professionals.... when there is a referral case from our health post but the health centre is not giving better services, then what is the difference between a health post and health centre? They have been using local "Kuraz" lighting [kerosene] as they do not even have a generator." (HEW, FGD).

Lack of proper training, skills and adequate care from health workers and HEWs

HEWs mentioned that some women who had been referred to facilities from the community had negative experiences, as the health professionals either did not respect them or provide quality health care. Part of the reason for this appeared to be the poor skills level and training of health workers at health centres.

> *"...the major problem I faced is at the health centre. They are not handling our referrals properly. I had an experience: I sent a woman to the health centre. They sent her back to her home, but she delivered on the road without getting support."* (HEW, FGD).

The quality of care at community level was criticised. *Woreda* HEP coordinators felt that the HEWs were not providing focused ANC, nor including all the components of care. This opinion was supported by others who felt that counselling by the HEWs during ANC visits was insufficient to encourage women to choose skilled attendance at delivery. HEWs themselves were critical about the quality of the delivery training they received to conduct safe and clean deliveries at health posts. Some reported having forgotten the basic delivery skills, because their training had no practical element, and they had little on-the-job experience partly due to a lack of necessary equipment for delivery at the health post. They also felt that the refresher training given to them had not improved their skills and confidence.

> *"We took delivery training in our initial training, but we forgot all things about it since we were not doing it in the health post." (HEW, FGD).*

Availability of staff at health facilities

The absence of HEWs from health posts is a common problem creating an unreliable supply of health services. Health posts should be staffed by two HEWs, but this is often not the case. If a HEW is on leave or attending training, the health post can be closed for days or weeks. Some women noted that they had not received full ANC and other maternal health services due to irregular opening hours of the health posts. For example:

"I didn't receive ANC until I gave birth, because I repeatedly went there (health post) and sometimes she (HEW) was not available... mostly the health post doesn't open for the beneficiary, it opens when they (the HEWs) have a meeting with the HDA and at the day of vaccinations." (FGD-Women).

Discussion

This is the first qualitative study to assess barriers to use of maternal primary health care services within the specific cultural context of Sidama. Below we synthesize the key findings under each level of delay, which aspects are unique to Sidama and then highlight the priorities for action to improve use of maternal health services and, ultimately, maternal health outcomes.

First phase delay

There were multiple intersecting factors that constituted the first delay within Sidama: lack of knowledge of the benefits of maternal health services and the danger signs of pregnancy, cultural and traditional beliefs that are specific to Southern Ethiopia, complex decision-making processes shaped by gendered interactions between husband and families, worry about culturally inappropriate practices in health facilities, and perceived costs of services. HDA volunteers – coordinated by HEWs – played an important role in addressing some of these barriers.

Studies carried out in Sekela and Banja districts of Amhara regional state and Sodo town of the Southern region of Ethiopia have also shown that women who lacked awareness and understanding of the benefits of maternal health services and danger signs of pregnancy and childbirth were also less likely to use the services [23, 24, 30]. Studies conducted in Ethiopia, Nigeria, and Bangladesh have shown that the tradition of hiding pregnancy at early stage affects timely booking for ANC [31–33]. It is not uncommon for Ethiopian pregnant women to book during their second or third trimester [21, 23, 25, 34, 35]. The main reason for not attending early ANC or publically revealing early pregnancy is a feeling of embarrassment experienced by pregnant women, because it is presumptuous to talk of pregnancy when miscarriage cannot be ruled out. It is important to consider how these social norms can be addressed with sensitivity so that complications are detected early and managed appropriately [36]. The culture of burying the placenta inside the home for good fortune means that mothers are reluctant to give birth at the health facilities, as generally health facilities don't provide the placenta for the families to take home. Similar findings have been observed in a study conducted in Kembata-Tembaro, South Ethiopia [37].

The place and time a woman should get maternal health services is influenced by a collective decision of the husband, mother-in-laws and other family members, and compounded by gender dynamics and poverty: not only are women often reliant on men for financial resources, but the local cultural norms mean that the views of mothers-in-law in Sidama need to be respected. Studies conducted in other parts of the country have documented similar findings [22, 38, 39]. Women who were able to decide themselves or jointly decide with their husbands were more likely to use maternal health services than those who were not able to decide themselves [26, 35, 40, 41].

Despite the availability of health professionals and HEWs nearby at the PHCU, TBAs were often the preferred choice to attend delivery over locally-based formal providers. Previous studies carried out in Ethiopia have confirmed that the majority of home deliveries were assisted by TBAs [34, 38, 42]. The community trust in TBAs – they provide services within the home and engage in traditional practices such as burying placentas inside home – meant they were often the first choice to provide maternal health care. This preference was compounded by concerns by some community members about the experience of HEWs, who were believed to be younger and less competent than TBAs. Even though HEWs had been trained to provide safe and clean delivery service, they often lacked basic knowledge and skills to carry it out, which deterred the community to use their services. Inadequate trust in the HEWs' capacity has been reported elsewhere in Ethiopia and may reflect a systemic problem with the HEW training package. In future the lack of trust related to delivery services might be less profound, since the government announced that HEWs should no longer be expected to conduct deliveries. In northern Ethiopia it was also found that HEWs had a low performance with respect to delivery and had poor knowledge about antenatal care counseling, danger signs and symptoms and complications of pregnancy [43].

Communication and coordination of maternal health services between the TBAs and the PHCU were limited. Other studies carried out in Afar regional state of Ethiopia recognized the importance of integrating TBAs with the formal health system in the light of human resource shortage for maternal health [44]. This is a challenging area given the government's resistance to the official inclusion of TBAs, and the sudden not well-communicated ban of TBA services, which can result in conflicts of interest between TBAs and HEWs.

This study and a number of other Ethiopian studies identified that women often pay for delivery services at hospitals and for routine pregnancy investigations and care at health centres. A study carried out in Addis Ababa identified that 91% of women paid for investigations (laboratory and ultrasound) or drugs during ANC visits in government health facilities [45]. The Ethiopian essential service package policy indicates that delivery service should be provided free of charge [46]. Several studies have documented that user fees for maternal health service have an impact on service use [37, 39, 47–50]. Other costs for transportation, food and lodging form also as challenges for using health services [22, 37, 39, 47]. Exemption of service fees improves use of the services. For instance in Kenya, a four-fold increase in hospital deliveries was observed among a study population who had both the cost of services and transport covered compared with a population where their costs were not covered [48].

Second phase delay

Lack of transport, distance, difficult topography, the cost of ambulance fuel, use of an ambulance for unintended purpose and uncooperative behavior of ambulance drivers affected the coordination of referrals within the PHCU and were the main factors with respect to delay two. Studies conducted in Ethiopia, Tanzania and Ghana have documented the problem of transport as a hindering factor for use of maternal health services [21, 22, 37, 39, 49, 50], but in this study, there are some specific hindrances that can be tackled locally. For example, some communities were affected by the improper use of the ambulance by local officials and the poor behavior of ambulance drivers.

Third phase delay

Lack of medical equipment, weak coordination, and management for referrals, health workers' unprofessional behaviour and absence of HEWs and health workers at health facilities were factors contributing to the third delay. This is consistent with other studies, one conducted in Tigray, Ethiopia, identifying that the majority of the health posts did not have medical equipment, water, and electricity supply [43].Other studies confirm that poor availability of drugs and supplies influences the use of maternal health services [37, 51, 52]. It will be necessary for health facilities and management teams in Sidama to address the poor availability of supplies and medical equipment at the PCHU if they are to increase the willingness of women to use formal local delivery services.

Towards improving use of maternal health services in Sidama

This study identified a number of challenges that are specific to local circumstances and some are amenable to locally developed solutions. Special attention to these challenges and local solutions is instrumental, as the current interplay of different factors makes many pregnant women decide still to deliver at home. The REACH Ethiopia NGO, in collaboration with Sidama zone health department through the REACHOUT consortium, has been implementing a quality improvement intervention to start the process of addressing key factors influencing the use of maternal health services in PHCU which will be reported elsewhere. The intervention facilitated local identification of priority problems that would lead to activities to bring about small, non-costly incremental changes to try to overcome them. The quality improvement cycle approach can facilitate which priority actions are needed and feasible to support coordination of and engagement with on maternal health at the community level. This approach attempts to works within existing systems and funding constraints.

This study found targeted awareness creation and community mobilization activities are needed to improve the knowledge of pregnant women and their families on danger signs of pregnancy and the benefits of maternal health services. Pregnant women also need to be identified at earlier stage of pregnancy by the HDAs and HEWs to enhance timely booking for ANC. Community based health programmes should include husbands and mothers in laws so that they will be aware of maternal health issues in order to support pregnant women in getting the services. Local leaders need to communicate clear directions how the TBAs can contribute to maternal health services and optimize their coordination with HEWs. The activities of 1 to 5 network should be strengthened to enhance access to maternal health services within the community.

Action is also required to improve the responsiveness, quality and cultural sensitivity of health facilities, and women's ability to get to these services. Ambulances should be used for the intended purpose and the government has to allocate a budget for fuel replenishment. The health system should take into account the cultural concerns of the community, like burying placenta inside home. Health facilities also need to be equipped with the necessary logistics and infrastructure, taking into account what is possible within available budgets. The government also needs to actively monitor the implementation of free maternal health services as per the regulation of the country.

Advocacy with local decision-makers and policy-makers on the importance and benefits of maternal health interventions, such as quality improvement cycles, is important for their sustainability. Ideally they need to be embedded in the health system from an early stage to ensure long term benefits.

Limitations

This study was part of a larger study looking at factors influencing the performance of maternal health services delivered by HEWs. Use of maternal health services at the PHCU level was an important emerging theme and from the women's perspective most factors related to delay 1 with relatively limited information on delays 2 and 3. Due to the recent ban on TBAs not to conduct delivery services, they were often reluctant to give detailed information.

Conclusions

Maternal health remains a priority in Ethiopia and strategies to improve maternal health outcomes that are contextually relevant are urgently required. In this study, we have used qualitative research to identify key barriers constraining use of maternal health care services in PHCUs in rural communities in Sidama. These have been framed within Thaddeus and Maine's three delays model; delays at the first and third phases emerged as particularly problematic in this study. There is a need to institute community based awareness creation and mobilization activities to address factors contributing to the first delay. Lack of logistics and supplies at health facilities and lack of proper training and skills of health workers need due attention from health system mangers and policy makers to address the third phase delay. The health system should also work towards more caring and compassionate health professionals. Action at these multiple intersecting levels will provide women with the quality and responsive health services they deserve to make progress towards the SDGs. One of the approaches that policy makers and local leaders can consider for doing this is quality improvement cycles.

Endnotes

[1]*Kebele* is the smallest unit of local government and can best be regarded as neighborhoods localized and delimited groups of people.

[2]'Clean and safe' deliveries are conducted by the HEW at the health post level and skilled deliveries are conducted by nurses and other health professionals at health centres and hospitals.

Abbreviations

ANC: Antenatal care; FGD: Focus group discussion; HDA: Health development army; HEP: Health extension programme; HEWs: Health extension workers; IDI: In-depth interview; MMR: Maternal mortality ratio; PNC: Postnatal care; TBAs: Traditional birth attendants

Acknowledgements

We would like to extend our appreciation to the regional health bureau, Sidama zone health department and the *woreda* health offices for cooperation and support provided to carry out this research project. Our warmest thanks go to the participants of the study and data collectors without whom this research would have been impossible.

Funding

We certify that all financial support for the conduct of this study was obtained from the European Commission through the European Union Seventh Framework Programme ([FP7/2007–2013] [FP7/2007–2011]) under grant agreement no 306090.

Author's contributions

AK, OT, DD and MK contributed towards study design. MK and AK were involved in data collection; data analysis was conducted by MK, AK, DD and OT. AK drafted the manuscript with significant input from OT, MK, ST and DD, and all authors critically reviewed and contributed towards the manuscript. All authors read and approved the final manuscript.

Ethics approval and consent to participate

The generic study protocol was approved by the Royal Tropical Institute Ethical Review Committee in Amsterdam. National approval was obtained from Research and Technology Transfer Core Process of South Nation Nationalities and Peoples Region Health Bureau, Ethiopia (*Ref. No pω6–19/ 17014, Date 26 June 2013*). Research and Technology Transfer Core Process is

a legal entity and responsible to assess research proposals and grant ethical approval for the studies conducted in South Nation Nationalities and Peoples Regional state. Permission to conduct the study was also obtained from Sidama zone health department and woreda health offices.
The ethics committee approved to obtain informed verbal consent from illiterate participants and hence we sought informed verbal consent from mothers, TBAs and male participants. Written informed consent was obtained from *Kebele* administrators, HEWs, health centre heads, delivery case team leaders and HEP coordinators at *woreda*, zonal health department and regional health bureau.

Competing interests

The authors declare that they have no competing interests.

Author details

[1]REACH Ethiopia, P.O. Box 303, Hawassa, Ethiopia. [2]Liverpool School of Tropical Medicine, Liverpool, UK. [3]Royal Tropical Institute, P.O. Box 95001, 1090, HA, Amsterdam, The Netherlands.

References

1. WHO, UNICEF, UNFPA, World Bank: Trends in maternal mortality 1990–2015, Geneva Switherland. 2015.
2. Thaddeus S, Maine D. Too far to walk: maternal mortality in context. Soc Sci Med. 1994;38(8):1091-110.
3. Ellis C, Schummers L, Rostoker J-F. Reducing maternal mortality in Uganda: applying the "three delays" framework. Int J Child Birth. 2011;1(4):218–26.
4. Shah N, Hossain N, Shoaib R, Hussain A, Gillani R, Khan NH. Socio-demographic characteristics and the three delays of maternal mortality. J Coll Physicians Surg Pak. 2009;19(2):95–8.
5. Thiri Win, Patama Vapattanawong, Vong-ek P. Three delays related to maternal mortality in Myanmar: a case study from maternal death review, 2013. J Health Res. 2015;29(3):179–87.
6. Saad El Gelany, Mohamed G. Mansour, Hassan MM. The three delays of maternal mortality in a public-sector tertiary teaching hospital: is there a paradigm shift? Gynecol Obstet Res Open J. 2015;2(2):52–6.
7. Abdella A. Maternal mortality trend in Ethiopia. Ethiop J Health Dev. 2010; 24(1):115–22.
8. Yifru Berhan, Asres Berhan: REASONS FOR PERSISTENTLY HIGH MATERNAL AND PERINATAL MORTALITIES IN ETHIOPIA: PART III–PERSPECTIVE OF THE "THREE DELAYS" MODEL. Ethiop J Health Sci 2014(Special Issue):137–148.
9. Pacagnella RC, Cecatti JG, Parpinelli MA, Sousa MH, Haddad SM, Costa ML, Souza JP, Pattinson RC, Morbidity atBNftSoSM, study group. Delays in receiving obstetric care and poor maternal outcomes: results from a national multicentre cross-sectional study. BMC Pregnancy Childbirth. 2014;14:159.
10. Sorensen BL, BruunNielsen B, Rasch V, Elsass P. User and provider perspectives on emergency obstetric care in a Tanzanian rural setting: a qualitative analysis of the three delays model in a field study. Afr J Reprod Health. 2011;15(2):117–30.
11. Austin A, Gulema H, Belizan M, Colaci DS, Kendall T, Tebeka M, Hailemariam M, Bekele D, Tadesse L, Berhane Y, et al. Barriers to providing quality emergency obstetric care in Addis Ababa, Ethiopia: healthcare providers' perspectives on training, referrals and supervision, a mixed methods study. BMC Pregnancy Childbirth. 2015;15:74.
12. Lubbock LA, Stephenson RB. Utilization of maternal health care services in the department of Matagalpa, Nicaragua. Rev Panam Salud Publica/Pan Am J Public Health. 2008;24(2):75–84.
13. Awoke W, Seleshi K. Maternal delays in utilizing institutional delivery services, Bahir Dar, Ethiopia. Health. 2013;5(6):1026–31.
14. Tarekegn SM, Lieberman LS, Giedraitis V. Determinants of maternal health service utilization in Ethiopia: analysis of the 2011 Ethiopian demographic and health survey. BMC Pregnancy Childbirth. 2014;14:161.
15. Gebrehiwot T, Sebastian MS, Edin K, Goicolea I. Health workers' perceptions of facilitators of and barriers to institutional delivery in Tigray, northern Ethiopia. BMC Pregnancy Childbirth. 2014;14:137.
16. Mbaruku G, van Roosmalen J, Kimondo I, Bilango F, Bergström S. Perinatal audit using the 3-delays model in western Tanzania. Int J Gynecol Obstet. 2009;106(1):85–8.
17. Andargie G, Berhane Y, Worku A, Kebede Y. Why is perinatal mortality higher among women delivered at health Facility in Rural Northwest Ethiopia? A qualitative study. Br J Med Med Res. 2014;4(29):4834–43.
18. Federal Ministry of Health: Health sector development Programme IV 2010/11–2014/15. 2010.
19. Ministry of Health: Health extension Programme in Ethiopia. 2007.
20. Ministry of Health: Health development Implimentation guideline 2011.
21. Central Statistical Agency Ethiopia, Ministry of health: Ethiopia mini demographic and health survey 2014.
22. Fikre A-A, Demissie M. Prevalence of institutional delivery and associated factors in Dodota Woreda (district), Oromia regional state, Ethiopia. Reprod Health. 2012;9:33.
23. Teferra A-S, Alemu F-M, Woldeyohannes S-M. Institutional delivery service utilization and associated factors among mothers who gave birth in the last 12 months in Sekela District, north west of Ethiopia: a community - based cross sectional study. BMC Pregnancy Childbirth. 2012;12:74.
24. Wolelie A, Aychiluhm M, Awoke W. Institutional delivery service utilization and associated factors in Banja District, Awie zone, Amhara regional sate, Ethiopia. Open J Epidemiol. 2014;4:30–5.
25. Tewodros B, G/Mariam A, Dibaba Y: Factors affecting antenatal care utlization in Yem special wored, southwestern Ethiopia. Ethiopia J Health Sci. 2009;19(1):45-51.
26. Ejeta E, Nigusse T. Determinants of skilled institutional delivery service utilization among women who gave birth in the last 12 months in Bako District, Oromia, Ethiopia, 2012/13 (case-control study design). J Gynecol Obstet. 2015;3(2):36–42.
27. Federal Democratic Republic of Ethiopia CSA: Population and housing census 2007.
28. Minstry of Culture and Tourism:, http://www.moct.gov.et: 2016.
29. Sidama zone health department: Annual zonal health department performance report 2013.
30. Feleke Hailemichael, Mirkuzie Woldie, Fikru Tafese: Predictors of institutional delivery in Sodo town, Southern Ethiopia. Afr J Prm Health Care Fam Med. 2013;5(1):1–8.
31. Yalem Tsegay, Tesfay Gebrehiwot, Isabel Goicolea, Kerstin Edin, Hailemariam Lemma, Sebastian MS: Determinants of antenatal care, institutional delivery and skilled birth attendant utilization in Samre Saharti District, Tigray, Ethiopia (thesis). 2010.
32. Islam MR, Odland JO. Determinants of antenatal and postnatal care visits among indigenous people in Bangladesh: a study of the Mru community. Rural Remote Health. 2011;11:1672.
33. Ndidi EP, Oseremen G. Reasons given by pregnant women for late initiation of antenatal care in the Niger Delta, Nigeria. Ghana Med J. 2010;44(2):47–51.
34. Birmeta K, Dibaba Y, Woldeyohannes D. Determinants of maternal health care utilization in Holeta town, Central Ethiopia. BMC Health Serv Res. 2013; 2013(13):256.
35. Abosse Z, Woldie M, Ololo S. Factors influencing antenatal care service utilization in Hadiya zone. Ethiop J Health Sci. 2010;20(2):75–82.
36. WHO, UNICEF. Antenatal care in developing countries: promises, achievements and missed opportunities. An analysis of trends, levels and differentials, 1990–2001. Switzerland: WHO Geneva; 2003.
37. Shiferaw S, Spigt M, Godefrooij M, Melkamu Y, Tekie M. Why do women prefer home births in Ethiopia? BMC Pregnancy Childbirth. 2013;13:5.
38. Juliet Bedford, Meena Gandhi, Metasebia Admassu, Anteneh-Girma: 'A Normal Delivery Takes Place at Home': A Qualitative Study of the Location of Childbirth in Rural Ethiopia. Matern Child Health J 2012.
39. Warren C. Care seeking for maternal health: challenges remain for poor women. Ethiopia J Health Dev. 2010;24(1):100–4.
40. Gurmesa-Tura, Mariam A-G. Safe delivery service utlization in Metekel zone north West Ethiopia Ethiopia. J Health Sci. 2008;17(4):213–22.
41. Hailemariam Alemayeh, Huruy Assefa, Yohannes Adama: Prevalence and Factors Associated with Post Natal Care Utilization in Abi-Adi Town, Tigray, Ethiopia: A Cross Sectional Study. IJPBSF International Journal of Pharmaceutical and Biological Sciences Fundamentals. 2014;08(01):23–35.
42. Nigussie M, Mariam DH, Mitike G. Assessment of safe delivery service utilization among women of childbearing age in North Gondar zone, north West Ethiopia. Ethiop J Health Dev. 2004;18(3):145–52.

43. Medhanyie A, Spigt M, Dinant GJ, Blanco R. Knowledge and performance of the Ethiopian health extension workers on antenatal and delivery care: a cross-sectional study. Hum Resour Health. 2012;10(44)
44. Temesgen TM, Umer JY, Buda DS, Haregu TN. Contribution of traditional birth attendants to the formal health system in Ethiopia: the case of afar region. Pan Afr Med J. 2012;13(Supp 1):15.
45. Jimalo AT. Why pregnant women delay to attend Pernatal care ? In: Cross sectional study on timing of first antenatal care booking at public health institutions in Addis Ababa (Addis Ababa University unpublished thesis); 2008.
46. Federal Ministry of Health: Essential health services package for Ethiopia. 2005.
47. Simkhada B, van Teijlingen ER, Porter M, Simkhada P. Factors affecting the utilization of antenatal care in developing countries: systematic review of the literature. J Adv Nurs. 2007;61(3):244–60.
48. Mwangome FK, Holding PA, Songola KM, Bomu GK. Barriers to hospital delivery in a rural setting in Coast Province, Kenya: community attitude and behaviours. Rural Remote Health. 1852;12:2012.
49. Exavery A, Kanté AM, Njozi M, Tani K, Doctor HV, Hingora A, Phillips JF. Access to institutional delivery care and reasons for home delivery in three districts of Tanzania. Int J Equity Health. 2014;13:48.
50. Reuben K. Esena, Mary-Margaret Sappor: Factors Associated With The Utilization Of Skilled Delivery Services In The Ga East Municipality Of Ghana Part 2: Barriers To Skilled Delivery. Int J Scientific Technol Res. 2013;2(8):195–207.
51. Francis Abugri AKUM. A qualitative study on factors contributing to low institutional child delivery rates in northern Ghana: the case of Bawku municipality. Community Med Health Educ. 2013;3:236.
52. Tetui M, Ekirapa EK, Bua J, Mutebi A, Tweheyo R, Waiswa P. Quality of antenatal care services in eastern Uganda: implications for interventions. Pan Afr Med J. 2012;13:27.

9

Association between skilled maternal healthcare and postpartum contraceptive use in Ethiopia

Gizachew Assefa Tessema[1,2*], Tensae Tadesse Mekonnen[3], Zelalem Birhanu Mengesha[1,4] and Katherine Tumlinson[5]

Abstract

Background: The postpartum period provides an important opportunity to address unmet need for contraception and reduce short birth intervals. This study aims to assess the association between skilled maternal healthcare and postpartum contraceptive use in Ethiopia.

Methods: Data for this analysis come from the 2011 to 2016 Ethiopian Demographic and Health Surveys (EDHS) and include nearly 5000 married women of reproductive age with a recent birth. Multivariate logistic regression was conducted to investigate the relationship between skilled maternal healthcare and postpartum contraceptive use.

Results: Between rounds of the 2011 and 2016 EDHS, the postpartum contraceptive prevalence increased from 15 to 23% and delivery in public facilities, use of skilled birth assistance, and skilled antenatal care also grew. In both survey rounds, educated women had approximately twice the odds of postpartum contraceptive use, compared with non-educated women, while an initially significant relationship between wealth and postpartum contraceptive use diminished in significance by 2016. Women with a desire to limit future pregnancy had five to six times the odds of postpartum contraceptive use in both survey rounds, and women in 2016 – unlike those in 2011 – with a desire to *delay* pregnancy were significantly more likely to use contraception (adjusted odds ratio (AOR) = 4.38, 95% CI: 1.46-13.18) compared to women who wanted another child soon. In 2011, no statistically significant associations were found between any maternal healthcare and postpartum contraceptive use. In contrast, in 2016, postpartum contraceptive use was significantly associated with an institutional delivery (AOR = 1.71, 95% confidence interval (CI): 1.12-2.62) and skilled antenatal care (AOR = 2.41, 95% CI: 1.41-4.10). No significant relationship was observed in either survey round between postpartum contraceptive use and skilled delivery or postnatal care.

Conclusions: A comparison of postpartum women in the 2011 and 2016 EDHS reveals increased use of both contraception and skilled maternal healthcare services and improved likelihood of contraceptive use among women with an institutional delivery or antenatal care, perhaps as a result of increased attention to postpartum family planning integration. Additionally, results suggest postpartum women are now using contraception to space future pregnancies, with the potential to help women achieve more optimal birth intervals.

Keywords: Postpartum, Family planning, Maternal healthcare, Ethiopia

* Correspondence: agizachew@gmail.com
[1]Department of Reproductive Health, Institute of Public Health, University of Gondar, Gondar, Ethiopia
[2]School of Public Health, The University of Adelaide, Adelaide, Australia
Full list of author information is available at the end of the article

Background

Approximately 20% of births in low-income countries are to women with fewer than 24 months since their previous birth, resulting in a significant number of birth intervals of short duration [1–3]. The critical public health importance of optimal birth intervals for women and children are well-documented. Birth intervals spanning two to five years are associated with improved child nutrition, reduced likelihood of preterm birth and low birth weight, and – subsequently – increased child survival [4–6]. Optimal child spacing may also reduce the likelihood of abortion, miscarriage, and stillbirth and reduces competition among siblings [1, 7]. In addition to these benefits for children and infants, women with healthy birth intervals are at reduced risk of maternal death and pregnancy-related morbidity [8]. As such, family planning programs have great potential to reduce maternal, child, and infant mortality in developing country settings by helping women achieve healthy birth intervals. Experts estimate nearly one third of all maternal deaths and close to 10 % of deaths to children under five years of age could be averted by eliminating short birth intervals [4, 9].

One key strategy for ensuring optimal birth intervals is the promotion of contraceptive use in the postpartum period [1]. Evidence suggests that the vast majority of women in developing countries wish to avoid pregnancy in the first year following a birth, but unmet need within this vulnerable group is consistently higher than in women outside of the extended postpartum period; some estimates of unmet need in the extended postpartum period are as high as 65% [10–13]. A variety of reasons may contribute to unmet need among postpartum women; yet several studies conducted in countries in Africa and Asia have demonstrated that use of maternal health services, such as pre- and postnatal care and institutional delivery, can enhance postpartum family planning use [14–18]. Therefore, the postpartum period provides a unique and critical opportunity to fulfil unmet need for contraceptives and to reduce the risks of closely spaced pregnancies [13]. Integration of family planning counselling with pre- and postpartum services has the potential to help motivated women achieve adequate birth spacing as well as limit unintended pregnancy. A recent study provides compelling evidence that the provision of information on family planning to women in the postpartum period resulted in significantly increased contraceptive use [19].

Ethiopia has a total population of 95 million people, nearly one quarter of which are women of reproductive age. The catchment area of primary health care facilities (public hospitals, health centres, and health posts) covers nearly 92% of the population [20]. Despite the potential to reach a vast majority of the Ethiopian population, in reality, a much smaller portion of the population utilise skilled maternal healthcare services in Ethiopia: in 2016, 26% of pregnant women delivered in a health facility, 62% of pregnant women received skilled antenatal care, and 17% received skilled postnatal care [21]. The current prevalence of modern contraceptive use in Ethiopia is approximately 25% of all women of reproductive age and 35% of married women of reproductive age; nearly one out of every four married women of reproductive age has an unmet need for family planning [21, 22]. An analysis of birth intervals in 44 low-income countries found 46% of parous women sampled in the 2005 Ethiopia Demographic and Health Survey (EDHS) reported birth intervals of less than two years. In comparison, among the 25 other African countries included in the analysis, the percent of women with a birth interval under two years ranged from 24 to 54% and, when compared with Ethiopia, only four African countries had a larger percentage of women with birth intervals under two years [5].

The 2011 Ethiopian national guidelines for family planning services mandate integration of family planning services with all skilled maternal healthcare services [23]. Government health policies also aim to increase the contraceptive prevalence rate among married women of reproductive age to 55% and to reduce unmet need to 10% by 2020 [24]. One key and promising national strategy being implemented in an effort to achieve these targets is promotion of postpartum contraceptive use through the scale-up of existing postpartum family planning services by expanding the services to district level health facilities and universal access of contraceptive methods in the immediate postpartum period in 2020 [24, 25]. Towards this end, additional information is needed to better understand whether use of skilled maternal healthcare services such as pre- and postnatal care and institutional delivery might impact subsequent postpartum contraceptive use in Ethiopia.

The present study uses large scale national datasets collected in 2011 and 2016 to examine the association between use of skilled maternal healthcare services and subsequent postpartum contraceptive use among married reproductive aged women in Ethiopia, and compares the findings between the two surveys. The findings of this study can inform policies and programs designed to improve postpartum family planning use, reduce unmet need, and reduce the prevalence of short birth intervals among Ethiopian women.

Methods

Study design and sample

The Ethiopian Demographic and Health Survey (EDHS) was first implemented in Ethiopia in 2000 and a total of four national surveys have been conducted as of 2016.

The present analysis uses data from the latest two rounds of the EDHS, collected in 2011 and 2016. The EDHS is a cross-sectional survey conducted every five to six years to measure the demographic and health-related characteristics of the population [26]. The EDHS 2011 survey was conducted from December 2010 to June 2011 and includes interviews with a total of 16,515 women of reproductive age [27]. The EDHS 2016 survey was conducted from January to June 2016 and includes a sample of 15,683 women of reproductive age [21]. A stratified, two-stage cluster sampling procedure was used to recruit the nationally representative sample in both surveys. The 11 administrative regions found in Ethiopia were initially stratified into urban and rural areas. Each stratum was subdivided into districts (*woredas),* and *woredas* were then subdivided into *kebeles* (the smallest administrative unit in Ethiopia). Finally each kebele was subdivided into Enumeration Areas (EAs) that served as sampling clusters. A total of 624 EAs were included in EDHS 2011 and 645 EAs were included in EDHS 2016. In the present analysis, we included married/in sexual union, non-pregnant women who gave birth in the 12 months prior to data collection. As a result, a total of 2545 married/in sexual union women in EDHS 2011 and 2386 married/in sexual union women in EDHS 2016 were included in our final analysis (Fig. 1). The analysis was restricted to married/in sexual union women to allow cross-country comparisons of contraceptive prevalence rate (CPR), which is often calculated only for married women and those in sexual union. Additionally, we excluded women who were not married or in sexual union because they are not considered at risk for pregnancy and therefore do not require methods of pregnancy prevention, the main outcome of interest in this analysis.

Postpartum contraceptive use

In this analysis the dependent variable is a binary variable for postpartum contraceptive use. Postpartum contraceptive use is defined as any self-reported use of a modern contraceptive method (modern methods reported in this sample included: female sterilization, implant, intrauterine device (IUD), injectable, oral contraceptive, emergency contraceptive, lactational amenorrhea method (LAM) or condom) at the time of data collection. Those women not reporting any modern method use and those reporting traditional method use (periodic abstinence or withdrawal) were classified as non-users.

Skilled maternal healthcare services

We examined the association between postpartum contraceptive use and four key maternal healthcare services, all coded as binary variables: institutional delivery, presence of a skilled birth attendant, skilled antenatal care, and skilled postnatal care. Institutional delivery was classified based on the place of delivery. A woman was defined as having an institutional delivery if she had given birth (the most recent time) at a hospital, health centre, or any private facility; otherwise women were classified as having a home delivery. Skilled attendance at birth was based on who attended the delivery irrespective of the place of delivery. Those women whose most recent birth was attended by a professional (doctor, midwife or nurse, health officer) possessing midwifery skills were classified as having skilled attendance at birth. Skilled antenatal care included any woman receiving one or more episodes of antenatal care by a skilled provider. Skilled postnatal care was based on health check-ups by skilled professionals (doctor, midwife or nurse, health officer) for women who

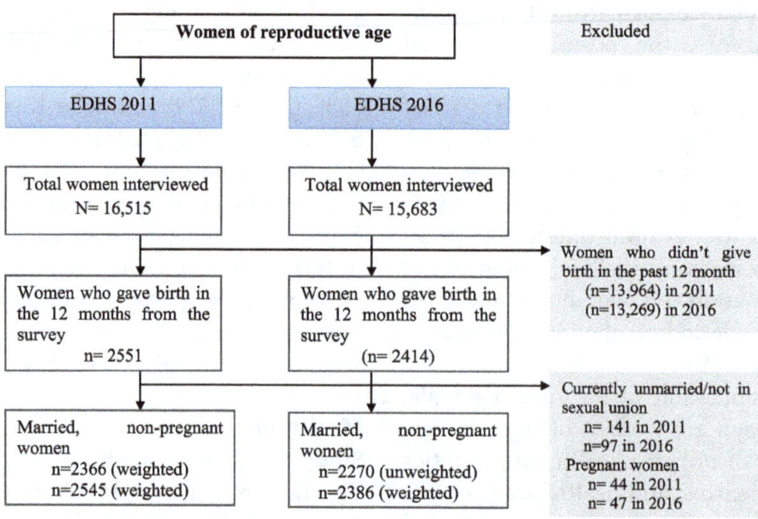

Fig. 1 Schematic presentation showing sampling in the 2011 and 2016 Ethiopia Demographic and Health Surveys (EDHS)

delivered in a health facility or at home within the first six weeks of the participant's most recent delivery.

Demographic and reproductive and maternal health variables

Demographic, reproductive health and other factors were also examined as potential covariates in this analysis. Demographic variables include age, rural versus urban residence, region, religion, participant's education, partner's education, employment status, wealth, and parity. Reproductive health and other factors include birth order, concordant family planning preferences, fertility preferences, women's decision-making, contraceptive knowledge (the ability to mention at least one method), any visit from a family planning worker in the last 12 months, and exposure to family planning media messages (newspaper, radio, television, or mobile SMS text) in the last few months. Women's decision making was defined by whether a woman reports that she can make decisions by herself or jointly with her partner about the following: decisions about health service utilisation, decisions about household purchases, and decisions to visit family or relatives. Specific categories for these variables are shown in Tables 1, 2, and 3.

Statistical analysis

We used STATA version 14.0 to conduct all the analysis. Descriptive statistics were calculated for all variables described above. Multivariate logistic regression was conducted to estimate adjusted odds ratios. Those demographic and reproductive health variables described above which had a *p*-value of less than 0.2 in the binary logistic regression analysis were included as covariates in our model. During EDHS 2011, some areas were oversampled in order to have regional estimates. Additionally, non-response was observed in the survey. In order to ensure the actual representativeness of survey results at the national level, all analyses in the present study were weighted. The complete sample weight computation is available with the dataset provided by ICF International.

Results

Socio-demographic characteristics

This analysis includes nearly 5000 married/in sexual union women of reproductive age with a birth in the 12 months preceding the survey; 2545 of these women participated in the 2011 EDHS while the remaining 2386 were participants in the 2016 survey. As seen in Table 1, about half of all women (47% in 2011 and 50% in 2016) were between the ages of 25 and 34, with a median age of 28 years. The majority of the respondents (87% in 2011 and 88% in 2016) were rural residents. Oromo and Amhara ethnic groups were the predominant groups in both rounds of the EDHS. With regard to the level of education, the proportion of women who did not have any formal education decreased from 67% in 2011 to 59% in 2016 and the proportion of women who completed secondary education more than doubled between surveys (4% in 2011 to 9% in 2016). Likewise, the proportion of participants whose partners completed secondary education nearly doubled between surveys from 9 to 15%. About 53% of these postpartum women were not working outside the home. When looking at the household wealth, 46% of participants in both surveys were in the poorest group, with no change between surveys in terms of the distribution of wealth.

Reproductive health characteristics of women in the postpartum period

As shown in Table 2, in both surveys, more than a third of women had between one and two children, more than a fourth had three to four children, and nearly a third had five or more children. For the majority of participants (80 to 85%), their most recent birth was not their first birth, although first-time deliveries increased by about 5 % when comparing the 2011 and 2016 samples. Few changes were seen between surveys in terms of family size concordance, with just about 40% of couples agreeing on ideal family size and approximately one in four women reporting that their partner wants a bigger family than they do. In both surveys, fertility preferences remained approximately stable, with only about six to 8 % of women reporting a desire for another child soon; about one third reported not wanting any more children and more than half reported wishing to delay their next pregnancy. Ability to mention at least one contraceptive method remained nearly universal in both survey rounds and exposure to family planning media messages stayed stable at around 25%. Notably, the percentage of women reporting some degree of decision-making power increased from 50 to 68%. Also of note, the percentage of women who reported a visit by a family planning worker in the preceding 12 months doubled between surveys from 16 to 33%.

Postpartum contraceptive and skilled maternal healthcare utilisation

In the last five years, the prevalence of contraceptive use increased by 53% from 15% in 2011 to 23% in 2016 (Table 3). In terms of the contraceptive method mix in both surveys, injectable contraception was the predominant method (Fig. 2). While there were little to no changes in the contribution to the national method mix by pills, female sterilization, condoms, and LAM, there was a notable change in the contribution of implants (10% in 2011 vs 16% in 2016) and IUD (1% in 2011 vs 4% in 2016) (Fig. 2).

Table 1 Sociodemographic characteristics in the 2011 and 2016 Ethiopia Demographic and Health Surveys (EDHS), among married/in sexual union women of reproductive age

Variables	EDHS 2011 (*N* = 2545)		EDHS 2016 (*N* = 2386)	
	Frequency	Percent	Frequency	Percent
Age in years				
15-24	833	32.7	745	31.2
25-34	1203	47.3	1194	50.0
35+	509	20.0	447	18.7
Mean age (SD)	27.68(±6.5)		27.63(6.3)	
Place of residence				
Urban	332	13.1	287	12.0
Rural	2213	86.9	2099	88.0
Region				
Tigray	139	5.5	168	7.0
Affar	22	0.9	23	1.0
Amhara	543	21.3	449	18.8
Oromiya	1136	44.6	1041	43.6
Somali	79	3.1	114	4.8
Benishangul-Gumuz	29	1.1	26	1.1
Southern Nation, Nationalities and People Region	525	20.6	488	20.4
Gambela	7	0.3	5	0.2
Harari	6	0.2	6	0.3
Addis Ababa	53	2.1	58	2.4
Dire Dawa	8	0.3	9	0.4
Religion				
Orthodox	908	35.7	792	33.2
Muslim	979	38.5	1042	43.7
Protestant	586	23.0	475	19.9
Other/missing	72	2.8	78	3.3
Highest educational status				
None	1703	66.9	1417	59.4
Primary	745	29.3	755	31.6
Secondary+	97	3.8	215	9.0
Partner highest educational status				
None	1223	48.0	1056	44.3
Primary	1100	43.2	969	40.6
Secondary+	223	8.7	361	15.1
Women occupation				
Not working	1355	53.2	1476	61.9
Working but not paid/paid in kind only	512	20.1	585	24.5
paid with cash	678	26.6	326	13.7
Wealth index				
Low	1160	45.6	1085	45.5
Middle	539	21.2	491	20.6
High	846	33.2	810	33.9

With respect to maternal healthcare, while only about one in ten women reported delivery in a health facility in 2011, more than a third of our 2016 sample reported delivery in a health facility. Use of public facilities became nearly universal within our 2016 sample, as compared to private facility use, among those women not delivering at home. Additionally we observed a threefold increase in the use of skilled assistance during delivery and a twofold increase in the number of women receiving skilled antenatal care, when comparing the two survey samples. We also observed modest increases in the number of women with four or more antenatal visits and skilled postnatal care (Table 3).

Factors associated with postpartum contraceptive use

In our 2011 sample of postpartum women, two demographic characteristics were strongly associated with postpartum family planning. Women in the highest wealth category had nearly three times the odds of postpartum contraceptive use compared to women in the lowest wealth category. In addition to wealth, education was strongly associated with postpartum contraceptive use in the 2011 sample; those with at least a primary education were nearly twice as likely to use contraception, compared to women with no education. In our 2016 sample of postpartum women, education remains associated with contraceptive use but the magnitude of the association between wealth and family planning use is greatly reduced and the result is only marginally significant (Tables 4 and 5).

In the 2011 sample of postpartum women, the strongest association with postpartum contraceptive use was seen among women who reported a desire to avoid future pregnancy. Women who wanted no more children had six times the odds of postpartum contraceptive use compared to women who would like to have a child soon. We did not find any relationship between women with a desire to delay pregnancy and contraceptive use in our 2011 sample of women. In the 2016 data, our sample of women also demonstrated a strong likelihood to use contraception in the postpartum period if they preferred no more children; in contrast with the 2011 data however, our 2016 sample of women were also significantly more likely to use contraception if they had a

Table 2 Reproductive health related characteristics in the 2011 and 2016 Ethiopia Demographic and Health Surveys (EDHS), among married/in sexual union women of reproductive age

Variables	EDHS 2011 (*N* = 2545)		EDHS 2016 (*N* = 2386)	
	Frequency	Percent	Frequency	Percent
Number of living children				
No child	24	0.9	15	0.6
1-2 child	942	37.0	939	39.4
3-4 child	746	29.3	653	27.4
5+	834	32.8	780	32.7
Birth order				
First	393	15.4	480	20.1
2-3 birth	848	33.3	749	31.4
4-5 birth	565	22.2	510	21.4
6+	739	29.0	647	27.1
Family size concordance				
Both want same	982	38.6	998	41.8
Husband wants more	662	26.0	580	24.3
Husbands wants fewer	187	7.4	147	6.1
Do not know/Missing	714	28.1	662	27.7
Fertility preference				
wants soon	151	5.9	187	7.8
wants later	1387	54.5	1298	54.4
wants no more	892	35.1	760	31.9
Undecided	115	4.5	142	5.9
Women's decision-making[b]				
Yes	1272	50.0	1623	68.0
No	1273	50.0	764	32.0
Knowledge of modern contraceptive				
Yes	2463	96.8	2351	98.5
No	82	3.2	35	1.5
Visited by FP worker in the last 12 months				
Yes	416	16.3	778	32.6
No	2129	83.7	1608	67.4
Exposure to family planning media[a]				
Yes	689	27.1	592	24.8
No	1856	72.9	1794	75.2

[a]Exposure to family planning media was determined by whether a woman reported she has heard/read about family planning from radio/television/ newspaper/ mobile SMS. [b]Women's decision-making was defined by whether a woman reported that she herself has made decisions (or made a joint decision with her partner) about her own health care, large household purchase, or visiting families/relatives

desire to *delay* a future pregnancy (AOR: 4.38, 95% CI: 1.46 – 13.18) (Tables 4 and 5).

Regarding use of skilled maternal healthcare, no statistically significant associations were found in the 2011 sample of women. Women who delivered in a health facility or with a skilled attendant were no more likely than women with home births or those without skilled attendance to use postpartum family planning. Similarly, women with antenatal care visits were no more likely to use postpartum family planning than those without such visits. We found only a marginally significant relationship between postnatal care and postpartum contraceptive use in the 2011 data. In contrast, delivery within a health facility as well as obtaining skilled antenatal care are both significantly associated with postpartum contraceptive use in the 2016 sample, with adjusted odds ratios of 1.71 (95% CI: 1.12-2.62) and 2.41 (95% CI: 1.41-4.10) respectively (Tables 4 and 5).

Table 3 Maternal healthcare services related characteristics in the 2011 and 2016 Ethiopia Demographic and Health Surveys (EDHS), among married/in sexual union women of reproductive age

Variables	EDHS 2011 (*N* = 2545)		EDHS 2016 (*N* = 2386)	
	Frequency	Percent	Frequency	Percent
Current contraceptive use				
Yes	378	14.9	553	23.2
No	2167	85.1	1834	76.8
Place of delivery				
Home	2272	89.3	1499	62.8
Health facility	273	10.7	887	37.2
Place of delivery by facility type[a]				
Public facility	234	85.7	864	97.4
Private facility	39	14.3	23	2.6
Who assisted delivery				
No assistance/ assisted by unskilled provider	2221	87.2	1478	62.0
Doctor	29	1.2	99	4.1
Nurse/midwife/HO	295	11.6	809	33.9
Skilled ANC				
Yes	820	32.2	1620	67.8
No	1725	67.8	766	32.7
Number of skilled ANC[b](*n* = 820)				
One times	117	14.3	126	7.8
2-3 times	356	43.4	677	41.8
4+ times	347	42.3	817	50.4
Skilled PNC use				
Yes	183	7.18	455	19.1
No PNC	2362	92.18	1931	80.9

ANC Antenatal care, *PNC* Postnatal care, *HO* Health officer
[a]*n* = calculated from facility delivery, [b]*n* = calculated from those who received skilled ANC

Discussion

This study describes the prevalence of postpartum contraceptive use and skilled maternal healthcare among

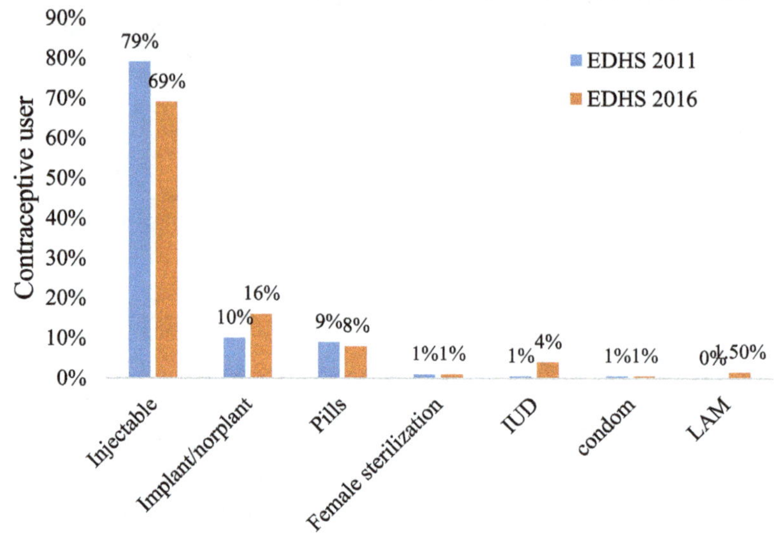

Fig. 2 Contraceptive method mix among postpartum women using modern contraceptive methods in 2011($n = 378$) and 2016 ($n = 553$) in the Ethiopia Demographic and Health Surveys (EDHS)

two representative samples (collected in 2011 and 2016) of married/in sexual union women in Ethiopia with a birth in the previous year. Our findings in both rounds are far lower than a finding from similar study in Indonesia (74%) [28]. In our 2011 sample, we found low contraceptive use; only 15% of women were protected from early pregnancy. This is much lower than the overall prevalence of modern method use reported by married women in the 2011 EDHS (approximately 27%), despite the increased health risks to women in the postpartum period [29]. Contraceptive use was much higher (23%) in our 2016 sample of married/in sexual union postpartum women, although still not keeping pace with the overall prevalence of modern method use among all married women of reproductive age in Ethiopia (35% in the 2016 EDHS). Additionally, when compared with the 2011 sample, women in our 2016 sample reported a higher prevalence of facility delivery, greater use of public facilities for delivery, higher prevalence of skilled assistance during delivery (especially nurse and midwife assistance), and a higher prevalence of receiving skilled ante- and postnatal care. In fact, the proportion of women reporting skilled birth assistance or pre- or postnatal care more than doubled and institutional births more than tripled during the five-year period. This growth between 2011 and 2016 in the prevalence of both contraceptive use and skilled maternal healthcare suggests government efforts to increase access to and use of these services are rapidly succeeding. However, the remaining large numbers of women giving birth at home and/or without assistance and without skilled postpartum care indicate the need for these efforts to continue.

In addition to increased uptake of both contraception and skilled maternal healthcare, we also noted a shift in the role played by both wealth and fertility intentions. In the 2011 data, residing in the highest wealth category was strongly associated with an increased likelihood of postpartum contraceptive use. In other words, among women in the 2011 sample, wealthier women were nearly three times more likely to use contraception compared to women in the lowest wealth category. This finding is consistent with studies conducted throughout Africa which have found that wealthier women were more likely to be using contraception compared to their poorer counterparts [17, 18, 30]. Although family planning services in Ethiopia are offered free of charge in public facilities, this finding could reflect indirect costs, such as transportation, which may prohibit access to family planning services. In the 2016 data however, wealth was only marginally significant in terms of its relationship with postpartum contraceptive use, with an adjusted odds ratio of far less magnitude (1.5 compared to 2.7 in 2011). This finding suggests that wealth may play a much smaller role in women's postpartum contraceptive behaviour compared to five years ago, perhaps as a result of increased outreach efforts; indeed, the proportion of participants reportedly visited by a family planning worker in the 12 months preceding the survey doubled between survey rounds. This finding is a promising indication that the prevalence of contraceptive use is not only rising, but that it is growing in ways that promote greater health equity.

Additionally, we saw in the 2011 data that women who didn't want any more children were significantly more likely to use family planning, compared to women

Table 4 Multivariate logistic regression examining factors associated with postpartum contraceptive use in Ethiopia, 2011 ($n = 2545$)

Variables	PPFP Use		OR (95% CI)			
	No	Yes	COR	95% CI	AOR	95% CI
Wealth index						
Low	1091	69	1		1	
Middle	479	61	2.01	1.16 - 3.50	1.55	0.89 - 2.72
High	597	249	6.61	4.20 - 10.39	2.74***	1.53 - 4.92
Age category (in years)						
15-24	642	191	1		1	
25-34	1055	148	0.47	0.32 - 0.69	0.82	0.51 - 1.31
35+	470	39	0.27	0.17 - 0.46	0.75	0.32 - 1.76
Residence						
Urban	186	147	6.77	4.55-10.07	1.89	0.93 - 3.84
Rural	1981	231	1		1	0.27-1.13
Access to family planning media						
No	1654	203	1		1	
Yes	513	175	2.79	1.94-4.00	1.41	0.91- 2.18
Women educational status						
No education	1564	139	1		1	
Primary	547	198	4.07	2.92 - 5.68	1.83*	1.22 - 2.77
Secondary or above	56	41	8.19	4.15 - 16.17	1.02	0.42 - 2.48
Partner education						
No education	1120	102	1		1	
Primary	893	207	2.54	1.67 - 3.84	1.23	0.73 - 2.06
Secondary or above	154	69	4.92	2.69 - 8.99	0.62	0.27 - 1.40
Women occupation						
Not working	1147	208	1		1	
Working but not paid	463	463	0.59	0.35 - 0.99	0.79	0.46 - 1.36
Working for paid	557	121	1.20	0.83 - 1.74	1.08	0.73 - 1.60
Number of living children						
No child	23	1	1		1	
1-2 child	703	239	8.69	1.89 - 40.03	2.68	0.40 - 17.83
3-4 child	652	93	3.64	0.77 - 17.40	1.35	0.19 - 9.78
5+ child	769	45	1.45	0.30 - 6.95	0.89	0.10 - 7.73
Decision making						
Not participated	1136	136	1		1	
Participated	1031	242	1.95	1.34 - 2.85	1.40	0.90 - 2.16
Fertility Preference						
Wants soon	144	7	1		1	
Wants later	1176	211	3.78	1.18 - 12.10	2.59	0.64 - 10.56
Wants no more	749	143	4.01	1.20 - 13.42	5.90*	1.43 - 24.44
undecided	98	17	3.69	0.93 - 14.52	4.58	1.00 - 21.02
Place of delivery						
Home	2009	264	1		1	
Health facility	158	115	5.53	3.68 - 8.30	0.63	0.18 - 2.19
Skilled attendance at birth						

Table 4 Multivariate logistic regression examining factors associated with postpartum contraceptive use in Ethiopia, 2011 ($n = 2545$) *(Continued)*

Variables	PPFP Use		OR (95% CI)			
	No	Yes	COR	95% CI	AOR	95% CI
No	2055	301	1		1	
Yes	112	77	6.13	4.24 - 8.88	2.07	0.69- 6.24
Skilled antenatal care						
No	1564	161	1		1	
Yes	603	217	3.48	2.40 - 5.03	1.16	0.72- 1.89
Skilled postnatal care						
No	2059	303	1		1	
Yes	108	75	4.74	3.02 - 7.45	1.86	0.94- 3.65
Birth order						
First	297	96	1		1	
2-3	653	195	0.93	0.60 - 1.43	1.09	0.61 - 1.94
4-5	515	50	0.31	0.17 - 0.54	0.59	0.25 - 1.41
6+	702	37	0.16	0.08 - 0.30	0.50	0.16 -1.60

PPFP Postpartum Family Planning, *COR* Crude Odds Ratio, *AOR* Adjusted Odds Ratio *** $p < 0.001$, *$p < 0.05$

with a desire to become pregnant again right away. This finding is unsurprising as we would expect greater contraceptive use among women who have already achieved (or possibly surpassed) their desired number of children, particularly when compared with women indicating a desire to have another child soon. However, women in the 2011 sample who wanted to delay (rather than avoid) their next pregnancy were no more likely to use family planning than women who wanted to become pregnant soon. In contrast, in the 2016 sample we see that women with a desire to delay their next pregnancy have more than 4 times the odds of family planning use compared to women who want a pregnancy soon. This suggests that postpartum women in Ethiopia are beginning to use contraception not just to avoid a future pregnancy but also to *delay* their next pregnancy; this increase in the use of contraception for birth spacing represents great promise in government efforts aimed at achieving optimal birth intervals and addressing unmet need for family planning.

Across both rounds of data collection and in agreement with numerous other studies [18, 31, 32], women's educational status was found to be associated with postpartum contraceptive use. In both samples, women who had at least some primary or secondary education had about twice the odds of contraceptive use as compared to non-educated women. Female education is widely thought to play an important role in fertility [33–35] and these findings support that conclusion.

Finally, this study investigated the association between several key maternal healthcare services and postpartum contraceptive use. Although numerous studies have shown a relationship between the use of some type of maternal healthcare service and postpartum contraceptive utilization, in the 2011 sample of women, these services did not show significant association. While these results may suggest no correlation between skilled maternal healthcare and subsequent postpartum contraceptive use in Ethiopia, we hypothesise two alternative explanations for this finding. First, it is possible that providers were offering family planning information to clients at the time they received one or more types of maternal healthcare services, but the amount or type of information provided may have been insufficient to result in actual contraceptive use. In other words, providers may have done a poor job of discussing information on a variety of methods or may have rushed through the information without verifying that women still recovering from labour and attending to a newborn are fully comprehending their contraceptive options and necessary next steps for obtaining their method of choice. Second, this finding could be the result of poor integration of family planning counselling and services during the provisions of skilled maternal healthcare. Services may be poorly integrated for a variety of reasons. Service providers may be poorly trained on integration protocols or may be simply unable to provide family planning information if experiencing a high case-load of clients. For example, a study in the capital city of Ethiopia showed that nearly two-third of pregnant women accessing antenatal care services did not receive any counselling about contraceptive methods [36]. Further, even those providers who are well-trained may lack sufficient motivation to follow integration protocol unless increased supervision or other accountability mechanisms are in place [37–40].

Table 5 Multivariate logistic regression examining factors associated with postpartum contraceptive use in Ethiopia, 2016 ($n = 2386$)

Variables	PPFP Use		OR (95% CI)			
	No	Yes	COR	95% CI	AOR	95% CI
Wealth index						
Low	933	152	1		1	
Middle	383	108	1.72	1.12 - 2.65	1.45	0.90 - 2.36
High	518	292	3.46	2.34 - 5.09	1.53	0.97 - 2.39
Age category (in years)						
15-24	538	208	1		1	
25-34	925	269	0.75	0.55 - 1.03	0.94	0.59 - 1.50
35+	371	76	0.53	0.33 - 0.86	1.18	0.57 - 2.42
Residence						
Urban	136	152	1		1	
Rural	1698	401	0.21	0.14 - 0.31	0.56	0.27-1.13
Access to family planning media						
No	1454	352	1		1	
Yes	380	200	2.17	1.54 - 3.06	0.95	0.64 - 1.40
Women educational status						
No education	1203	213	1		1	
Primary	523	232	2.51	1.79 - 3.50	1.32	0.90 - 1.93
Secondary or above	107	107	5.63	3.58 - 8.85	2.03*	1.09 - 3.78
Partner education						
No education	899	158	1		1	
Primary	710	259	2.08	1.44 - 3.02	1.36	0.95 - 1.96
Secondary or above	225	136	3.44	2.24 - 5.30	0.75	0.41 - 1.37
Number of living children						
No child	8	7	1		1	
1-2 child	640	299	0.56	0.10 - 3.12	0.22	0.04 - 1.30
3-4 child	507	145	0.34	0.06 - 1.82	0.21	0.03 - 1.28
5+ child	678	102	0.18	0.03 - 1.02	0.15	0.02 - 1.00
Visited by FP worker in the past 12 months						
No	1289	319	1		1	
Yes	545	233	1.73	1.24 - 2.40	1.40	0.99 - 1.99
Fertility Preference						
Wants soon	172	15	1		1	
Wants later	955	343	4.23	1.70 - 10.55	4.38**	1.46 - 13.18
Wants no more	589	171	3.42	1.28 - 9.09	5.14**	1.59 - 16.59
undecided	117	24	2.43	0.77 - 7.67	3.44	0.97 - 12.17
Place of delivery						
Home	1289	210	1		1	
Health facility	545	342	3.85	2.81 - 5.23	1.71*	1.12 - 2.62
Skilled attendance at birth						
No	1689	436	1		1	
Yes	144	117	3.15	2.15 - 4.62	1.28	0.81 - 2.01
Skilled antenatal care						
No	706	61	1		1	

Table 5 Multivariate logistic regression examining factors associated with postpartum contraceptive use in Ethiopia, 2016 ($n = 2386$) *(Continued)*

Variables	PPFP Use		OR (95% CI)			
	No	Yes	COR	95% CI	AOR	95% CI
Yes	1128	492	5.08	3.01 - 8.46	2.41**	1.41 - 4.10
Skilled postnatal care						
No	1558	373	1		1	
Yes	276	180	2.72	1.96 - 3.75	1.03	0.68 - 1.56
Birth order						
First	321	159	1		1	
2-3	528	221	0.85	0.58 - 1.24	1.02	0.63 - 1.64
4-5	416	94	0.46	0.30 - 0.70	0.83	0.38 - 1.81
6+	569	79	0.49	0.17 - 0.46	0.69	0.25 - 1.94

PPFP Postpartum Family Planning, *COR* Crude Odds Ratio, *AOR* Adjusted Odds Ratio ** $p < 0.01$, *$p < 0.05$

In contrast to the null findings in our 2011 sample regarding skilled maternal healthcare and postpartum contraceptive use, within our 2016 sample, we found that both delivery within a health care facility and receipt of skilled antenatal care approximately doubled the odds of postpartum contraceptive use. These findings are in line with previous studies investigating the impact of postpartum family planning integration on subsequent contraceptive use [15–19, 31]. The fact that these associations did not exist in the 2011 sample lends some weight to our hypothesis that postpartum family planning messages and services were not well integrated in Ethiopia in 2011 compared to 2016. The new associations emerging in the 2016 data suggest that the Ethiopian ministry of health is succeeding in their demonstrated efforts to integrate contraceptive messages and services during the prenatal period as well as at some point before the patient exits the facility after giving birth. In other words, not only are women having more skilled care before, during, and after delivery, our findings suggest that women may also receive more exposure to family planning services during this critical time; It appears that facilities are capitalising on the convenience of reaching women with family planning messaging while they are already at the facility giving birth.

Importantly, despite remarkable progress in postpartum contraceptive use and increased use of skilled maternal healthcare in Ethiopia, there are still large numbers of women giving births at home, without benefit of skilled antenatal care or skilled delivery, and without skilled postnatal care following their birth. These findings suggest the Ethiopian government would benefit from examining the variety of factors that may be keeping skilled care beyond the reach of large numbers of women, for example the quality of family planning counselling provided during outreach to rural women in their residential homes. Currently, the Ethiopian government has an ambitious plan to achieve nearly universal coverage for ante- and postnatal care and skilled birth attendance [25]. There is much progress remaining in obtaining this goal and the government should continue to prioritize and reinforce efforts to expand and improve maternal healthcare, postpartum contraceptive use, and integration of family planning into all reproductive health services.

This study is not without limitations. First, the data used in this analysis are self-reported and therefore may bias results if participants felt the need to alter their responses based on perceived preferences of the enumerators. Second, while participants report on whether or not they received various types of maternal healthcare services, they did not report on the content of those services and – as we suggest above – it may be the case that not all service providers adhere to national guidelines that mandate family planning integration into reproductive healthcare services. Additionally, it is possible that some women may have started a contraceptive method at some point following their most recent birth but may have discontinued that method prior to being interviewed. In this case, it is possible that some women with some postpartum contraceptive use would have been misclassified as non-users. However, the majority of contraceptive users selected injectable contraception which has a duration of three months following each injection; we would not expect discontinuation rates to be high in the short period of time between contraceptive initiation and the date of interview, particularly among those women who did not immediately initiate contraception following birth and/or those whose last birth preceded the interview date by only a few months. In this regard, for instance, the present analysis shows that nearly two thirds of our participants commence contraceptive six months after delivery. Finally, participants vary in terms of the amount of time since their recent birth, with the time between birth and interview ranging from one to 12 months. Those with fewer months since their recent birth may differ from those with more distant births, and this heterogeneity may warrant further exploration in subsequent analyses.

Conclusion

In conclusion, the present study revealed that postpartum contraceptive use in Ethiopia is low but increased between 2011 and 2016. Unsurprisingly, educational obtainment and the desire to avoid future pregnancy were positively associated with postpartum contraceptive use in both survey rounds; however 2016 saw a diminished role of wealth as a key correlate of contraceptive use and an emerging association among women with a desire to delay their next pregnancy. Within our 2011 sample, several key maternal healthcare services such as antenatal care and institutional delivery had no association with postpartum contraceptive use, but these null findings became positive associations in the 2016 sample. These results suggest national efforts to strengthen the integration of family planning counselling and services with skilled maternal healthcare services are succeeding, allowing health care facilities to reduce missed opportunities for increasing contraceptive use among this critical population within Ethiopia. Efforts should continue given the large numbers of women in Ethiopia still delivering at home and without the benefit of skilled pre- and postnatal care.

Abbreviations

AOR: Adjusted odds ratio; CI: Confidence interval; CPC: Carolina Population Center; CPR: Contraceptive prevalence rate; DHS: Demographic and health survey; EA: Enumeration area; EDHS: Ethiopian demographic and health survey; EHNRI: Ethiopian Health Nutrition Research Institute; FP: Family planning; IUD: Intrauterine device; LAM: Lactational amenorrhea method; NICHD: National Institute of Child Health & Human Development; NRERC: National Research Ethics Review Committee; PPFP: Postpartum family planning

Acknowledgements

We thank DHS Program for giving us permission to use the EDHS 2011 and EDHS 2016 data for this analysis.

Funding

We are grateful to the Carolina Population Center (CPC) (R24HD050924) for general support and to a career development grant (4R00HD086270-04) from the National Institute of Child Health & Human Development (NICHD) to the manuscript's senior author. However, beyond the general and career support to the manuscript's senior author, the funders did not have any role in the design of the study and collection, analysis, and interpretation of data and in writing the manuscript. The contents of this article are solely the responsibility of the authors and do not necessarily represent the official views of CPC or NICHD.

Authors' contributions

Initially conceived and designed the study: GAT, TTM and ZBM. Conducted the analysis: GAT. Wrote the paper and made revisions: GAT, KT. Reviewing the manuscript critically: TTM, ZBM. All authors read and approved the manuscript.

Ethics approval and consent to participate

Authorisation for using the data in the current study was granted from the DHS program upon presenting the aims of the study and the research plan. This analysis uses secondary, de-identified data made publicly available by ICF International and the EDHS. Ethical review for the primary data collection activities conducted by the EDHS was performed by the Review Board of the Ethiopian Health Nutrition Research Institute (EHNRI), the National Research Ethics Review Committee (NRERC) at the Ministry of Science and Technology, the Institutional Review Board of ICF International, and the United States Center for Disease Control. Detailed information on the data collection procedures employed by EHDS has been published as a full report elsewhere [21, 27].

Competing interests

The authors declare that they have no competing interests.

Author details

[1]Department of Reproductive Health, Institute of Public Health, University of Gondar, Gondar, Ethiopia. [2]School of Public Health, The University of Adelaide, Adelaide, Australia. [3]Department of Midwifery, Tseda Health Science College, Gondar, Ethiopia. [4]Centre for Health Research, Western Sydney University, Sydney, Australia. [5]Department of Maternal and Child Health, Gillings School of Global Public Health, University of North Carolina at Chapel Hill, Chapel Hill, USA.

References

1. Ahmed S, Ahmed S, McKaig C, Begum N, Mungia J, Norton M, Baqui AH. The effect of integrating family planning with a maternal and newborn health program on postpartum contraceptive use and optimal birth spacing in rural Bangladesh. Stud Fam Plan. 2015;46(3):297–312.
2. Rutstein SO, Winter R. The effects of fertility behavior on child survival and child nutritional status: evidence from demographic and health surveys, 2006-2012. In: DHS Analystical studies no 37. Rockville: ICF International; 2014.
3. World Health Organization (WHO). Report of a WHO technical consultation on birth spacing. Geneva: WHO; 2005.
4. Cleland J, Bernstein S, Ezeh A, Faundes A, Glasier A, Innis J. Family planning: the unfinished agenda. Lancet. 2006;368(9549):1810–27.
5. Rutstein SO. Further evidence of the effects of preceding birth intervals on neonatal, infant, and under-five-years mortality and nutritional status in developing countries: evidence from the demographic and health surveys. DHSWorking papers no. 41. Calverton: Macro International; 2008.
6. Zhu BP, Rolfs RT, Nangle BE, Horan JM. Effect of the interval between pregnancies on perinatal outcomes. N Engl J Med. 1999;340(8):589–94.
7. DaVanzo J, Hale L, Razzaque A, Rahman M. The effects of pregnancy spacing on infant and child mortality in Matlab, Bangladesh: how they vary by the type of pregnancy outcome that began the interval. Popul Stud. 2008;62(2):131–54.
8. Conde-Agudelo A, Rosas-Bermudez A, Kafury-Goeta AC. Effects of birth spacing on maternal health: a systematic review. Am J Obstet Gynecol. 2007;196(4):297–308.
9. Cleland J, Conde-Agudelo A, Peterson H, Ross J, Tsui A. Contraception and health. Lancet. 2012;380(9837):149–56.
10. Tegegn M, Arefaynie M, Tiruye TY. Unmet need for modern contraceptives and associated factors among women in the extended postpartum period in Dessie town, Ethiopia. Contracept Reprod Med. 2017;2:21.
11. Ross JA, Winfrey WL. Contraceptive use, intention to use and unmet need during the extended postpartum period. Int Fam Plan Perspect. 2001;27(1):20–7.
12. MacQuarrie Kerry LD. Unmet need for family planning among young women: levels and trends. DHS comparative reports no. 34. Rockville: ICF International; 2014.
13. Gaffield ME, Egan S, Temmerman M. It's about time: WHO and partners release programming strategies for postpartum family planning. Glob Health Sci Pract. 2014;2(1):4–9.
14. Do M, Hotchkiss D. Relationships between antenatal and postnatal care and post-partum modern contraceptive use: evidence from population surveys in Kenya and Zambia. BMC Health Serv Res. 2013;13:6.

15. Abera Y, Mengesha ZB, Tessema GA. Postpartum contraceptive use in Gondar town, Northwest Ethiopia: a community based cross-sectional study. BMC Womens Health. 2015;15:19.
16. Achyut P, Mishra A, Montana L, Sengupta R, Calhoun LM, Nanda P. Integration of family planning with maternal health services: an opportunity to increase postpartum modern contraceptive use in urban Uttar Pradesh, India. J Fam Plann Reprod Health Care. 2016;42(2):107-15.
17. Akinlo A, Bisiriyu A, Esimai O. Influence of use of maternal health care on postpartum contraception in Nigeria. DHSWorking papers no. 92. Calverton: ICF International; 2013.
18. Rutaremwa G, Kabagenyi A, Wandera SO, Jhamba T, Akiror E, Nviiri HL. Predictors of modern contraceptive use during the postpartum period among women in Uganda: a population-based cross sectional study. BMC Public Health. 2015;15:262.
19. Tappis H, Kazi A, Hameed W, Dahar Z, Ali A, Agha S. The role of quality health services and discussion about birth spacing in postpartum contraceptive use in Sindh, Pakistan: a multilevel analysis. PLoS One. 2015; 10(10):e0139628.
20. Teklehaimanot HD, Teklehaimanot A. Human resource development for a community-based health extension program: a case study from Ethiopia. Hum Resour Health. 2013;11:39.
21. CSA [Ethiopia] and ICF International. Ethiopia demographic and health survey 2016. Addis Ababa and Rockville: CSA [Ethiopia] and ICF International; 2016.
22. Ethiopia: Commitment Maker Since 2012 [http://www.familyplanning2020.org/entities/56].
23. Ethiopia Ministry of Health. National Guideline for family planning Services in Ethiopia. Addis Ababa: Federal Democratic Republic of Ethiopia Ministry of Health; 2011.
24. FMOH. Health sector transformation plan (HSTP) 2015/16 - 2019/20. Addis Ababa: Federal Ministry of Health (FMOH); 2015.
25. FMOH. Draft National Reproductive Health Strategy (2016 – 2020). Addis Ababa: Federal Ministry of Health (FMOH); 2016.
26. The DHS data collection [http://dhsprogram.com/data/data-collection.cfm].
27. Central Statistics Agency (CSA) of Ethiopia and ICF International. Ethiopian demographic and health survey report 2011. Addis Ababa, Ethiopia and Calverton: Central Statistical Agency and ICF International; 2012.
28. Wilopo SA, Setyawan A, Pinandari AW, Prihyugiarto T, Juliaan F, Magnani RJ. Levels, trends and correlates of unmet need for family planning among postpartum women in Indonesia: 2007-2015. BMC Womens Health. 2017; 17(1):120.
29. Population Reference Bureau (PRB): Family planning worldwide 2013 data. Washington DC: PRB; 2013. https://www.prb.org/family-planning-worldwide-2013/.
30. Kandala NB, Lukumu FK, Mantempa JN, Kandala JD, Chirwa T. Disparities in modern contraception use among women in the democratic republic of Congo: a cross-sectional spatial analysis of provincial variations based on household survey data. J Biosoc Sci. 2015;47(3):345–62.
31. Abraha TH, Teferra AS, Gelagay AA. Postpartum modern contraceptive use in northern Ethiopia: prevalence and associated factors. Epidemiol Health. 2017;39:e2017012.
32. Mahmood SE, Srivastava A, Shrotriya VP, Shaifali I, Mishra P. Postpartum contraceptive use in rural Bareilly. Indian J Commun Health. 2011;23(2):56–7.
33. Hahn Y, Islam A, Nuzhat K, Smyth R, Yang H-S. Education, marriage and fertility: long-term evidence from a female stipend program in Bangladesh. Melbourne: Monash University; 2015.
34. Becker SO, Cinnirella F, Woessmann L. Does women's education affect fertility? Evidence from pre-demographic transition Prussia. Eur Rev Econ Hist. 2013;17(1):24–44.
35. Lam D, Sedlacek G, Duryea S. Increase in women' s education and fertility decline in Brazil. Anais. 2016:89–118.
36. Teshome A, Birara M, Rominski SD. Quality of family planning counseling among women attending prenatal care at a hospital in Addis Ababa, Ethiopia. Int J Gynaecol Obstet. 2017;137(2):174–9.
37. Das J, Hammer J, Leonard K. The quality of medical advice in low-income countries. J Econ Perspect. 2008;22(2):93–114.
38. Mohanan M, Vera-Hernandez M, Das V, Giardili S, Goldhaber-Fiebert JD, Rabin TL, Raj SS, Schwartz JI, Seth A. The know-do gap in quality of health care for childhood diarrhea and pneumonia in rural India. JAMA Pediatr. 2015;169(4):349–57.
39. Tumlinson K, Okigbo CC, Speizer IS. Provider barriers to family planning access in urban Kenya. Contraception. 2015;92(2):143–51.
40. Tumlinson K, Speizer IS, Curtis SL, Pence BW. Accuracy of standard measures of family planning service quality: findings from the simulated client method. Stud Fam Plan. 2014;45(4):443–70.

10

Mobility patterns and associated factors among pregnant internal migrant women in China

Ying Ji[1], Xiaoping Zhao[2], Zhili Wang[3], Shenglan Liu[1], Yang Shen[1] and Chun Chang[1*]

Abstract

Background: Residential instability during pregnancy has been linked to poor health outcomes. As a first step toward providing better health care to pregnant migrant women, the size and characteristics of this population and factors associated with mobility during pregnancy should be studied.

Methods: Using the "Monitoring Data of Chinese Migrants" for 2012, from the Chinese National Population and Family Planning Commission, this study explored mobility patterns during pregnancy and associated factors among migrants within China. From a library of 158,556 participants, two subsamples were selected. Percentages, with chi-squared tests, and means and standard deviations, with ANOVAs, were adopted to describe mobility patterns during pregnancy (*always staying in sending area, mainly staying in sending area, mainly staying in receiving area,* and *always staying in receiving area*) and delivery location choice. Logistic regression analysis was used to explore the associated factors.

Results: We found that the percentage of migrants always or mainly staying in receiving areas during pregnancy rose from nearly 40% in 1985 to more than 80% in 2012, while the percentage of migrants who were mobile between receiving and sending areas during pregnancy fluctuated between 30 and 40% before 1995, and between 40 and 45% after 1995, decreasing to around 40% after 2008. The percentage of respondents who chose to deliver in receiving areas fluctuated but increased from 10% in 1985 to more than 50% in 2011. Among respondents who had delivered during the last year of the survey period, families with older pregnant women (OR = 1.09, 95% CI 1.05–1.13), their own housing (OR = 5.66, 95% CI 2.45–13.05), longer time in the receiving area (OR = 1.14, 95% CI 1.09–1.20), and strong will to integrate (OR = 1.32, 95% CI 1.15–1.51) always stayed in the receiving area during pregnancy, rather than the sending area, and families with broadly similar characteristics were inclined to choose the receiving area for their delivery.

Conclusions: The mobility patterns of pregnant migrant women in China have been changing in recent years, with the percentage of them staying in receiving areas during pregnancy and delivering there increasing. Individual and family characteristics were also associated with mobility patterns and delivery location choice.

Keywords: Mobility during pregnancy, Internal migrant, Maternal health, Social integration, Delivery location

* Correspondence: changchun@bjmu.edu.cn
[1]Department of Social Medicine and Health Education, School of Public Health, Peking University, Beijing, China
Full list of author information is available at the end of the article

Background

Pregnancy is a critical period for the health of both mothers and infants, and mobility during pregnancy raises public health concerns given that residential instability has been linked to poor health outcomes of children and mothers. First, mobility during pregnancy brings environmental change that may be associated with congenital anomalies and children with asthma [1–5]. Second, mobility during pregnancy may lead to decreased use of maternal health care services due to less knowledge and information, financial barriers, or other barriers to accessibility of services [6–11], although it is important from the outcomes perspective to utilize and maintain regular contact with health services during pregnancy to reduce the risk of low birth weight, preterm births, and perinatal deaths [6, 12–15]. Third, mobility during pregnancy is detrimental to health care provision. Failure to address the scale and traits of these populations and their specific demands impedes appropriate service provision [7, 16–20]. In addition to these factors, in China, inadequate health information tracing and discontinuity of pregnancy health records contribute much to the difficulties of service provision. Given the deficiency of referral mechanisms in China, pregnant women might choose any accessible hospital for their delivery, which might lead to considerable unexpected pressure on large hospitals. Therefore, describing the trends of and factors affecting mobility during pregnancy is necessary.

Internal migrants are a special population in China. "Migrant" is an identity applied to those leaving their residence for a certain period without changing their household registration, or *hukou*. The *hukou* system in China has segregated the rural and urban populations in geographical terms. Established in the late 1950s, it was initially a primary means of controlling population mobility and determining eligibility for public services and welfare, such as access to local public schools, pension plans, and public housing. *Hukou* conversion, meaning change from the rural to the urban category or from a small city to a large one, was controlled and permitted only under limited conditions [21]. After the mid-1980s, however, large-scale rural-to-urban migration became possible. A relaxation in the implementation of *hukou* laws and the re-commodification of many basic goods meant that the rapidly growing urban private sector was able to absorb large numbers of laborers from small cities and the countryside. An unprecedented wave of large-scale migration had begun. Although the mobility of people is no longer tightly regulated and migrants without local *hukou* in receiving areas can access to more public welfare than before, transfer of *hukou* status is still subject to strict policy and quota controls, especially in large cities [22]. Although the *hukou* system is specific to China, internal migrants have other characteristics in common with migrants in China and other developing countries, such as low education, rural origins, and heavy work stress [18, 22–25]. Among migrants in developing countries, the utilization of antenatal care services in receiving areas is inadequate [18, 26, 27]. The reasons for low utilization rates of maternal health care by migrants are various, including poor health knowledge and awareness, financial or cultural barriers, and provider factors [7, 16, 18–20, 23]. This population migration has brought increased attention to the issue of migrant health, as illustrated for example by the World Health Organization's calling upon its member states to promote migrant-sensitive health policies, equal access to health promotion, and disease prevention, especially for migrant women and children [28].

As mentioned above, both mobility behavior during pregnancy and the identity characteristics of migrants can influence their health care utilization and provisions. In our study, we define *migrant* as an identity applied to those leaving their residence for a certain period without changing their household registration, and *mobility* as a migrant's travel behavior between sending and receiving areas. During pregnancy and delivery, migrants may either go back to their original registration area (sending area), stay in the receiving area, or move to a new area (new receiving area). Therefore, as a first step to providing better health care to pregnant migrant women, policymakers should familiarize themselves with the scale, characteristics, and change trends of the target population and the factors associated with their movements. Many studies from developed countries have explored mobility during pregnancy in the general population [1, 2, 29, 30], and family and individual characteristics have been analyzed to detect associated factors [1, 8, 29]. However, few studies have explored mobility during pregnancy among internally migrant population in developing countries.

In this context, the purpose of this study was to analyze mobility patterns in China's internal migrant population during pregnancy, including factors associated with it.

Methods

Data source

Cross-sectional data were obtained from the 2012 "Monitoring Data of Chinese Migrants" survey conducted in China and published by the National Population and Family Planning Commission (containing data for 2011). Inclusion criteria for the survey were males and females living in their local area for 1 month or longer without local household registration and aged between 15 and 59 years as of May 2012. Exclusion criteria were those having a spouse or child from a local household (those whose spouse or child holds local household registration are not deemed migrants, as their families can access local public welfare services, such as entering public school and applying for public housing) or those who were part of the temporary floating population at railway stations, docks, airports, hotels, and hospitals. Only one person in each household was surveyed. The survey contained items for respondents' demographic characteristics and those of their family members, employment, housing, health care, marital status, obstetrical status, and level of social integration. This adopted stratified sampling for migrants from each province and a three-stage sampling method with probability proportional to unit size within the province (town/subdistrict, village/community, and individual). The samples were representative nationally as well as for each province [31]. (See Additional file 1).

The sample size of the survey was 158,556 people. The survey method used was face-to-face interviews, with community staff filling out questionnaires and importing data through an electronic system. The study has been granted an exemption from the Peking University Institutional Review Board (No. IRB00001052–16011).

Selection of samples for analysis

From the library of 158,556 individual samples, 29,720 cases (18.74%) who were married, had borne children, and had had migration experience before the conception of their first child were chosen. Within the shortlisted cases, 185 cases who had had children between 1970 and 1984 were excluded due to their relatively small number, as their inclusion may have led to data instability. Furthermore, 771 cases who had given birth between January and May of 2012 and thus did not have a full year of data available were excluded, leaving 28,764 cases from which to analyze the mobility patterns of migrants during the gestational and peripartum period of their first child. Thus, from the library of 158,556 samples, 4176 cases (2.63%) who were married and had borne children between June 2011 and May 2012, the last year of the survey period, were chosen; they were mothers who had had migration experience before conception, and thus were a fitting sample from which to analyze the mobility characteristics of migrants during pregnancy. The respondents selected were women aged 17–49.

Measures

Based on previous studies, we hypothesized that the socioeconomic status (SES) of the family, family migration characteristics, parity (that is, first or not first child), and social integration situation were associated with mobility during pregnancy.

Family SES includes the *education level of the pregnant woman*, the family *Engel coefficient* (hereafter EC, the percentage of household expenditure devoted to food), *whether they have their own house in the receiving area*, and *whether family members have urban employee medical insurance*. The EC was considered to be a measure of effective wealth; since the income gaps between provinces in China are big and the levels of consumption are different, it is difficult to compare absolute value of income. In our study, two questions were used to calculate EC: "How much does your family spend monthly (in RMB) on local food?" and "What is your monthly household income (in RMB)?" The minimum EC value was 0.01 and the maximum value was 1.00, with a mean of 0.55 (medium value 0.56) and a standard deviation of 0.19. In other studies, EC has been used as an indirect reflection of SES [32, 33]; as demand for food is inelastic, poorer families have a higher EC.

Owning a house in the receiving area was considered as a covariate. In the late 1990s, with development of the market economy in China, owning a house ceased to be strictly limited by the household registration system—that is, people could buy a house without local household registration. Since 2010, however, to control the rapidly increasing price of houses, some local governments in big cities have imposed restrictions on buying houses for people without a local household registration, even though migrants might have their own houses owing to the different housing policies among cities. For example, in Beijing migrants are eligible to buy houses if they have been working in Beijing for more than 5 years, provided they submit certification of continuous income taxes. Some types of houses are unrestricted, such as houses used for both commerce and living (*ShangzhuLiangyong*). Given this background, owning a house reflects the following choices: whether a migrant family bought a house early (before 2010), whether they worked in the city for a long time, and/or whether they became rich enough to buy a permitted house.

Family migration characteristics include *rural household registration, range of migration* (cross-province, cross-city within province, cross-district within city), and *migration time* (time since the person migrated into the local area). The *hukou* system in China has segregated not only the rural and urban populations but also various geographical populations at levels as small as subdistrict (urban)/town (rural). In our study, we used "*rural household registration*" (yes or no) to demonstrate rural–urban or urban–urban migration status (for our survey carried out in cities, no urban–rural or rural–rural migration was included) and adopted *migration range* (cross-province, cross-city within province, cross-district within city) as another variable demonstrating migration status.

Status of social integration (*SSI*) was determined by eight questions (see Table 1). Factor analysis was adopted, and two factors were extracted to explain the 50.3% variance, with $KMO = 0.816$ and $p < 0.001$ for Bartlett's test. "Participation in local activities" and "With whom do you have the most contact?" were the two

Table 1 Eight questions to measure status of social integration

	Items	Assignment methods
1	Have you or your family participated in cultural and sports activities, social activities, family planning association activities, health education activities, and elections in the local community this year?	A score from 0 to 5 based on participation in these five items
2	During your spare time, with whom do you have the most contact, locally?	Rarely have contact with people = 0, fellow villagers whose household registration is still in sending areas = 1, fellow villagers who are registered permanent residents in the local area = 2, and locals = 3; range from 0 to 3
3	I like the city I am living in presently	The answers "completely disagree," "disagree," "somewhat agree," and "completely agree," respectively assigned values 1, 2, 3, and 4
4	I pay attention to the changes in the city I am living in	
5	I am willing to blend in with the locals	
6	I think locals are willing to accept me	
7	I feel that locals despise outsiders	The answers "completely disagree," "disagree," "somewhat agree," and "completely agree," respectively assigned values 4, 3, 2, and 1
8	Compared to the sending area, do you feel happy now?	The answers "very happy," "happy," "so-so," "unhappy," and "very unhappy," respectively assigned values 5, 4, 3, 2, and 1

items that contributed more to Factor 1; we named these factors together the *level of participation*. The other six items demonstrated the feelings of migrants in the receiving areas and contributed more to Factor 2. We viewed this factor as a good proxy for will to integrate and named it accordingly as *will to integrate*. The Cronbach's alpha of the overall SSI factor was 0.71, with 0.54 for *level of participation* and 0.75 for *will to integrate*. In the factor analysis, the means and standard deviations of the original variables were standardized to 0 and 1, respectively; higher scores indicated better integration status.

Mobility during pregnancy was assessed by investigating mobility patterns and selection of delivery location. Mobility patterns were grouped into *always staying in the sending area* (AS), *mainly staying in the sending area* (MS), *mainly staying in the receiving area* (MR), and *always staying in the receiving area* (AR). Delivery locations included *receiving area* (RA) and *sending area* (SA).

Data analysis

Categorical variables were described using percentages and underwent a chi-squared test. Continuous variables were described using means and standard deviations and underwent an analysis of variance (ANOVA) with thresholds of $a = 0.05$ and $p < 0.05$. Logistic regression analysis demonstrated the influence of factors associated with mobility patterns and delivery location choice. Analyses were carried out using SPSS 13.0 (SPSS Inc., Chicago, IL).

Results

Retrospective analysis of 28,764 respondents' mobility during pregnancy with their first child and of their delivery location

As Fig. 1 indicates, for respondents expecting their first child, the rate of AS decreased and the rate of AR increased, while MS continually occupied a very low percentage, mostly less than 5%, and the rate of MR fluctuated while gradually increasing, only to decrease slightly after 2010. Meanwhile, it was found that the percentage of respondents who stayed in the receiving area (including AR and MR) increased from nearly 40% in 1985 to more than 80% in 2012. The percentage of migrants who were mobile during pregnancy (including MR and MS) fluctuated between 30 and 40% before 1995 and between 40 and 45% after 1995, decreasing to just under 40% after 2008.

As Fig. 2 indicates, the percentage of respondents choosing to deliver in receiving areas increased each year; in 1985, only 10% of pregnant women delivered in a receiving area, but by 2011, this number had reached more than 50%.

Respondents' mobility patterns during pregnancy and choice of delivery location, among 4176 respondents who bore children between June 2011 and may 2012

Table 2 indicates that among these 4176 respondents, two-thirds had an education level below junior high school and an average EC of more than 50%. Only a few people had their own housing and/or urban medical insurance. The vast majority were from rural sending areas with rural household registration, and more than half of the children were the first child. Cross-provincial migration was the type of migration engaged in by 70.4% of respondents, and the average migration time was 3.77 years. Families with older pregnant women (compared with younger), their own housing (compared with not), from urban *sending areas* (compared with rural ones), whose children were not the first child (compared with the first child), and who had a cross-district *migration range* (compared with cross-province and cross-city), a longer *migration time* (compared with shorter), and/or a higher

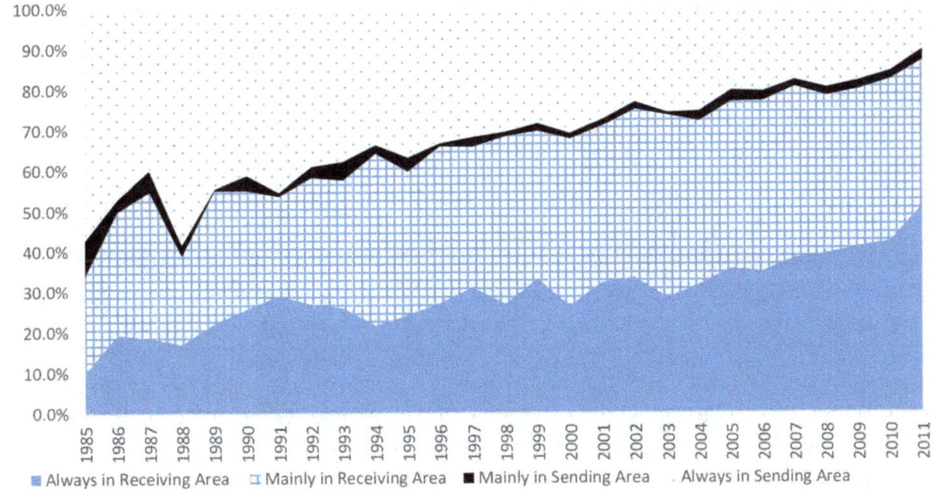

Fig. 1 Mobility patterns during pregnancy among migrants in China (1985–2011)

level of *participation* (compared with lower) had a higher rate of AR and a higher rate of delivery in the receiving area. Conversely, people with no *housing of their own* in the receiving area (compared with housing of their own), from rural *sending areas* (compared with urban areas), in their first *parity* (compared with not the first child), whose *migration range* was cross-city within the province or cross-province (compared with a merely cross-district migration range), having a moderate *migration time* (compared with shorter or longer), and with a moderate level of *participation* (compared with lower or higher) had a higher rate of mobility during pregnancy (including MR and MS).

As Table 3 indicates, *will to integrate* was the only consistently significant factor associated with staying in the receiving area during pregnancy, mobility during pregnancy, and choosing to deliver in the receiving area. Other factors were only significant in some models. Families with older *age of pregnant women* (OR = 1.09, 95% CI 1.05–1.13), having their *own housing* (OR = 5.66, 95% CI 2.45–13.05), with a longer *migration time* (OR = 1.14, 95% CI 1.09–1.20), and with a higher level of *will to integrate* (OR = 1.32, 95% CI 1.15–1.51) were more likely to stay in the receiving area rather than the sending area during pregnancy. Among the associated factors, having one's own housing had the greatest impact. Families with older

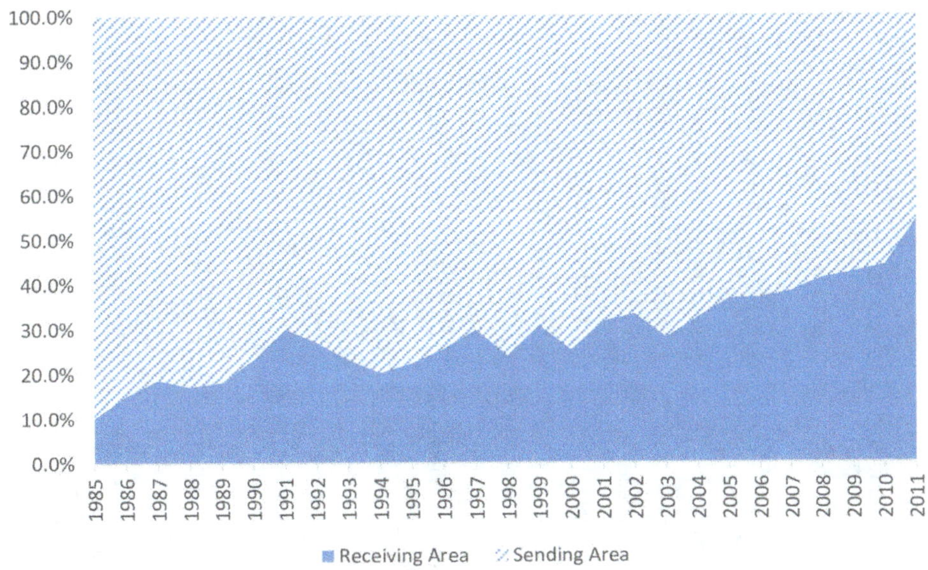

Fig. 2 Choices of delivery location among migrants in China (1985–2011)

Table 2 Characteristics of respondents; comparison of migrant mobility patterns during pregnancy and delivery locations (n (%), $m \pm SD$)

		Mobility patterns					Delivery locations			Total
		AS	MS	MR	AR	p	RA	SA	p	$N = 4176$
		$N = 305$	$N = 80$	$N = 1329$	$N = 2461$		$N = 2585$	$N = 1591$		
Age (years)		25.90 ± 4.10	26.82 ± 4.23	27.16 ± 4.39	27.90 ± 4.88	< 0.001	27.89 ± 4.82	26.87 ± 4.43	< 0.001	27.50 ± 4.70
Education Level	Junior high school and below	214(7.7)	59(2.1)	878(31.4)	1641(58.8)	0.22	1719(61.6)	1073(38.4)	0.45	2793(67.0)
	Senior high school and above	87(6.3)	21(1.5)	447(32.6)	817(59.5)		862(62.8)	511(37.2)		
Engel Coefficient		0.54 ± 0.19	0.60 ± 0.21	0.54 ± 0.19	0.55 ± 0.19	0.03	0.55 ± 0.19	0.54 ± 0.19	0.24	0.55 ± 0.19
Own housing in RA	Yes	7(1.5)	7(1.5)	70 (14.8)	388(82.2)	< 0.001	403(85.0)	71(15.0)	< 0.001	473(11.3)
	No	297(8.0)	73(2.0)	1258(34.0)	2073(56.0)		2182(58.9)	1521(41.1)		
Urban employee Insurance	Yes	66(6.9)	22(2.3)	296(31.1)	569(59.7)	0.66	597(62.6)	357(37.4)	0.62	954(22.8)
	No	239(7.4)	52(1.8)	1032(32.0)	1892(58.7)		1988(61.7)	1234(38.3)		
Rural household registration	Yes	251(7.5)	64(1.9)	1099(33.0)	1916(57.5)	0.002	2006(60.2)	1325(39.8)	< 0.001	3331(80.1)
	No	50(6.1)	16(1.9)	225(27.2)	535(64.8)		569(68.9)	257(31.1)		
First parity	Yes	202(8.1)	52(2.1)	815(32.7)	1424(57.1)	0.017	1500(60.2)	992(39.8)	0.012	2493(59.7)
	No	103(6.1)	28(1.7)	513(30.5)	1037(61.7)		1084(64.4)	599(35.6)		
Range of migration	Cross-province	214(7.4)	54(1.9)	890(30.9)	1720(59.8)	< 0.001	1819(63.2)	1059(36.8)	< 0.001	2878(70.4)
	Within province cross-city	60(6.6)	13(1.4)	343(37.8)	491(54.1)		508(56.0)	399(44.0)		907(22.2)
	Within city cross-district	16(5.2)	7(2.3)	67(21.9)	216(70.6)		227(74.4)	78(25.6)		
Migration time	(years)	2.33 ± 3.00	2.94 ± 3.40	3.39 ± 3.54	4.17 ± 3.94	< 0.001	0.08 ± 1.02	−0.12 ± 0.96	< 0.001	3.77 ± 3.79
Level of participation		−0.09 ± 0.91	−0.06 ± 0.94	−0.05 ± 0.97	0.04 ± 1.03	0.03	4.14 ± 3.91	3.16 ± 3.50	< 0.001	0.00 ± 1.00
Will to integrate		− 0.31 ± 0.96	0.23 ± 1.03	− 0.05 ± 0.97	0.06 ± 1.01	< 0.001	0.03 ± 1.02	−0.05 ± 0.96	0.02	0.00 ± 1.00

AS **always staying in the sending area,** ***MS*** **mainly staying in the sending area,** ***MR*** **mainly staying in the receiving area,** ***AR*** **always staying in the receiving area,** ***RA*** **receiving area,** ***SA*** **sending area**

Table 3 Logistic regression analysis of mobility patterns during pregnancy and delivery location choice

		Mobility pattern (AS = 0)						AR = 0		Delivery locations	
		MS		MR		AR		MR		(SA = 0)	
		OR	95% C.I.	OR	95% C.I.	OR	95% C.I.	OR	95% C.I.	OR	95% C.I.
Age (years)	continuous	1.05	0.98, 1.12	1.06**	1.02, 1.10	1.09**	1.05, 1.13	0.98**	0.96, 0.99	1.04**	1.02, 1.06
Educational years	continuous	0.94	0.72, 1.23	1.08	0.93, 1.24	1.01	0.88, 1.15	1.07	0.99, 1.15	0.96	0.90, 1.03
Engel Coefficient	continuous	8.31**	1.97, 35.01	1.23	0.62, 2.45	1.45	0.74, 2.83	0.84	0.58, 1.22	1.12	0.79, 1.59
Own housing in RA	NO = 0	2.96	0.91, 9.69	1.81	0.76, 4.29	5.66**	2.45, 13.05	0.32**	0.24, 0.43	3.47**	2.60, 4.64
Urban Employees Insurance	NO = 0	1.23	0.65, 2.33	0.84	0.60, 1.19	0.71*	0.55, 0.99	1.18	0.43, 1.98	0.79*	0.66, 0.94
Rural household registration	NO = 0	1.04	0.47, 2.28	1.29	0.86, 1.94	1.06	0.71, 1.56	1.21	0.97, 1.50	0.83	0.68, 1.03
The first parity	NO = 0	1.25	0.65, 2.40	1.03	0.74, 1.42	1.02	0.75, 1.40	1.00	0.85, 1.19	0.99	0.85, 1.17
Range of migration	Cross-province	0.99	0.36, 2.69	1.19	0.66, 2.13	0.83	0.48, 1.44	1.42*	1.05, 1.91	0.73*	0.55, 0.97
Cross-district = 0	Cross-city	0.70	0.23, 2.15	1.54	0.82, 2.89	0.70	0.39, 1.28	2.17**	1.05, 1.91	0.46**	0.34, 0.62
Migration time	continuous	1.05	0.96, 1.15	1.10**	1.05, 1.16	1.14**	1.09, 1.20	0.96**	0.94, 0.98	1.05**	1.03, 1.07
Level of participation	continuous	0.98	0.75, 1.28	1.01	0.88, 1.16	1.08	0.94, 1.24	0.93	0.87, 1.00	1.06	0.99, 1.14
Will to integrate	continuous	1.89**	1.43, 2.49	1.26**	1.10, 1.45	1.32**	1.15, 1.51	0.95	0.89, 1.03	1.14**	1.06, 1.21

AS always staying in the sending area, *MS* mainly staying in the sending area, *MR* mainly staying in the receiving area, *AR* always staying in the receiving area, *RA* receiving area, *SA* sending area

$*p < 0.05$, $**p < 0.01$

age of pregnant women (OR = 1.06, 95% CI 1.02–1.10), a longer *migration time* (OR = 1.10, 95% CI 1.05–1.16), and a higher level of *will to integrate* (OR = 1.26, 95% CI 1.10–1.45) were more likely to spend most of their time during pregnancy in the receiving area or to be mobile between the sending area and receiving area, instead of staying in the sending area all or most the time, and *will to integrate* had stronger impact on them than on other families. Similarly, families with their *own housing*, a smaller *range of migration*, a longer *migration time*, and a higher level of *will to integrate* more often chose to deliver in the receiving area instead of the sending area; however, having their own housing was still the factor that had the most impact.

Patterns of mobility during pregnancy and choice of delivery location were not statistically related to the *education level* of the pregnant woman, *rural residency*, *parity*, or level of *participation*.

Discussion

This study found that of 28,764 respondents who had their first child between 1985 and 2011, the percentage always or mainly staying in receiving areas during pregnancy (AR and MR) increased over the years, while the percentage mobility during pregnancy (MS and MR) first increased and then decreased. The percentage of respondents who chose to deliver in receiving areas increased, reaching more than 50% in 2011.

Among the 4176 respondents who gave birth in the last year of the survey, families with older *age of pregnant women*, longer *length of stay in the receiving area*, and a stronger *will to integrate* were more likely to be AR or MR than others, but not AS. Similarly, families with older *age of pregnant women*, their *own housing*, small *migration range*, longer *length of stay in the receiving area*, and a stronger *will to integrate* chose the receiving area instead of the sending area as their delivery place. *Owning housing* in RA remained the factor with the most impact throughout.

Studies from other countries have indicated that 10–30% of pregnant women from the general population will be mobile during pregnancy [1, 2, 11]. The present study focused on people who had already had migration experience in China and demonstrated that the percentage of pregnant women who were mobile has been between 30 and 45% over the past 30 years, higher than among the general population in most other countries. However, because different countries' backgrounds vary, the data are not appropriate for comparison. We speculate that in China, once women have migration experience, they prefer to be mobile during pregnancy in order to receive better family care or save on costs. Furthermore, we have little data from the Chinese general population, and our conclusion that the percentage of pregnant migrant women who are mobile is higher than that of pregnant women in general needs to be confirmed. Our results might surprise clinicians who had experience with a much higher mobility rate during pregnancy among migrants, and an environmental risks evaluation and prenatal examination reminders might be provided to the target population to provide better care.

Our results showed that migrant mobility patterns during pregnancy have been shifting from going back to sending areas once pregnant to staying in receiving areas for a longer time, even for the whole duration of the pregnancy. The rate of mobility during pregnancy (including MR and MS) began to fall in 2008, and the percentage of respondents choosing to deliver in receiving areas increased. Health care demands (such as antenatal and delivery care) decreased in sending areas but increased in receiving areas, since there were more and more pregnant migrants staying in receiving areas. As demonstrated in the last column in Table 2, rural residents accounted for 80.1%, and cross-provincial migration reached 70.4% of all respondents. Further analysis showed that 80.7% of cross-provincial migrants moved to eastern areas from central and western areas. In general, health resources quality and quantity are better in eastern China than in central and western areas (as is as economic level), as most health resources were allocated referring to the population distribution, especially to the household registration population, rather than all residents (household registration population and migrants) in China. More and more migrants inclining to give birth in receiving areas might bring challenges for health care provision, especially for overloaded hospitals in big cities. For example, according to 2012 health statistics, daily visits per doctor in China were 9.0, 5.6, and 6.7 for eastern, central, and western areas, respectively [34]. Gathering more information on the size and change trends of the population of pregnant migrant women is essential for policymakers and health care providers to make health care plans.

It has been shown that women who are young or who have fewer children, a lower level of education, lower household income, and do not own their own housing are more likely to be mobile during pregnancy [1, 8, 29]. The logistic regression analysis conducted in this study also confirmed that in internal migrant populations, young women without their own housing in RA are more likely to be mobile, similar to the findings of previous studies. The results should be used by clinicians to take note of pregnant women with these characteristics because of their higher possibility of mobility. In our results, though the mean differences in age were statistically significant, the value was between 25.90 and 27.90, thus with only limited clinical implications. In our analysis, contrary to the previous studies, it was also found that the education level of pregnant women and whether they were having their first child were not statistically significant. Furthermore, based on EC results, poor families are more likely to be mobile instead of staying in the sending area during pregnancy. Urban employee medical insurance is one of the three types of medical insurance the Chinese government provides for employees; having this insurance indicates that the family is of a high SES. This study showed that people with this insurance in RA were more likely to stay in their hometown or deliver in their hometown; this result did not match our expectation and needs further analysis.

In migrant populations, SSI's impact on health and health behaviors has been demonstrated [35–37]. However, the definitions of SSI used by these studies have not been uniform. Different studies have evaluated social integration in terms of language, economic characteristics, activity participation, inflow time, housing situation, and other indicators [24, 38, 39]. The present study measured SSI in two dimensions from a factor analysis of eight questions and found that a stronger *will to integrate* had a significant positive impact on mobility during pregnancy and delivery in receiving areas, while *level of participation* did not show a significant impact. Since 2000, the Chinese government has been trying to promote social integration and decrease social exclusion for migrants by providing them more social welfare, insurance, and a generally migrant-friendly environment in the receiving areas. With resulting social integration, we expect an increase in pregnant migrants staying in receiving areas for most of their pregnancy period and giving birth there.

The World Health Organization believes it is necessary to make public health service delivery more migrant-friendly [40], and the right to health care for internal migrants has been raised in many developing countries [41, 42]. In 2012, the number of domestic migrants in China was approximately 236 million [25]. Pregnant migrant women's health, which relates to the health of two generations, should thus be a focus of attention; however, there is still a gap between health care provision for pregnant migrants and those for local household–registered populations, as well as in health care utilization between them [43, 44]. Given this background, the results of this study should remind maternal health service providers to pay more attention to the increasing number of pregnant migrant women spending most of their pregnancy and/or giving birth in receiving areas. Maternal health resources should be allocated with consideration to the size and shifting trends in this population, especially for those who are inclined to stay in receiving areas during most or all of their pregnancy and those who choose receiving areas as delivery locations (who are in general also those who have their own housing, those migrating on only a small scale, those with longer migration time, and those with a strong will to integrate), since more attention has been paid to the size and demands of the household registered population to date [43, 44] . For younger women without their *own housing*, with a cross-province or cross-city *migration range*, and who have high mobility during pregnancy (MR and MS), the integrity and continuity of medical records between sending and receiving areas need to be improved (remembering that medical record systems are a general challenge for the efficiency of health care in many developing countries [45, 46]).

This study has some limitations that should be reflected here. First, the power of cause–effect relationships in a cross-sectional study is low. Our study could not securely demonstrate causal effects but does give clues as to the characteristics of migrant women with high mobility during pregnancy. Second, the study may have some selection bias. The sample is from a migrant population in 2012, based on which we reviewed the trends of the migrants' mobility during the pregnancy and delivery locations of their first child between 1985 and 2011. Families that migrated in the early years but returned to their registered household in recent years were not included in the sampling frame. The lack of these families' information may cause bias.

This study analyzed mobility patterns during pregnancy as well as selection of delivery locations among migrants in China using cross-sectional data for a large population. To the best of our knowledge, this is the first study to describe the changing patterns of mobility during pregnancy based on representative large-scale national population data from China. Moreover, the study focused on internally migrating pregnant women who may face higher risks of adverse pregnancy outcomes due to less health care utilization in the perinatal period. As we know, without prenatal examinations, a pregnant woman's conditions such as hypertension, hyperglycemia, and some infectious diseases cannot be diagnosed, not to mention treated in time, and fetus position and health status cannot be assessed. The present study described the scale, characteristics, and change trends of the population in China, which can provide a reference for maternal health service providers in developing countries.

Conclusions

Our research indicated that the percentage of migrants always or mainly staying in receiving areas during pregnancy rose steadily between 1985 and 2011 in China. The percentage of migrants who were mobile during pregnancy increased and then decreased, while the percentage of respondents who chose to deliver in receiving areas increased. Individual and family characteristics, including age, owning housing, rural/urban sending areas, migration range, migration time, and will to integrate were extensively associated with mobility patterns and delivery location choice. Maternal health care providers might consider the size and change trends of this population.

Abbreviations

AR: Always staying in the receiving area; AS: Always staying in the sending area; EC: Engel coefficient; MR: Mainly staying in the receiving area; MS: Mainly staying in the sending area; RA: Receiving area; SA: Sending area; SES: Socio-economic status; SSI: Status of social integration

Acknowledgments

We thank the Department of Family Planning Service and Management for Migrants, National Health and Family Planning Commission of the People's Republic of China, for their support in providing access to the database (2012 Migrant Dynamics Monitoring Survey in China) used in the study.

Authors' contributions

YJ had primary responsibility for the conception of the analysis and preparation of the manuscript; XZ drafted the manuscript and incorporated critical revisions; ZW assisted with data cleaning and analysis; SL and YS contributed to the interpretation of the results and revised successive versions of the article; CC was responsible for oversight and interpretation of the data and critical revisions of the manuscript. All authors contributed to the interpretations of results, revised the manuscript critically for intellectual content, and approved the final manuscript.

Competing interests

The authors declare that they have no competing interests.

Author details

[1]Department of Social Medicine and Health Education, School of Public Health, Peking University, Beijing, China. [2]Service Center for Immigrant of National Health and Family Planning Commission of China, Beijing, China. [3]China Population and Development Research Center, Beijing, China.

References

1. Hodgson S, Shirley M, Bythell M, Rankin J. Residential mobility during pregnancy in the north of England. BMC Pregnancy Childbirth. 2009;9:52.
2. Bell ML, Belanger K. Review of research on residential mobility during pregnancy: consequences for assessment of prenatal environmental exposures. J Expo Sci Environ Epidemiol. 2012;22:429–38.
3. Jones RC, Hughes CR, Wright D, Baumer JH. Early house moves, indoor air, heating methods and asthma. Respir Med. 1999;93:919–22.
4. Briggs DJ. Exposure assessment. In: Elliott P, Wakefield J, Best NG, Briggs D, editors. Spatial epidemiology. Oxford: Oxford University Press; 2000. p. 335–59.
5. Dolk H, Vrijheid M. The impact of environmental pollution on congenital anomalies. Br Med Bull. 2003;68:25–45.
6. Barros H, Tavares M, Rodrigues T. Role of prenatal care in preterm birth and low birthweight in Portugal. J Public Health Med. 1996;18:321–8.
7. Boerleider AW, Wiegers TA, Mannien J, Francke AL, Deville WL. Factors affecting the use of prenatal care by non-western women in industrialized western countries: a systematic review. BMC Pregnancy Childbirth. 2013;13:81.
8. Tunstall H, Pickett K, Johnsen S. Residential mobility in the UK during pregnancy and infancy: are pregnant women, new mothers and infants 'unhealthy migrants'? Soc Sci Med. 2010;71:786–98.
9. Kirby JB, Kaneda T. Access to health care: does neighborhood residential instability matter? J Health Soc Behav. 2006;47:142–55.
10. Duchon LM, Weitzman BC, Shinn M. The relationship of residential instability to medical care utilization among poor mothers in new York City. Med Care. 1999;37:1282–93.
11. Fell DB, Dodds L, King WD. Residential mobility during pregnancy. Paediatr Perinat Epidemiol. 2004;18:408–14.
12. Heaman MI, Newburn-Cook CV, Green CG, Elliott LJ, Helewa ME. Inadequate prenatal care and its association with adverse pregnancy outcomes: a comparison of indices. BMC Pregnancy Childbirth. 2008;8:15.
13. Petrou S, Kupek E, Vause S, Maresh M. Antenatal visits and adverse perinatal outcomes: results from a British population-based study. Eur J Obstet Gynecol Reprod Biol. 2003;106:40–9.
14. Reime B, Lindwedel U, Ertl KM, Jacob C, Schucking B, Wenzlaff P. Does underutilization of prenatal care explain the excess risk for stillbirth among women with migration background in Germany? Acta Obstet Gynecol Scand. 2009;88(11):1276–83.
15. Sherraden MS, Barrera RE. Prenatal care experiences and birth weight among Mexican immigrant women. J Med Syst. 1996;20(5):329–50.
16. Oropesa RS, Landale NS, Inkley M, Gorman BK. Prenatal care among Puerto Ricans on the United States mainland. SocSci Med. 2000;51(12):1723–39.
17. Blondel B, Marshall B. Poor antenatal care in 20 French districts: risk factors and pregnancy outcome. J Epidemiol Community Health. 1998;52(8):501–6.
18. Kusuma YS, Kumari R, Kaushal S. Migration and access to maternal healthcare: determinants of adequate antenatal care and institutional delivery among socio-economically disadvantaged migrants in Delhi, India. Trop Med Int Health. 2013;18(10):1202–10.
19. Li Y. Understanding health constraints among rural-to-urban migrants in China. Qual Health Res. 2013;23(11):1459–69.
20. Gawde NC, Sivakami M, Babu BV. Utilization of maternal health services among internal migrants in Mumbai. India J Biosoc Sci. 2016;48(6):767–96.
21. Chan KW. The household registration system and migrant labor in China: notes on a debate. Popul Dev Rev. 2010;36(2):357–64.
22. Goodburn C. Learning from migrant education: a case study of the schooling of rural migrant children in Beijing. Int J Edu Dev. 2009;29(5):495–504.
23. Islam MM, Gagnon AJ. Use of reproductive health care services among urban migrant women in Bangladesh. BMC Womens Health. 2016;16:15.
24. Ford K, Chamratrithirong A, Apipornchaisakul K, Panichapak P, Pinyosinwat T. Social integration, AIDS knowledge and factors related to HIV prevention among migrant workers in Thailand. AIDS Behav. 2014;18:390–7.
25. National Population and Family Planning Commission of China. 2013 report on China's migrant population development. Beijing: Population Publishing House; 2013.
26. Heaman M, Bayrampour H, Kingston D, Blondel B, Gissler M, Roth C, et al. Migrant women's utilization of prenatal care: a systematic review. Matern Child Health J. 2013;17:816–36.
27. Shaokang Z, Zhenwei S, Blas E. Economic transition and maternal health care for internal migrants in shanghai, China. Health Policy Plan. 2002;17(Suppl):47–55.
28. World Health Organization. The 61st world health assembly. Health of migrants. WHA61.17. 2008.
29. Saadeh FB, Clark MA, Rogers ML, Linkletter CD, Phipps MG, Padbury JF, et al. Pregnant and moving: understanding residential mobility during pregnancy and in the first year of life using a prospective birth cohort. Matern Child Health J. 2013;17:330–43.
30. Hodgson S, Lurz PW, Shirley MD, Bythell M, Rankin J. Exposure misclassification due to residential mobility during pregnancy. Int J Hyg Environ Health. 2015;218:414–21.
31. National Population and Family Planning Commission. Handbook of dynamic monitoring on migrants in China (2012). Beijing: National Population and Family Planning Commission; 2012.
32. Uchino S. Regional analysis of fertility changes. Jinko Mondai Kenkyu. 1979;151:37–41.
33. Chen TJ, Modin B, Ji CY, Hjern A. Regional, socioeconomic and urban-rural disparities in child and adolescent obesity in China: a multilevel analysis. Acta Paediatr. 2011;100(12):1583–9.
34. National Population and Family Planning Commission of China. Health Statistics Annuals 2013. http://www.nhfpc.gov.cn/htmlfiles/zwgkzt/ptjnj/year2013/index2013.html. Accessed 21 Oct 2017.
35. Bail KM, Foster J, Dalmida SG, Kelly U, Howett M, Ferranti EP, et al. The impact of invisibility on the health of migrant farmworkers in the southeastern United States: a case study from Georgia. Nurs Res Pract. 2012; https://doi.org/10.1155/2012/760418.
36. Tarricone I, Atti AR, Salvatori F, Braca M, Ferrari S, Malmusi D, et al. Psychotic

symptoms and general health in a socially disadvantaged migrant community in bologna. Int J Soc Psychiatry. 2009;55:203–13.
37. Umberson D. Family status and health behaviors: social control as a dimension of social integration. J Health Soc Behav. 1987;28:306–19.
38. Garcia-Ramirez M, de la Mata ML, Paloma V, Hernandez-Plaza S. A liberation psychology approach to acculturative integration of migrant populations. Am J Community Psychol. 2011;47:86–97.
39. Schmiedebach HP, Beddies T, Schulz J, Priebe S. Housing and work as criteria of the "social integration" of the mentally ill - development in Germany between 1900 and 2000. Psychiatr Prax. 2002;29:285–94.
40. Ghent A. Overcoming migrants' barriers to health. Bull World Health Organ. 2008;86:583–4.
41. Akinola AB, Krishna AK, Chetlapalli SK. Health equity for internal migrant labourers in India: an ethical perspective. Indian J Med Ethics. 2014;11(4):232–7.
42. Mirkuzie AH. Exploring inequities in skilled care at birth among migrant population in a metropolitan city Addis Ababa, Ethiopia; a qualitative study. Int J Equity Health. 2014;13:110.
43. Cheung NF, Pan A. Childbirth experience of migrants in China: a systematic review. Nurs Health Sci. 2012;14:362–71.
44. You X, Tan H, Hu S, Wu J, Jiang H, Peng A, et al. Effects of preconception counseling on maternal health care of migrant women in China: a community-based, cross-sectional survey. BMC Pregnancy Childbirth. 2015;15:55.
45. Watkinson-Powell A, Lee A. Benefits of an electronic medical records system in rural Nepal. J Nepal Med Assoc. 2012;52(188):196–200.
46. Osaki K, Hattori T, Kosen S. The role of home-based records in the establishment of a continuum of care for mothers, newborns, and children in Indonesia. Glob Health Action. 2013;6:1–12.

11

Understanding the consumption of folic acid during preconception, among Pakistani, Bangladeshi and white British mothers in Luton, UK

Rebecca Garcia[1*], Nasreen Ali[2], Malcolm Griffiths[3] and Gurch Randhawa[2]

Abstract

Background: To review the similarities and differences in Pakistani, Bangladeshi and White British mothers health beliefs (attitudes, knowledge and perceptions) and health behaviour regarding their consumption of folic acid pre-conception, to reduce the risk of neural tube defects.

Methods: Our study used a descriptive qualitative research approach, implementing face-to-face focus group discussions with Pakistani, Bangladeshi or White British mothers (normal birth outcomes and mothers with poor birth outcomes) and semi-structured interviews or focus groups with service providers using semi-structured topic guides. This method is well suited for under researched areas where in-depth information is sought.
There were three sample groups:

1. Pakistani, Bangladeshi and White British mothers with normal birth outcomes (delivery after 37 weeks of gestation, in the preceding 6 to 24 months, weighing 2500 g and living within a specified postcode area in Luton, UK).
2. Pakistani Bangladeshi and white British bereaved mothers who had suffered a perinatal mortality (preceding 6 to 24 months, residing within a specificied postcode area).
3. Healthcare professionals working on the local maternity care pathway (i.e. services providing preconception, antenatal, antepartum and postpartum care).

Transcribed discussions were analysed using the Framework Analysis approach.

Results: The majority of mothers in this sample did not understand the benefits or optimal time to take folic acid pre-conception. Conversely, healthcare professionals believed the majority of women did consume folic acid, prior to conception.

Conclusions: There is a need to increase public health awareness of the optimal time and subsequent benefits for taking folic acid, to prevent neural tube defects.

Keywords: Folic acid, Neural tube defects, South Asian, Pakistani, Indian Bangladeshi white British

* Correspondence: Rebecca.Garcia@beds.ac.uk
[1]The School of Healthcare Practice, University of Bedfordshire, Putteridge Bury, Hitchin Road, Luton, Luton LU2 8LE, England
Full list of author information is available at the end of the article

Background

Folic acid consumption pre-conception is necessary for optimal embryogenesis [1, 2]; the benefits are well documented and include reducing the incidence of neural tube defect (NTD) [3–7] in addition to other structural congenital anomalies [8]. NTD are a significant congenital anomaly which account for the second leading cause of infant mortality and also results in high rates of morbidity [9]. Current guidance in the United Kingdom (UK) idenitifies certain women at higher risk of having an infant with NTDs; for instance, a family history of NTD, medical conditions such as diabetes, or thalassemia or women identified with a body mass index (BMI) of > 30 kg/m^2 [10].

Public health surveillance has shown that there is an increasing prevalence of NTD [2], while trends for consumption of folic acid have decreased [11, 12]. Estimates of consumption rates range from 10.4–35% of pregnancies, with estimates for South Asian women (i.e. Indian, Pakistani, Bangladeshi or Sri Lankan) are even lower (20%) [11, 13, 14]. Figures have also shown there is an ethnic variation to the incidence of congenital anomalies; the leading cause of death in South Asian infants death being congenital anomalies, however in White infants it related to fetal maturity [15]. Furthermore, it has been estimated that only half of all pregnancies are actually planned [16], suggesting that increasing trends of NTD and high numbers of unplanned pregnancies indicate that many women have poor health literacy on the benefits of folic acid consumption before pregnancy occurs. In the U.K., folic acid may be prescribed at a higher dose (5 mg) by General Practitioners under certain circumstances (e.g. risk or previous history of NTD, consumption of anti-epilepsy medication, history of coeliac, diabetes mellitus, sickle cell anaemia or thalassemia, or obesity, [10]), alternatively women can readily purchase folic acid supplements (400mcg) from pharmacies.

Maternal attitudes, knowledge and perceptions have been found to be more indicative of birth outcome than deprivation [17], with a recent study providing evidence demonstrative of various barriers to consuming folic acid, including poor knowledge, unplanned pregnancy and poor memory as a result of leading complex lives [18]. Moreover, inadvertent disadvantage may occur with (some) mothers, as a consequence of lower educational attainment, reduced health literacy, language barriers, in addition to pre-existing assumptions made by healthcare staff and services that the homogenous maternity population properly understands the benefits and timing of consuming folic acid, prior to conception [19, 20].

There is a dearth of evidence exploring similarities and differences in Pakistani, Bangladeshi and White British women's attitudes, knowledge and perceptions of the association between folic acid consumption and reducing the risk of NTD, in addition to understanding healthcare professionals views [19]. This study addresses this gap; seeking to identify similarity and differences between the participant groups, to further understand this modifiable problem.

Methods

Aim

To review the similarities and differences in Pakistani, Bangladeshi and White British mothers health beliefs (attitudes, knowledge and perceptions) and health behaviour regarding their consumption of folic acid pre-conception, to reduce the risk of neural tube defects.

Design

Our study used a descriptive qualitative research approach, implementing face-to-face focus group discussions with Pakistani, Bangladeshi or White British mothers (normal birth outcomes and mothers with poor birth outcomes) and semi-structured interviews or focus groups with service providers using semi-structured topic guides. This method is well suited for under researched areas where in-depth information is sought [21].

The findings in this paper form part of a larger mixed-methods study, which sought to identify similarities and differences in health beliefs and health behaviours of Pakistani, Bangladeshi and White British women, and how these contributed to perinatal mortality. The results and findings are published elsewhere [22, 23]. This paper concentrates reports on the findings of womens' attitudes and experiences in using folic acid in the preconception period.

Setting

Purposive sampling from Pakistani, Bangladeshi or White British mothers who had a normal birth outcome were recruited from local Children's Centres to participate in focus group discussions [24]. They were eligible to take part if they had delivered a live-born baby after 37 weeks of gestation, in the preceding 6 to 24 months, weighing 2500 g and resided within a specified postcode area. Luton is a town with high rates of deprivation [25]. RG and NA held discussions with Children's Centre managers and representatives from the local Luton community requested non-English speaking mothers were included in the study, as it was believed that non-English speaking mothers maternity experiences is disadvantaged; Therefore women were eligible to take part even if they did not speak English. Exclusions included women who had delivered infants before 37 weeks of gestation, outside the date range, who did not reside within the specified postcode area and his baby was under 2500 g, women from other ethnic groups and presence of gynaecological cancer or women who conceived through assistive reproduction techniques [26].

Recruitment methods included face-to-face invitation, poster advert and snowballing. The focus groups took place in community centres and church halls, in the proximity of the children centres from where they were recruited.

The second sample consisted of Pakistani Bangladeshi and white British bereaved mothers, who were invited to participate in semi-structured face-to-face interviews. These included women who had suffered a perinatal mortality in the preceding 6 to 24 months, his baby was either delivered stillborn or was classified as a neonatal death (0–7 days), residing within a specific postcode area. Women were eligible to participate if they did not speak English. Exclusions were women whose infant death occurred outside the preceding 6–24 months range specified; they failed to reside in the postcode area stated, women from other ethnic groups and presence of gynaecological cancer or women who conceived through assistive reproduction techniques [26]. The recruitment method used a gatekeeper (senior midwife) at the Luton and Dunstable University Hospital NHS Foundation Trust, to protect patient confidentiality and minimise distress [27]. The hospital sent potential participants a recruitment pack with a reply paid opt-in or opt-out contact sheet. Non-English speaking women were also invited using translators, who informed them about the studys' purpose. The bereaved mothers were given the choice of the venue before the interview as their own home, a room in the community centre or a room at the University.

The third sample consisted of healthcare professionals (midwives ($n = 2$), community midwives ($n = 14$), key workers ($n = 4$), student midwives ($n = 2$), practice nurses ($n = 1$), GP ($n = 1$), and Health Visitors ($n = 1$) who were working on the local maternity care pathway (i.e. services providing preconception, antenatal, antepartum and postpartum care) were invited by poster, verbal invitation or letter to take part in focus groups or semi-structured interviews. The interviews for focus groups were held in staff offices or training rooms.

Recruitment took place between December 2014 and March 2016. Before commencement of any focus groups or interviews, participants were provided written information sheet detailing the purpose and aims of the research (including dissemination of results), and were encouraged to discuss any queries regarding participation in this study, prior to providing informed and signed consent. and. RG (who is a female, mature, research student and registered nurse who undertook NHS' '*Good Clinial Practice*' training as a condition of the ethic approval for this study) conducted the majority of the interviews or focus groups. Prior to the FG/interview, RG did not know the participants and had only met (some) of them during initial face to face recruitment and to respond to any enquires regarding taking part in the research. Two groups were held in Urdu and these were conducted by RM (with RG present) and two were conducted in Slyheti conducted by RS, (with RG present). The Focus groups or interviews were audio recorded and lasted between 62 and 132 min. Recruitment ceased when data saturation occurred and no new themes emerged from the transcripts [28].

Ethics approval was provided by University of Bedfordshire Institute for Health Research, (IHRREC442, November 2014) and NHS ethics committee (15/EE/0181: 157751, June 2015). Funding - The Steel Trust has provided funding to the University of Bedfordshire for RG to undertake research at Institute for Health Research, University of Bedfordshire, under the direction of NA and GR. The funders have no involvement in the research or publication.

Materials

The topic guides for the focus groups and semi-structured interviews were developed in the same way for each participant group and were informed through a review of the existing literature and by the research aim (see Additional files 1 and 2 for copies of the topic guides). Each one built on existing themes in the literature that could be utilised flexibly during the focus group, interview and analysis stage, with probes that were grounded within the current evidence base. Several iterations were produced and piloted, prior to the final drafts. Piloting is a valuable method to ascertain whether the interview or focus group tool constrains participants and facilitates discussions on the intended topics [29]. The main themes of the topic guides are shown in Table 1.

A bio-questionnaire was utilised with mothers who had a normal birth outcome and healthcare professionals to record demographic data, while bereaved mothers were asked these questions on commencement of the recorded interview, forming part of the rapport building.

Data analysis

The demographic data from the bio-questionnaires and interview transcripts for all participant groups (normal birth outcome, bereaved mothers and healthcare professionals) was entered into Microsoft Excel to determine participant characteristics. RG produced verbatim transcripts for the English speaking focus groups or interviews; however, for the Urdu and Slyheti focus groups or interviews a university approved translator translated. Also, a second translator back-translated to ensure consistency of transliteration [30, 31]. NA reviewed the codes, themes and sub-themes until consistency was achieved between RG and NA. Additionally, four transcripts were presented back to participants for further verification of the accuracy of the transcript, ensuring trustworthiness was achieved [31–33]. Framework

Table 1 Main themes for each topic guide, by participant group

Mothers with a normal birth outcome	Bereaved mothers	Healthcare professionals
Perceptions of pregnancy	Rapport building	Information about maternity services
Knowledge and information	Mothers story, background and context	Using maternity services
Views on low birthweight, still birth and infant mortality	Mothers experience of maternity services and healthcare professionals	Providing services to diverse ethnic groups
Experiences of current services and maternity healthcare professionals	Knowledge and information	Views on high-risk pregnancies
Service improvements	Views on stillbirth	Service improvements
	Service improvements	

analysis is considered an appropriate method of analysing large amounts of qualitative data consequently is efficient in dealing with large amounts of data and contributes to the reliability and trustworthiness of the findings [29, 34]. RG and NA read the transcripts many times to become submerged and familiar with the narrative, this then allowed emergent themes to become evident, in addition to pre-existing themes from the topic guide. Next, the data was indexed and charted, using Microsoft Excel [35], which allowed the data to be organised and interpreted [34, 36].

Results

The characterisitcs of the focus groups and interviews are shown in Table 2. The interviews with the six bereaved mothers were all conducted in participants' homes. All the bereaved mothers had experienced a stillbirth and five out of six bereaved mothers were born and grew up in the UK, while the remaining Pakistani mother had been settled in the UK for 15 years. None of the mothers (normal birth outcome or bereaved) had smoked or consumed alcohol during their pregnancy. A number of themes and subthemes emerged from the narrative, which is organised by 'mothers' (i.e. normal birth outcome and bereaved mothers) and 'healthcare professionals'.

Findings from mothers

Limited knowledge on risk factors associated with adverse outcomes

The mothers discussed their limited knowledge of pregnancy and understanding of risks associated with causes of infant death. While the consumption of folic acid during pregnancy emerged from the narrative of all focus groups, it was evident that very few mothers were aware of the importance of taking folic acid before conception. This is seen in the following narratives;

> Well you hear in the media that taking folic acid, that is not just the first 12 weeks but they recommend that you take it 3 months prior to conception, as well - so if you are planning, so I had been taking folic acid for 12 months before falling pregnant this time (White British mother).

> Vitamins, folic acid they say is very important - important for the baby's mental development. Before conceiving and after, we should continue taking it, as the mother's and baby's body becomes stronger (Bangladeshi mother).

> When I went to the doctors, they told me that when I was trying... To take folic acid so I did throughout my pregnancy (Bangladeshi mother).

Conversely, the majority of mothers explained that they only commenced taking folic acid after receiving explicit advice from their GP or midwife, during their first appointment with the health professional.

> You find out, as soon as you register yourself really, that is when they prescribe it [folic acid] when you take it is the first three months isn't it? (Bangladeshi mother).

> I started taking it [folic acid] as soon as I found out I was pregnant. I spoke to the midwife, and they gave me like a prescription to go and get erm, folic acid (White British mother).

The narratives revealed that mothers, regardless of their ethnicity were uncertain about the benefits of taking folic acid during the antenatal period. Discussions centred on ideas that pregnant women should not be taking 'medication' during pregnancy, or whether the folic acid was 'pure' enough for pregnant women. These ideas are evident in the following narratives:

> I was a bit scared taking folic acid tablets and all the tablets for pregnancy; I was a bit scared of that, just in case like, I dunno, like there are all these scary (White British mother).

> I think, psychologically I can't take any medication when I'm pregnant I just feel it is better for the baby (White British mother).

Table 2 Focus group or interview participant characterisitcs

Stratification	Focus group/ interview	Participants (N)	Lanugage of FG/interview	Ethicity	Duration of FG/interview	Lowest education level	Highest education level	Age range
Mothers with normal birth outcome	FG1	5	English	WB	70	GCSE	NVQ – level 2	23–42
	FG2	5	English	WB	69	GCSE	A Level	25–40
	FG3	4	English	Pakistani	84	NVQ level 2	Masters	28–38
	FG4	6	English	Pakistani	134	BSc	MBA	27–40
	FG5	4	English	Bangladeshi	73	BSc	MSc	24–39
	FG6	3	English	Pakistani	88	A level	MSc	32–41
	FG7	4	Slyheti	Bangladeshi	81	GCSE	BSc	26–32
	FG8	8	Slyheti	Bangladeshi	64	GCSE	BA (hons)	26–42
	FG9	7	Urdu	Pakistani	62	Year 8	MPA	23–49
Bereaved mothers	B1	1	English	WB	135		B-Tec	
	B2	1	English	Pakisani	49		A level	
	B3	1	English	Pakistani	32		GCSE	
	B4	1	English	Pakistani	40		A level	
	B5	1	English	WB	124		A level	
	B6	1	English	Bangladeshi	102		B-Tec	
	Focus group/ interview	Participants (N)	Staff role	Ethnicty				
Health care professionals	FG1	2	Hospital Midwives	WB				
	FG2	10	Community midwives	WB				
	FG3	9	Community midwives,	WB, Pakistani				
	Interview 1	1	Health visitor	WB				
	Interview 2	1	Practice Nurse	Black African				
	Interview 3	1	GP	Pakistani				

> The other thing with science, my sister-in-law is expecting, and my brother-in-law is really into his science stuff, and he doesn't agree with folic acid because he says it's not pure enough he said it's got folate or something, or something else which I don't know about, anyway but that is the thing, it depends on how deeply you go into things and you always find alternatives and things that are better but you have to read up on it don't you? (Pakistani mother).

Mothers' awareness of genetic risk factors

The mothers discussed their understanding of genetic influences and risks of congenital anomalies on adverse birth outcomes. Pakistani, Bangladeshi and WB participants spoke specifically about how they believed Downs Syndrome was heritable, although they did not discuss NTD, or any extra chromosomes. The following extracts show this;

> It's [Downs Syndrome] in your genes as well, isn't it? (Pakistani mother).

> I have got, like.... Back in Bangladesh, like quite a few members of my family are disabled and they have Down syndrome, and all of that, so you do... You do think it could become passed down (Bangladeshi mother).

Interestingly, adverse risks associated with genetic factors was discussed by two Pakistani mothers, but was in relation to consanguineous marriage and not folic acid. This is evident from the following narrative;

> Lots of people saying that [cousin marriage increases risk of genetic problems] to be honest, but we are cousin married as well (Pakistani mother).

> I think they [cousins] have more genetic problems, don't they? (Pakistani mother).

Barriers to consuming folic acid

The mothers' narrative revealed several barriers to preconception consumption of folic acid. Several mothers explained the reasons why they did not consider taking folic acid at all, which included a lack of information;

> It [folic acid] is not something that example a 16-year-old would even think about; I don't think there's that much information out there (Pakistani mother).

In addition, the mothers demonstrated misunderstandings of the causes of adverse birth outcomes and they showed limited understanding of the benefit of folic acid supplementation;

> Because my mum took folic acid and she lost her baby so you can't really say can you? Do you know I mean? There is people that take it and they have problems (White British mother).

> No, I mean I could get the vouchers for it [folic acid] because I get the appropriate benefits, but I just never, I didn't really know how to do it or how to apply for it. So I just didn't bother it seemed pointless (White British mother).

This is seen in the following;

> For me I didn't know [I was pregnant], I had a fall, went to the hospital. They asked me if I was pregnant I said I don't know if I had missed my periods... I said I don't know. They checked – I was pregnant! My mum had figured it out by me being reluctant to eat certain foods. I was happy but felt embarrassed too (Bangladeshi mother).

One mother described consuming Marmite as an alternative to tablets when she forgot her tablet;

> My step-dad was looking up on the Marmite, and you know that it said folic acid on there and erm, so I was a bit scared...so then I was taking it, and then if I forgot to take a tablet, I'd have a bit of marmite. (White British mother).

Findings from healthcare professionals

Staff perceptions of mothers awareness of risk factors for NTD The analysis revealed that there were conflicting opinions between healthcare professionals whether local mothers actually consumed folic acid *before* conception; some participants did not think the mothers did, as seen in the following:

> It's interesting because not lots of them take the folic acid, though ...(White British).

> Preconceptually? – no [folic acid] ... (White British mother).

Conversely, other healthcare professionals believed that the majority of pregnant women did consume folic acid, prior to conception:

> Yes, most people have [taken folic acid] (White British mother).

> I think that they do, [take folic acid] – I mean from the diabetic perspective I am aware that we need to prescribe it because they are meant to have a high dose of folic acid ... I think that that awareness is there (Practice Nurse, White British).

It was evident that health care professionals were aware of the confusion some mothers experience in respect of consuming folic acid in the early weeks. This is seen in the following extract;

> ...but the folic acid they have that in the first few weeks, most of the time they would have had it before we go in, but when I'm doing my assessment. I go through that, I say, 'have you had you folic acid?' some of them don't remember what they've had, they having their pregnancy vitamin (HV1).

Using maternity services

Furthermore, the Practice Nurse reported that she believed local South Asian women had a good understanding of preconception care, because of delivering a previous baby;

> I think that is quite likely, [taking folic acid] because ...I think that a lot of the Asian ladies that we see it is not always the first child or they are not necessarily first generation Asian that are over here so basically they are British Asian as they were born here... so therefore the Asians may have a good concept of the services that are provided by the NHS (Practice Nurse, White British).

The community midwives explained that eligible mothers could receive vitamin and folic acid supplements; this is seen in the following;

> No not everyone. Just the healthy start. They get the vitamin C and folic acid - is all in the healthy start (MW).

Discussion

Main findings

The majority of the findings in the study identified similarities in the mothers' understanding of the benefits of folic acid consumption, irrespective of the mothers' ethnicity or birth outcome. This study identified that very few women consumed folic acid before conception, nor did they understand the benefits of consumption, which would otherwise prevent congenital anomalies, including NTD in the early weeks of meiosis [16]. Moreover, only a few mothers described alternate sources of folic acid through alternate foods, such as leafy vegetables, which is commensurate with the findings of Yeasmin and Regmi [37].

Conversely, this study found that the majority of healthcare staff believed most women did commence folic acid consumption prior to conception, showing an important mismatch between women's actual health behaviour in consuming folic acid, contrasted with health professionals perception of women's health behaviour and subsequent understanding regarding pregnant women's risk reduction for NTD. Importantly, this study also highlights that the majority of women consider Downs Syndrome (specifically) when discussing genetic factors, and fail to mention risks associated with NTD (e.g. spina bifida), suggesting a poor understanding of genetic factors and a need for increased public health awareness.

The common explanation for higher rates of congenital anomalies in Pakistani infants is consanguinity [38–40]. Interestingly, this study did highlight that Pakistani mothers associated congenital anomalies with consanguineous unions, as opposed to other known risk factors for congenital anomalies such as poor nutrient intake [41, 42], (including folic acid), diabetes and obesity [43–45]. Moreover, consanguinity contributes to autosomal recessive disorders, whereas NTDs are related to suboptimal folic acid consumption, although few studies make this distinction, which may obscure the precise aetiology behind congenital anomalies [46].

Current estimates suggest less than a third of women consume folic acid prior to conception [11, 13, 14], and the last decade has shown a trend in declining figures of consumption [3], meanwhile increasing trends have been observed in the prevalence of NTD [2]. This indicates more reseach is required to understand the reasons behind this pnenomenon better, and this study contributes to this necessary body of knowledge.

Strengths and limitations

This study has a number of limitations. Luton is a deprived town and the findings may reflect lower educational levels as shown in the demographic profile of the town. More research is needed to determine an accurate prevalence rate for Luton, since this finding was obtained through a small number of self-reports and will identify the scope of the problem. There were also a number of strengths. This is the first study to identify similarities and differences between Pakistani, Bangladeshi and White British mothers understanding of consuming folic acid. In addition, much time and attention was given to recruiting representative women from the local community, including non-English speaking mothers. This process was time-consuming and involved the kind support and collaboration of many members of the community, Children's Centres and local NHS Trust in supporting the focus groups and ensuring women's experiences were documented. Consequently, since several distinct samples were used, this has facilitated triangulation of the data which increases the trustworthiness of the converged findings [47].

Interpretation

Taken together, it appears that there is a need for increasing health literacy on the benefits of folic acid consumption (including the timing of commencing supplementation prior to pregnancy) for women regardless of ethnicity or ability to speak English which is perhaps best aimed at teenagers in formal educational environments, before they become pregnant.

Conclusion

Few Pakistani, Bangladeshi or WB women understood the benefit of taking folic acid for optimising meiosis and reducing risks associated with NTD, while staff wrongly believed mothers supplement folic acid during the recommended preconception period. There is clearly a need to increase public health awareness, regarding the optimal time and benefits of consuming folic acid.

Additional files

Additional file 1: Topic guide for lay mothers. This topic guide was the final approved version, after pilot revisions were made and used with mothers in focus groups, stratified by ethnicity and who had a normal birth outcome (see methods section for further description).

Additional file 2: Topic guide for bereaved mothers. This topic guide was used with mothers who suffered a perinatal bereavement in face-to-face interviews (see Method section for a full description).

Abbreviations

FG: Focus group; NA: Nasreen Ali; NHS: National Health Service; NTD: Neural tube defect; P: Participnat; RG: Rebecca Garcia; RM: Riffat Mahmood; RS: Rukia Saalem; UK: United Kingdom

Acknowledgments

The authors would like to thank the mothers and staff who generously participated in this research and Catherine Hudson who assisted with recruiting bereaved mothers from the Luton and Dunstable University Hospital NHS Trust. Also, thanks to Riffat Mahmood and Rukia Saalem who assisted with translations and transliteration of the transcripts.

Funding

The Steel Trust provided funding to the University of Bedfordshire to undertake PhD research on adverse birth outcomes. They have no contribution to the study design, findings or dissemination. The Steel Trust has provided funding to the University of Bedfordshire for RG to research at Institute for Health Research, University of Bedfordshire, under the direction of NA and GR. The funders have no involvement in the research or publication.

Authors' contributions

RG and NA conceived the study; MG assisted with identification of participants, RG and NA conducted the framework analyses, RG, GR, MG and NA contributed to earlier drafts of the manuscript. All authors read and approved the final manuscript.

Competing interests

The authors declare that they have no competing interests.

Author details

[1]The School of Healthcare Practice, University of Bedfordshire, Putteridge Bury, Hitchin Road, Luton, Luton LU2 8LE, England. [2]The Institute For Health Research, University of Bedfordshire, Putteridge Bury, Hitchin Road, Luton, Luton LU2 8LE, England. [3]Luton & Dunstable University Hospital NHS Foundation Trust, Lewsey Rd, Luton LU4 0DZ, England.

References

1. The National Institute for Health and Care Excellence: Antenatal Care; Clinical Guideline 62. 2010.
2. Khoshnood B, Loane M, de Walle H, Arriola L, Addor M-C, Barisic I, Beres J, Bianchi F, Dias C, Draper E, Garne E, Gatt M, Haeusler M, Klungsoyr K, Latos-Bielenska A, Lynch C, McDonnell B, Nelen V, Neville AJ, O'Mahony MT, Queisser-Luft A, Rankin J, Rissmann A, Ritvanen A, Rounding C, Sipek A, Tucker D, Verellen-Dumoulin C, Wellesley D, Dolk H. Long term trends in prevalence of neural tube defects in Europe: population based study. BMJ (Clinical research ed). 2015;351:h5949.
3. Lassi ZS, Salam RA, Haider BA, Bhutta ZA. Folic acid supplementation during pregnancy for maternal health and pregnancy outcomes. Review. 2013;(3): CD006896.
4. Jessa F, Hampshire AJ. Use of folic acid by pregnant British Pakistani women: a qualitative pilot study. Health Educ J. 1999;58:139–45.
5. Hodgetts V, Morris R, Francis A, Gardosi J, Ismail K. Effectiveness of folic acid supplementation in pregnancy on reducing the risk of small-for-gestational age neonates: a population study, systematic review and meta-analysis. BJOG : An Int J Obstetrics and Gynaecol. 2015;122:478–90.
6. Yakoob MY, Menezes EV, Soomro T, Haws RA, Darmstadt GL, Bhutta ZA. Reducing stillbirths: behavioural and nutritional interventions before and during pregnancy. BMC Pregnancy Childbirth. 2009;9(Suppl 1):S3.
7. De-Regil L, Pena-Rosas J, Fernandez-Gaxiola A, Rayco-Solon P. Effects and safety of Periconceptional folate Supplementaion for preventing birth defects. Review. 2015;(12):CD007950.
8. Czeizel A. Prevention of congenital abnormalities by Periconceptional multivitamin supplementation. BMJ : British Med J. 1993;306:1645–8.
9. Morris JK, Rankin J, Draper ES, Kurinczuk JJ, Springett A, Tucker D, Wellesley D, Wreyford B, Wald NJ. Prevention of neural tube defects in the UK: a missed opportunity. Arch Dis Child. 2015;101:604–7.
10. Pre-conception - advice and management [https://cks.nice.org.uk/pre-conception-advice-and-management].
11. Tort J, Lelong N, Prunet C, Khoshnood B, Blondel B. Maternal and health care determinants of preconceptional use of folic acid supplementation in France: results from the 2010 National Perinatal Survey. BJOG: An Int J Obstetrics and Gynaecol. 2013;120:1661–7.
12. British Isles Network of Congenital Anomaly registers: British Isles Network of Congenital Anomaly Registers. 2014(December).
13. Bestwick JP, Huttly WJ, Morris JK, Wald NJ: Prevention of neural tube defects: A cross-sectional study of the uptake of folic acid supplementation in nearly half a million women. PLoS ONE. 2014;9:1–6.
14. Nilsen RM, Vollset SE, Magnus P, Meltzer HM, Haugen M, Ueland PM. Patterns and predictors of folic acid supplement use among pregnant women: the Norwegian mother and child cohort study. Am J Clin Nutr. 2007;84:1134–41.
15. Office for National Statistics: Childhood Mortality in England and Wales: 2015. 2017.
16. Wellings K, Jones KG, Mercer CH, Tanton C, Clifton S, Datta J, Copas AJ, Erens B, Gibson LJ, Macdowall W, Sonnenberg P, Phelps A, Johnson AM. The prevalence of unplanned pregnancy and associated factors in Britain: findings from the third National Survey of sexual attitudes and lifestyles (Natsal-3). Lancet. 2013;382:1807–16.
17. Hauck FR, Tanabe KO, Moon RY. Racial and ethnic disparities in infant mortality. Semin Perinatol. 2011;35:209–20.
18. Barbour RS, Macleod M, Mires G, Anderson AS. Uptake of folic acid supplements before and during pregnancy: focus group analysis of women's views and experiences. J Hum Nutr Diet. 2012;25:140–7.
19. Mazza D, Chapman A. Improving the uptake of preconception care and periconceptional folate supplementation: what do women think? BMC Public Health. 2010;10:1–6.
20. Temel S, Erdem Ö, Voorham TAJJ, Bonsel GJ, Steegers EAP, Denktaş S. Knowledge on preconceptional folic acid supplementation and intention to seek for preconception care among men and women in an urban city: a population-based cross-sectional study. BMC Pregnancy and Childbirth. 2015;15:340.
21. Holloway I, Wheeler S. Qual Res For Nurses. Oxford: Blackwell Publishers; 1996.
22. Garcia R, Ali N, Guppy A, Griffiths M, Randhawa G: A comparison of antenatal classifications of 'overweight' and 'obesity' prevalence between white British, Indian, Pakistani and Bangladeshi pregnant women in England. An analysis of retrospective data. BMC Public Health. 2017;17:1–7.
23. Garcia R, Ali N, Guppy A, Griffiths M, Randhawa G. Differences in the pregnancy gestation period and mean birth weights in infants born to Indian, Pakistani, Bangladeshi and white British mothers in Luton, UK: a retrospective analysis of routinely collected data. BMJ Open. 2017;7:e017139.
24. Bryman A. Social research strategies. In: Social Research Methods. 4th edn. Oxford: Oxford University Press; 2012. p. 18–44.
25. Research and Geospatial information: 2015 Indices of multiple deprivation: Luton. 2015(November).
26. Flenady V, Koopmans L, Middleton P, Frøen JF, Smith GC, Gibbons K, Coory M, Gordon A, Ellwood D, McIntyre HD, Fretts R, Ezzati M. Major risk factors for stillbirth in high-income countries: a systematic review and meta-analysis. Lancet. 2011;377:1331–40.
27. Sque M, Walker W, Long-Sutehall T. Research with bereaved families : a framework for ethical decision-making. Nurs Ethics. 2014;21:946–55.
28. Strauss A, Corbin J. Grounded theory methodology, an overview. In: Denzin N, Lincoln Y, editors. Handbook of Qualitative Research. London: Sage Publications; 1994. p. 273–85.
29. Ritchie J, Lewis J. Qualitative research practice: a guide for social science students and researchers. London: Sage Publications; 2003.
30. Regmi K, Naidoo J, Pilkington P. Understanding the processes of translation and transliteration in qualitative research. Int J Qual Methods. 2010;9:16–26.
31. Temple B, Young A. Qualitative research and translation dilemmas. Qual Res. 2004;4:161–78.
32. Stainton-Rogers W. Logics of Enquiry. In: Potter S, Keynes M, editors. In Doing Post Graduate Research. Second ed. Milton Keynes: Open University Press; 2006. p. 73–92.
33. Shenton AK. Strategies for ensuring trustworthiness in qualitative research projects. Educ Inf. 2004;22:63–75.
34. Srivastava A, Thompson SB. Framework analysis: a qualitative methodology for applied policy research. JOAAG. 2009;4:72–9.
35. Gale NK, Heath G, Cameron E, Rashid S, Redwood S. Using the framework method for the analysis of qualitative data in multi-disciplinary health research. BMC Med Res Methodol. 2013;13:117.
36. Richie J, Spencer L. Qualitative data analysis for applied policy research. In: Bryman A, Burgess R, editors. Analyzing Qualitaive Data. London: Routledge; 1995. p. 173–95.
37. Yeasmin SF, Regmi K. A qualitative study on the food habits and related beliefs of pregnant British Bangladeshis. Health Care for Women Int. 2013;34:395–415.
38. Bittles A, Grant J, Shami S. Consanguinity as a determinant of reproductive behaviour and mortality in Pakistan. Int J Epidemiol. 1993;22:463–7.
39. Grant J, Bittles A. The comparative role of consanguinity in infant and childhood mortality in Pakistan. Ann Hum Genet. 1997;61:143–9.
40. Ali N, McLean C, Rehman H. Faulty genes: consanguinity in the Pakistani community. Ethnicity and Inequalities in Health and Social Care. 2012;5:43–51.
41. Roseboom TJ, van der Meulen JHP, Ravelli ACJ, Osmond C, Barker DJP, Bleker OP. Effects of prenatal exposure to the Dutch famine on adult disease in later life: an overview. Mol Cell Endocrinol. 2001;185:93–8.
42. Tahrani AA, Ball A, Shepherd L, Rahim A, Jones AF, Bates A. The prevalence

of vitamin D abnormalities in south Asians with type 2 diabetes mellitus in the UK. Int J Clin Pract. 2010;64:351–5.
43. Macintosh M, Fleming K, Bailey J, Doyle P, Modder J, Acolet D, Golightly S, Miller A. Perinatal mortality and congenital anomalies in babies of women with type 1 or type 2 diabetes in England, Wales, and Northern Ireland: population based study. BMJ Clinical Research Ed. 2006;333:177.
44. Penn N, Oteng-Ntim E, Oakley LL, Doyle P. Ethnic variation in stillbirth risk and the role of maternal obesity: analysis of routine data from a London maternity unit. BMC pregnancy and childbirth. 2014;14
45. Lindam A, Johansson S, Stephansson O, Wikström AK, Cnattingius S. High maternal body mass index in early pregnancy and risks of stillbirth and infant mortality - a population-based sibling study in Sweden. Am J Epidemiol. 2016;184:98–105.
46. Chisholm J, Bittles A. Consanguinity and the developmental origins of health and disease. J Evol Med. 2015;3:1–4.
47. Hammersley M. Troubles with triangulation. In: Bergman M, editor. Advances in mixed method research. London: Sage Publications; 2008. p. 22–36.

12

A multicenter survey on toxoplasmosis knowledge among pregnant women in Poland (the TOWER study)

Jacek Smereka[1], Lukasz Szarpak[2*], Kurt Ruetzler[3], Yehoshua Schacham[3], Adam Smereka[4], Marek Dabrowski[5], Marzena Terpilowska[6], Lukasz Terpilowski[1] and Ishag Adam[7]

Abstract

Background: The seroprevalence of *Toxoplasma gondii* ranges widely in different areas of the world and different populations. Although toxoplasmosis is typically benign and asymptomatic, it induces major complications in immunocompromised individuals and during pregnancy. Prevention of maternal primary infection constitutes the major tool for avoiding congenital *T. gondii* infections and toxoplasmosis complications. The preventive measures depend on the women's knowledge about toxoplasmosis. The aim of the study was to assess the knowledge on toxoplasmosis among pregnant women in Poland.

Methods: The study was conducted between October 2016 and January 2017 in 3 Polish cities. During a visit in a hospital outpatient clinic, pregnant women aged > 16 years fulfilled a previously validated questionnaire. The questions concerned personal data (age, parity, educational level, place of residence), toxoplasmosis knowledge (etiology, routes of transmission, symptoms, sequelae), and sources consulted to collect information.

Results: Overall, 465 pregnant women participated in the survey; 439 (94.4%) were aware of toxoplasmosis. Toxoplasmosis was perceived as a zoonotic disease by 77.4%, as a parasitic disease by 41.7%, as a disease transmitted through poor hand hygiene by 8.6%, as a childhood illness by 4%, and as a congenital disease by 0.4%. Regarding the transmission route, 84.5% of women pointed at a domestic cat, 46.7% at eating raw or undercooked meat. The total of 84.3% did not know toxoplasmosis symptoms, and 12.0% stated that they did not present the symptoms. In multivariate analysis, younger age (OR, 2.74; 95% CI, 1.67–4.49; $p < 0.001$), city residence (OR, 13.45; 95% CI, 3.12–57.89; $p < 0.003$), and higher education level (OR, 6.81; 95% CI, 3.69–12.59; $p < 0.001$) were significantly associated with better knowledge of toxoplasmosis, and the number of children (OR, 0.32; 95% CI, 0.22–0.48; $p < 0.001$) – with higher knowledge of the symptoms.

Conclusions: Among pregnant women in Poland, the basic knowledge on toxoplasmosis is very high (94.4%). Younger age, city residence, higher education level, and the number of children turned out significantly associated with better knowledge of *T. gondii* and toxoplasmosis symptoms.

Keywords: Toxoplasmosis, Pregnancy, Toxoplasma gondii, Awareness

* Correspondence: lukasz.szarpak@gmail.com
[2]Faculty of Medicine, Lazarski University, 43 Swieradowska Str., 02-662 Warsaw, Poland
Full list of author information is available at the end of the article

Background

Toxoplasma gondii is an obligate intracellular protozoan parasite transmitted to humans through ingestion of food containing infectious oocysts that had been contaminated by feline feces (the definitive host), or ingestion of tissue cysts in undercooked meat of intermediate hosts, e.g. pork or lamb [1–3]. The seroprevalence of *T. gondii* ranges widely in different areas of the world and different populations, from ≤10% to almost 100% [4, 5]. Although toxoplasmosis is typically benign and asymptomatic, it induces major complications in immunocompromised individuals and during pregnancy, where it can lead to miscarriage and congenital disease [6]. Congenital toxoplasmosis is a substantial burden for public health worldwide [7]. A previous report showed that about 41% and 5% of Polish pregnant women had specific IgG and IgM antibodies, respectively, and estimated that 1.5/1000 neonates were infected in utero [8].

Since there is no vaccine against *T. gondii*, prevention of maternal primary infection constitutes the major tool for avoiding congenital *T. gondii* infections and their complications. The preventive measures mostly depend on the women's knowledge about toxoplasmosis, its transmission, and origin. Previous studies have shown different levels of pregnant women's knowledge regarding the risk and consequences of toxoplasmosis infection during pregnancy. It remains controversial, however, if improved knowledge and access to reliable information about sources of infection are suitable to consequently change women's behavior during pregnancy [9, 10]. Nevertheless, the aim of the study was to assess the toxoplasmosis knowledge of pregnant women in Poland.

Methods

The study was approved by the Institutional Review Board of the Polish Society of Disaster Medicine (approval No. 14.09.2016.IRB) and by the administrations of the healthcare institutions participating in the study. All data were anonymously collected and safely stored.

This cross-sectional, multicenter study was conducted between October 2016 and January 2017 in third-level hospitals in 3 Polish cities: Wroclaw, Warsaw, and Poznan. Pregnant women aged above 16 years who had a regular antenatal clinic visit in an outpatient clinic were asked to participate in the study. Once a patient agreed, written consent was obtained and the patient was interviewed in accordance with the pre-defined questionnaire by 2 of the researchers.

Questionnaire

The questionnaire was previously prepared by 2 researchers and validated in a pilot study conducted in September 2016 in Wroclaw, Poland. The comments of the participating pregnant women were used to improve the wording of some items in the questionnaire and eliminate redundant questions. The pilot study also allowed to determine the time needed to complete the questionnaire.

The questions addressed the following issues: personal data (age, parity, educational level, place of residence), knowledge about *T. gondii* (etiology, routes of transmission, symptoms, and sequelae), and sources consulted to collect information (Additional file 1).

Only closed-ended questions were used: dichotomous (e.g. gender, presence of children), nominal (e.g. educational level, marital status, knowledge of items) or multiple choice (e.g. sources of information).

Statistical analysis

Statistical analysis was performed with the Statistica version 13.1EN software (StatSoft, Tulsa, OK, USA). Descriptive statistics were used to summarize the demographic variables. Demographics were categorized by gender, age (≤ 19, 20–25, 26–35, 36–45, > 45 years), education (did not graduate from middle school, graduated from middle school, graduated from secondary school, university degree), place of residence (city, village), and number of pregnancies (1, 2, ≥ 3).

The differences between the groups were analyzed with chi-square tests for categorical data and either an independent *t*-test or Mann-Whitney U test for continuous data. Pearson's correlation coefficient was used to evaluate the correlations between variables. Linear regression was performed with the stepwise method to identify the variables most likely to predict a high level of knowledge regarding *T. gondii* among the pregnant women. The Durbin-Watson test was applied to identify an auto-correction in the regression analysis in which a value close to 2 indicated no first-order serial correlation. Multivariate logistic regression analyses allowed to identify factors associated with toxoplasmosis knowledge. Variables with $p < 0.2$ in univariate analyses were included in the multivariate analysis.

The p-value of < 0.05 was regarded as statistically significant.

Results

The total of 500 pregnant women were asked to participate in the survey. Of those, 465 agreed, which resulted in the participation rate of 93%. The demographic data of all the 465 subjects are shown in Table 1.

The education level of the study participants varied - 53 (11.4%) did not graduate from middle school, 111 (23.9%) graduated from middle school, 249 (53.5%) graduated from secondary school and 52 (11.2%) had university degree. Near half of the study participants - 231 (49.7%) reside in urban area and 234 (50.3%) in rural area. Number of pregnancies of study participants varied

Table 1 Demographic characteristics of pregnant women participating in the survey

Characteristics	N = 465
Age (years):	
≤ 19 years	25 (5.4%)
20–25 years	105 (22.6%)
26–30 years	137 (29.5%)
31–35 years	113 (24.3%)
36–40 years	83 (17.8%)
> 40 years	2 (0.4%)
Educational level	
did not graduate from middle school	53 (11.4%)
graduated from middle school	111 (23.9%)
graduated from secondary school	249 (53.5%)
university degree	52 (11.2%)
Place of residence	
Urban area	231 (49.7%)
Village	234 (50.3%)
Number of pregnancies:	
1	126 (27.1%)
2	218 (46.9%)
≥ 3	121 (26.0%)

– 1 pregnancy was reported in 126 study participants (27.1%), 2 in 218 (46.9%) and 3 and more in 121 (26.0%).

Overall, 439 (94.4%) of the 465 included pregnant women were aware of the existence of toxoplasmosis. Among the most common sources providing information about toxoplasmosis, the following were reported: medical doctors (76.1%), the Internet (45.6%), television (41.3%), books (12.0%), and mother, family, or friends (1.9%).

According to 77.4% of the pregnant women, toxoplasmosis was a zoonotic disease, 41.7% believed that it was a parasitic disease, 8.6% were convinced that toxoplasmosis was transmitted through poor hand hygiene, 4% maintained that toxoplasmosis was a childhood illness, and 0.4% stated that it was a congenital disease.

Regarding the question about the transmission route of *T. gondii*, 84.5% of women responded that it was transmitted via a domestic cat, and 46.7% pointed at eating raw or undercooked meat. Only 0.6% of the participants thought the parasite was spread through insect bites and 5.2% did not have knowledge on the subject.

The total of 84.3% of the surveyed did not know toxoplasmosis symptoms, and 12.0% stated that they did not present any symptoms of the disease. The pregnant women reported that the symptoms of toxoplasmosis included enlarged lymph nodes (3.4%), diarrhea (1.3%), and constipation (0.4%).

Among the preventative measures against toxoplasmosis, the respondents most frequently enumerated: avoiding contact with cats (83.9%), personal hygiene (46.0%), avoiding consumption of raw meat (45.8%), avoiding sandy beaches (4.9%), and avoiding contact with previously infected patients (0.4%).

In general, 83.2% of the participants believed that toxoplasmosis might be dangerous during pregnancy and according to 49.9% infection with the parasite could cause premature labor or miscarriage. When asked whether toxoplasmosis was a cause of any developmental defects in children (epilepsy, hypopigmentation, cataract, hydrocephalus, or heart defects), the vast majority of respondents (84.7%) reported no knowledge; 13.1% indicated heart defects as a potential consequence of toxoplasmosis, 11.4% pointed at hydrocephalus, 3.9% at epilepsy, and 1.3% at smallpox.

In the studied group, 83% did not know which trimester of pregnancy was associated with the greatest fetal risk related to the disease, whereas 17% indicated the first trimester.

Out of all the participants, 93.3% admitted that more emphasis should be put on health education related to toxoplasmosis prevention, 100% said that physicians should pay more attention to women at risk; 60.3% believed that the issue should be addressed in childbirth classes; 17.2% maintained that it should also be discussed by nutritionists.

To identify potential associations between high knowledge of *T. gondii* and socio-demographic characteristics, multivariate logistic regression analysis was conducted (Table 2). Younger age (OR, 2.74; 95% CI, 1.67–4.49; $p < 0.001$), city residence (OR, 13.45; 95% CI, 3.12–57.89; $p < 0.003$), and higher education level (OR, 6.81; 95% CI, 3.69–12.59; $p < 0.001$) turned out significantly associated with better knowledge of toxoplasmosis, and the number of children (OR, 0.32; 95% CI, 0.22–0.48; $p < 0.001$) – with higher knowledge of the symptoms.

Discussion

The main finding of the current study was a high (94.4%) basic knowledge on toxoplasmosis among the studied pregnant women in Poland. This correlates with the recent results that pregnant women in Geneva, Switzerland had a high (87%) knowledge about toxoplasmosis [11], and about 75.3% of Dutch women had been exposed to information concerning toxoplasmosis [12]. These outcomes contrast with previous worldwide findings reporting a generally low level of knowledge about toxoplasmosis, risk factors, prevention, and consequences of the disease among pregnant women [13]. Ogunmodede et al. reported that less than half of pregnant women in the USA had heard about toxoplasmosis, and that higher education levels were significantly

Table 2 Results of the logistic regression

	OR	95% CI	*p*
Have you ever heard of toxoplasmosis? (YES)			
Advanced age	2.74	1.67–4.49	< 0.001
Place of residence, Urban area	13.45	3.12–57.89	< 0.001
Higher education level	6.81	3.69–12.59	< 0.001
Higher number of pregnancies	1.33	0.77–2.32	0.305
Do you know what symptoms are associated with toxoplasmosis? (YES)			
Advanced age	1.29	0.92–1.80	0.140
Place of residence, Urban area	4.75	2.60–8.67	< 0.001
Higher education level	5.97	3.65–9.77	< 0.001
Higher number of pregnancies	0.32	0.22–0.48	< 0.001
Do you think that toxoplasmosis can be dangerous to the fetus? (YES)			
Advanced age	1.46	1.07–1.99	0.015
Place of residence, Urban area	8.28	4.24–16.20	< 0.001
Higher education level	3.20	2.33–4.40	< 0.001
Higher number of pregnancies	0.75	0.54–1.05	0.095
Do you think that toxoplasmosis can cause premature labor or miscarriage? (YES)			
Advanced age	1.07	0.85–1.36	0.556
Place of residence, Urban area	3.50	2.39–5.13	< 0.001
Higher education level	2.14	1.66–2.74	< 0.001
Higher number of pregnancies	0.52	0.40–0.67	< 0.001
Do you think that infection with toxoplasmosis can cause one of the following developmental defects in the child? (KNOWS)			
Advanced age	1.05	0.75–1.46	0.779
Place of residence, Urban area	6.90	3.51–13.54	< 0.001
Higher education level	6.98	4.16–11.72	< 0.001
Higher number of pregnancies	0.26	0.17–0.40	< 0.001
In which trimester of pregnancy do you think the fetus is most at risk f or toxoplasmosis? (KNOWS)			
Advanced age	1.05	0.76–1.44	0.763
Place of residence, Urban area	4.17	2.37–7.33	< 0.001
Higher education level	12.5	6.91–22.69	< 0.001
Higher number of pregnancies	0.24	0.16–0.37	< 0.001

associated with knowledge of the disease [14]. In Sri Lanka, *T. gondii* awareness among pregnant women equaled only 4.4%. Health personnel and media were the sources of information in 46.2% and 53.8%, respectively [15]. Likewise, it was reported that 3/4 of 400 pregnant Saudi women had never heard of toxoplasmosis, and those who lacked that knowledge were at 4.04 times higher risk of toxoplasmosis [16]. Interestingly, only 27.8% of the studied pregnant women in Niterói, Rio de Janeiro claimed to know about toxoplasmosis. Those who were conscious of *T. gondii* had a significantly lower probability of being seropositive to *T. gondii* IgG [17].

Previous studies reported that health education of pregnant women might help reduce the risk of congenital toxoplasmosis [10, 18]. Another study performed in Belgium indicated that health education led to a 63% reduction in T. gondii seroconversion [19]. Toxoplas mosis-related ducation of pregnant women in Poland increased their knowledge about the disease and its prevention twice in a 4-year period [20].

The total of 2598 pregnant women from Malaysia, Philippines, and Thailand were randomly surveyed in order to determine their knowledge and practices regarding *T. gondii* infection. Only 11% of them had read, heard, or seen information regarding toxoplasmosis and only 3.5% were aware of having been tested for the infection [21].

The practical implication of our study is the necessity to improve the knowledge of *T. gondii* and toxoplasmosis symptoms in pregnant women especially in rural areas or with lower education level.

The limitation of our study is the use of close questions in the questionnaire the free-form response was not allowed. Our study included only participants from several centers and certain geographic area and it may not reflect the whole country. The strength of our study is a high number of participants and the fact that it was to our best knowledge the first study on knowledge on toxoplasmosis among the pregnant women in Poland.

Conclusions

Among pregnant women in Poland, the basic knowledge on toxoplasmosis is very high (94.4%). Younger age, city residence, higher education level, and the number of children turned out significantly associated with better knowledge of *T. gondii* and toxoplasmosis symptoms.

Abbreviations

CI: Confidence interval; OR: Odds ratio; *T.gondii*: *Toxoplasma gondii*

Acknowledgements

We are grateful to all the persons who participated in this study.

Funding

Funding was not received for this work.

Authors' contributions

JS, AS, MT, LT, LS recruited the patients, collected the data, performed preliminary data analysis and drafted the manuscript. JS and LS performed detailed statistical analysis and prepared the Fig. JS, KR, IA, LS, MD and YS participated in the discussion and improved the manuscript. JS, IA, LS made substantial contributions to the original idea and design, analyses and interpretation of data as well as revising the manuscript. LS is the corresponding author and is responsible for the finalization of the manuscript. All authors have read and approved the final manuscript.

Competing interests

The authors declare that they have no competing interest.

Author details

[1]Department of Emergency Medical Service, Laboratory of Experimental Medicine and Innovative Technology, Wroclaw Medical University, Wroclaw, Poland. [2]Faculty of Medicine, Lazarski University, 43 Swieradowska Str., 02-662 Warsaw, Poland. [3]Department of Outcomes Research, Anesthesiology Institute, Cleveland Clinic, Cleveland, OH, USA. [4]Department of Clinic of Gastroenterology and Hepatology, Wroclaw Medical University, Wroclaw, Poland. [5]Chair and Department of Medical Education, Poznań University of Medical Sciences, Poznan, Poland. [6]Division of Neonatology, Department of Pediatrics, Faculty of Health Sciences, Wroclaw Medical University, Wroclaw, Poland. [7]Faculty of Medicine, University of Khartoum, Khartoum, Sudan.

References

1. Cook AJ, Gilbert RE, Buffolano W, Zufferey J, Petersen E, Jenum PA, Foulon W, Semprini AE, Dunn DT. Sources of toxoplasma infection in pregnant women: European multicentre case-control study. European research network on congenital toxoplasmosis. BMJ. 2000;321(7254):142–7.
2. Hill D, Dubey JP. Toxoplasma gondii: transmission, diagnosis and prevention. Clin Microbiol Infect. 2002;8(10):634–40.
3. Dabritz HA, Conrad PA. Cats and toxoplasma: implications for public health. Zoonoses Public Health. 2010;57(1):34–52.
4. Tenter AM, Heckeroth AR, Weiss LM. Toxoplasma gondii: from animals to humans. Int J Parasitol. 2008;30(12–13):1217–58.
5. Jones JL, Kruszon-Moran D, Elder S, Rivera HN, Press C, Montoya JG, McQuillan GM. Toxoplasma gondii infection in the United States, 2011-2014. Am J Trop Med Hyg. 2018;98(2):551–7.
6. Flegr J. Influence of latent toxoplasma infection on human personality, physiology and morphology: pros and cons of the toxoplasma-human model in studying the manipulation hypothesis. J Exp Biol. 2013;216(Pt 1):127–33.
7. Torgerson PR, Mastroiacovo P. The global burden of congenital toxoplasmosis: a systematic review. Bull World Health Organ. 2013;91(7):501–8.
8. Nowakowska D, Stray-Pedersen B, Spiewak E, Sobala W, Małafiej E, Wilczyński J. Prevalence and estimated incidence of toxoplasma infection among pregnant women in Poland: a decreasing trend in the younger population. Clin Microbiol Infect. 2006;12(9):913–7.
9. Di Mario S, Basevi V, Gagliotti C, Spettoli D, Gori G, D'Amico R, Magrini N. Prenatal education for congenital toxoplasmosis. Cochrane Database Syst Rev. 2015;(10):CD006171. https://doi.org/10.1002/14651858.CD006171.pub4.
10. Gollub EL, Leroy V, Gilbert R, Chêne G, Wallon M, European Toxoprevention Study Group (EUROTOXO). Effectiveness of health education on toxoplasma-related knowledge, behaviour, and risk of seroconversion in pregnancy. Eur J Obstet Gynecol Reprod Biol. 2008;136(2):137–45.
11. Willame A, Blanchard-Rohner G, Combescure C, Irion O, Posfay-Barbe K, Martinez de Tejada B. Awareness of cytomegalovirus infection among pregnant women in Geneva, Switzerland: a cross-sectional study. Int J Environ Res Public Health. 2015;12(12):15285–97.
12. Pereboom MT, Manniën J, Spelten ER, Schellevis FG, Hutton EK. Observational study to assess pregnant women's knowledge and behaviour to prevent toxoplasmosis, listeriosis and cytomegalovirus. BMC Pregnancy Childbirth. 2013;13:98.
13. Jones JL, Ogunmodede F, Scheftel J, Kirkland E, Lopez A, Schulkin J, Lynfield R. Toxoplasmosis-related knowledge and practices among pregnant women in the United States. Infect Dis Obstet Gynecol. 2003;11(3):139–45.
14. Ogunmodede F, Scheftel J, Jones JL, Lynfield R. Toxoplasmosis prevention knowledge among pregnant women in Minnesota. Minn Med. 2005;88(2):32–4.
15. Chandrasena N, Herath R, Rupasinghe N, Samarasinghe B, Samaranayake H, Kastuririratne A, de Silva NR. Toxoplasmosis awareness, seroprevalence and risk behavior among pregnant women in the Gampaha district, Sri Lanka. Pathog Glob Health. 2016;110(2):62–7.
16. Elsafi SH, Al-Mutairi WF, Al-Jubran KM, Abu Hassan MM, Al Zahrani EM. Toxoplasmosis seroprevalence in relation to knowledge and practice among pregnant women in Dhahran, Saudi Arabia. Pathog Glob Health. 2015;109(8):377–82.
17. Millar PR, Moura FL, Bastos OM, Mattos DP, Fonseca AB, Sudré AP, Leles D, Amendoeira MR. Toxoplasmosis-related knowledge among pregnant and postpartum women attended in public health units in Niterói, Rio de Janeiro, Brazil. Rev Inst Med Trop Sao Paulo. 2014;56(5):433–8.
18. Carter AO, Gelmon SB, Wells GA, Toepell AP. The effectiveness of a prenatal education programme for the prevention of congenital toxoplasmosis. Epidemiol Infect. 1989;103(3):539–45.
19. Foulon W, Naessens A, Derde MP. Evaluation of the possibilities for preventing congenital toxoplasmosis. Am J Perinatol. 1994;11(1):57–62.
20. Pawlowski ZS, Gromadecka-Sutkiewicz M, Skommer J, Paul M, Rokossowski H, Suchocka E, Schantz PM. Impact of health education on knowledge and prevention behavior for congenital toxoplasmosis: the experience in Poznań, Poland. Health Educ Res. 2001;16(4):493–502.
21. Andiappan H, Nissapatorn V, Sawangjaroen N, Khaing SL, Salibay CC, Cheung MM, Dungca JZ, Chemoh W, Xiao Teng C, Lau YL, Mat Adenan NA. Knowledge and practice on toxoplasma infection in pregnant women from Malaysia, Philippines, and Thailand. Front Microbiol. 2014;5:291.

13

Perceived causes of adverse pregnancy outcomes and remedies adopted by Kalenjin women in rural Kenya

Roselyter Monchari Riang'a[1,2*], Anne Kisaka Nangulu[1,3] and Jacqueline E. W. Broerse[2]

Abstract

Background: There have been few studies about the basis on which women in developing regions evaluate and choose traditional rather than western maternal care. This qualitative study explores the socio-cultural perceptions of complications associated with pregnancy and childbirth and how these perceptions influence maternal health and care-seeking behaviours in Kenya.

Methods: Kalenjin women ($n = 42$) aged 18–45 years, who were pregnant or had given birth within the last 12 months, were interviewed. A semi-structured interview guide was used for data collection. A further nine key informant interviews with Traditional Birth Attendants (TBAs) who were also herbalists ($n = 6$), community health workers (CHWs) ($n = 3$) and a Maternal and Child Health (MCH) nursing officer ($n = 1$) were conducted. The data were analysed using MAXQDA12 software and categorised, thematised and analysed based on the symbolic dimensions of Helman's (2000) ill-health causation aetiologies model.

Results: Pregnancy complications are perceived as the consequence of pregnant women not observing culturally restricted and recommended behaviour during pregnancy, including diet; physical activities; evil social relations and spirits of the dead. These complications are considered to be preventable by following a restricted and recommended diet, and avoiding heavy duties, funerals, killing of animals and eating meat of animal carcasses, as well as restricting geographical mobility, and use of herbal remedies to counter evil and prevent complications.

Conclusion: Delay in deciding to seek maternal care is a result of women's failure to recognise symptoms and maternal health problems as potential hospital cases, and this failure stems from culturally informed perceptions of symptoms of maternal morbidity and pregnancy complications that differ significantly from biomedical interpretations. Some of the cultural maternal care and remedies adopted to prevent pregnancy complications, such as restriction of diet and social mobility, may pose risks to the pregnant woman's health and access to health facilities whereas other remedies such as restricting consumption of meat from animal carcasses and heavy duties, as well as maintaining good social relations, are cultural adaptive mechanisms that indirectly control the transmission of disease and improve maternal health, and thus should not be considered to be exclusively folk or primitive.

Keywords: Pregnancy, Perceptions, Care-seeking behaviour, Maternal health, Kalenjin, Uasin-Gishu, Kenya

* Correspondence: monchari2002@yahoo.com; r.m.rianga@vu.nl
[1]School of Arts and Social Sciences, Moi University, P.O. Box 3900-30100, Eldoret, Kenya
[2]Athena Institute, Faculty of Science, Vrije Universiteit Amsterdam, De Boelelaan 1085, 1081 HV Amsterdam, The Netherlands
Full list of author information is available at the end of the article

Background

Utilization of professional maternal health services is crucial in improving maternal, foetal and newborn health outcomes. It is estimated that 90% of pregnancy-related maternal deaths can be prevented with timely medical interventions during Antenatal Care (ANC) appointments, emergency obstetric care, safe abortion, delivery and Postnatal Care (PNC) period [1]. As a result, the World Health Organization (WHO) recommends at least four ANC visits, postnatal check-ups within 2 days of birth, and that all deliveries be attended delivered by skilled health providers and that ANC begin as soon as a woman becomes pregnant for essential interventions to be effectively administered [2].

However, maternal deaths remain high in low- and middle-income countries (LMICs) with a maternal mortality rate (MMR) of 239 per 100,000 live births [3]. Untimely, underuse or lack of professional medical interventions have been established as the main contributing factors [4, 5]. Globally, during the period 2007–2014, 64% of pregnant women attended the WHO-recommended minimum of four ANC contacts, with 78% of births being attended by a skilled health professional [6]. Low access to professional maternal care services is worse in LMICs. The Kenya Demographic Health Survey (KDHS) statistics, for instance, indicated that although nearly 90% of women seek ANC in health facilities, 58% of pregnant women made four or more ANC visits, while 20% made their first visit within the first trimester [7]. Many women wait until the last trimester to do this while others make only one visit, thus limiting the benefits that would have been extended to them under the free government maternal care programme [8–10]. Overall, 44% of births in Kenya are attended by skilled birth attendants [11]. The underuse of professional maternal health services is reportedly higher in rural areas [7] and the situation is worse in some parts of the country. For instance, in Uasin Gishu County of Kenya (where this study was conducted), only 22% of pregnant women attended at least four ANC sessions, while only 30% of all births are attended by skilled health staff [12].

In contrast to the limited uptake of professional maternal health services in Kenya and other LMICs, most women make extensive use and reliance on traditional maternal care and remedies, even when they are suffering serious emergency obstetric complications. A study by Kaingu et al. [10] in Machakos County Kenya, for instance, identified a total of 10 pregnancy-related complications and symptoms, including being threatened spontaneous abortion, labour complications and post-partum haemorrhage that are being managed at the mother's home by Traditional Birth Attendants (TBAs). They further identified 55 plant species that were being used as medicinal herbs for the management and treatment of pregnancy complications. TBAs, mothers-in-law and older female relatives are important community resource persons whom pregnant women routinely consult throughout the course of pregnancy and childbirth, especially in rural areas in LMICs [7, 8, 11]. The situation is made particularly challenging by the fact that most informal maternal care providers, especially in the rural areas, have no formal training in maternal care and child delivery, instead they rely on their traditional knowledge, which is not well known in the literature. There is little evidence that this situation will soon improve because even when mothers seek care at the health facilities, studies indicate that they tend to integrate both western and indigenous knowledge in their understanding of health and medicine [13].

Indigenous knowledge is an integral part of life in rural communities. This knowledge has a great influence on how communities perceive health, illness, causes of disease and consequently their care-seeking behaviours [14, 15]. These traditional healthcare practices could be useful or detrimental. Rather than ignoring and condemning it, this knowledge should be explored, strengthened through research and scientific evidence, documented and disseminated, especially to healthcare providers, so that they can be informed about the actual practices in which women engage during pregnancy and childbirth. To this end, the present study aims to gain insight into traditional antenatal care practices adopted by pregnant women and their implications for maternal health and access to biomedical care interventions. Examining the socio-cultural context of pregnancy and childbirth is important to understanding maternal mortality and health-seeking behaviours.

Theoretical framework

This study was guided by symbolic interaction and functionalist perspectives. The research findings are analysed through the lens of symbolic interactionism in order to understand how the Kalenjin perceive and respond to adverse pregnancy outcomes. It was established that the Kalenjin women's responses and behaviours regarding pregnancy complications are directed by the meanings they attribute to these complications. These meanings are constructed and learned through social interactions with other members of society. What is important to realise, however, is that these meanings are based on what is culturally believed to be true and not what is 'objectively true' from the perspective of western biomedical models. Hence, these meanings may override and conflict with biomedical realities of health and thus require contextualised interpretations and interventions. Women act in ways that accord with the meaning that they attribute to adverse pregnancy outcomes. Understanding these symbolic meanings, therefore, will assist in comprehending the Kalenjin women's responses and behaviour towards adverse pregnancy outcomes.

The discussion of the research results was also guided by the functionalist perspectives. These cultural explanatory models of illness, even if based on scientifically incorrect premises, frequently have an internal logic and consistency, which often helps the victim of illness to "make sense" of what has happened, why it has happened and the appropriate disease prevention and treatment therapy to adopt. On the other hand, some of these causal explanations of pregnancy-related illness are deliberate attempts to reduce pregnancy complications but are based on an understanding of disease transmission that differs from the western biomedical models. When the underlying unconscious adaptive significance is effective, these pregnant women will continue adopting the practice even though they may not be aware of the adoptive value of what they are doing, which contributes to the selective retention of these prevention and treatment remedies. For this reason, it is necessary to take into account these unintended, adaptive benefits of various pregnancy practices and belief systems in any attempt to unravel complex patterns of treatment during pregnancy.

However, ethnomedical explanatory models of illness are not always in people's best interest. Some belief systems and ritual practices appear to have maladaptive effects, which pose medical risks to those practising them. It is therefore important to understand these practices in any given intervention.

Methods

Study setting and data collection

The major focus of this qualitative study was on the cultural interpretation of pregnancy complications and the preventive and treatment remedies adopted. This study is part of broader research investigating the socio-cultural context of maternal nutrition and health in rural Uasin Gishu County in western Kenya. Data were collected between April and August 2015 from Kalenjin women, either pregnant or with a child of less than 1 year, seeking care at the government health facilities in the Maternal and Child Health (MCH) care section.

The Kalenjin is the main ethnic population in Uasin Gishu County and comprises eight sub-ethnic groups (the Kipsigis, Nandi, Tugen, Keiyo, Marakwet, Pokot, Sabaot and the Terik) that share a common dialect and similar cultural traits. Among the Kalenjin speakers, each sub-ethnic group has its own distinctive dialect. The Nandi occupies the largest settlement in Uasin Gishu County, followed by the Keiyo.

All 90 public health facilities in the county were included in the sampling frame. Quota and purposive sampling techniques were employed in the selection of a representative sample of health facilities for the study. The selection criteria included ensuring that the health facilities in all the six-quotas (sub-counties) are proportionately represented in the sample. All the health facilities must be in the rural area (outside the municipality territory) and have a catchment population mainly comprising at least 90% Kalenjin patients to enhance cultural homogeneity. This means that areas dominated by other non-Kalenjin ethnic groups and those within the municipal boundaries were eliminated. The last criterion is that the selected facilities should be spatially distributed from each other to diversify responses. In the end, a total of 23 health facilities were sampled for the study.

All the Kalenjin women who come for routine antenatal and post-partum child welfare check-ups in the sampled health facilities were included in the sampling frame. They were recruited at the MCH clinics and in maternity wards. Eligibility criteria for the study participants depended on: being pregnant or having given birth within the last year, a Kalenjin by birth, willing and able to participate in the study, able to give informed consent [16] and willing to be audio recorded. This selection criterion eliminated non-Kalenjin women and those not willing to be audio recorded. Data were collected until the information reached saturation at a sample size of 42 women [17].

Nine key informants, including six TBAs who are also herbalists, one CHW, and one nursing officer in charge of MCH, were also selected for an interview. Quota sampling and purposive sampling techniques were used in the selection of key informants [17]. One TBA from each of the six sub-counties, who was highly mentioned by women respondents who had given birth at home or took herbal remedies during pregnancy, was selected and they could be reached at home or in the market centre. The CHW and nursing officer were selected from one of the largest rural facilities in the county because they are likely to encounter a wide range of pregnancy experiences and challenges given their large catchment area. In total, six TBAs who were also herbalists, one nursing officer offering MCH care, and one CHW were recruited.

Data collection

An open-ended interview guide (Additional file 1), divided into four sections, was used to elicit the information from the Kalenjin women. The first section presented demographic characteristics of the respondents including age, educational level, parity, ethnic affiliation and gestational age at the first ANC visit, marital status, and tribal affiliation among others. The other sections contained questions about food restrictions, recommended food, activities restricted and activities encouraged during pregnancy. Every practice mentioned was probed to obtain an insight into the underlying reasons. The respondents were further questioned about their opinions regarding these cultural practices and whether they indeed practised them.

Face-to-face individual interviews were conducted in a private room. Each woman was interviewed once and the interview lasted between 30 and 60 min, depending on her responses. Key informant interviews (KIIs) followed later to provide clarity on the issues raised during the interviews. The KIIs lasted between an hour and 2.5 h. They were also questioned about the kind of advice they give pregnant women and health challenges they face when providing care to pregnant women. Important notes were taken and at the same time responses were audio recorded.

Ethical considerations

The study was approved by the National Commission for Science, Technology and Innovation (NACOSTI) in Kenya and a research clearance permit number: NACOSTI/P/15/2335/5353 dated 2 April 2015 was issued to facilitate the research process. As approved by NACOSTI, the permit was then presented to the Uasin-Gishu County Commissioner, County Director of Education and County Director of Health, for their approval to conduct the study in the County. Further, appointments were booked with the respective officers in charge of the various facilities visited. Participation was voluntary. The respondents were informed of the aim of the research, confidentiality and anonymity of their responses, and then gave their signed consent to participate. Permission to audio record the interview sessions was sought from each respondent. Only voices for those who consented were recorded.

Analysis

Recorded responses were transcribed and, together with field notes, were studied by way of content analysis using MAXQDA 12.0.3 software. Helman's [15] classification of lay-illness aetiologies model was adopted as the initial coding guide. Meanings attributed to various adverse pregnancy outcomes were established in the data and were classified into four major categories based on Helman's [15] symbolic classification of lay-illness causation aetiologies model: individual, natural, social and supernatural, as illustrated in Fig. 1. The categories were further classified into sub-categories and themes as interpreted below.

Individual causes These include lay theories that locate the meaning of pregnancy complications in the individual woman for "not taking care" of herself in terms of diet, dress, hygiene, lifestyle, relationships, sexual behaviour, smoking and drinking habits, physical exercise, emotions or doing something abnormal or incorrect. An adverse pregnancy outcome is, therefore, evidence of "carelessness" and the woman should feel guilty and responsible for causing it. However, in some rare circumstances, individual causes can result from external forces over which the victim had no control such as bad luck, economic power or hereditary factors.

Natural causes In this category, an adverse pregnancy outcome is thought to be caused by the natural environment, both living and inanimate. Common in this group are climatic conditions, such as excess cold, heat, wind, rain, snow, damp, cyclones, tornadoes, eclipse or severe storms. Others include accidental injuries which originate from the "natural environment", or are caused by animals, birds, insects, or infections caused by micro-organisms, such as germs, bugs or viruses.

Social causes This category involves blaming other people for causing adverse pregnancy outcomes and is a common feature of non-industrialised and smaller-scale societies, where interpersonal conflicts are frequent. The common forms of these are witchcraft, sorcery and "evil eyes". In witchcraft, certain people are believed to possess a mystical power to harm others and this power is inherited, either genetically or by membership of a particular kinship group. Sorcery, as defined by Helman

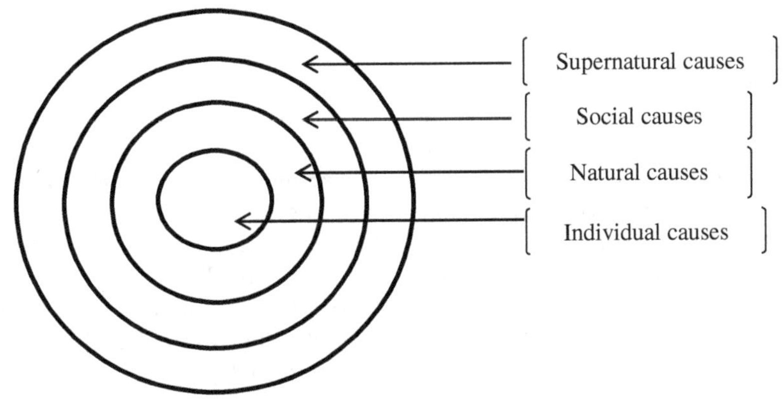

Fig. 1 Sites of illness aetiology (Helman, 2000:120)

[15], is the power to manipulate and alter natural and supernatural events with the proper magical knowledge and performance of rituals, and this is different from witchcraft. Sorcery is often practised among one's social world of friends, family or neighbours, and is often based on envy. Evil eyes, or a "wounding eye", relates to the fear of envy in the eyes of the beholder. The possessors of evil eye are usually believed to harm unintentionally and are often unaware of their powers and are unable to control them. The influence of evil eye, as explained by Helman [15], is avoided or counteracted by means of devices calculated to distract its attention, and by practices of sympathetic magic. The social aetiology of illness also includes physical injuries, such as poisoning or battle wounds, inflicted by other people. Furthermore, it can be stress or actions caused by spouse, children, friends, employer or colleagues and neighbours. It can also be contagious diseases transmitted by other people.

Supernatural causes Here a pregnancy complication is ascribed to the direct actions of supernatural entities, such as gods, spirits or ancestral shades. In the gods aetiology, illness is described as a reminder from God for a behavioural lapse or sinful behaviour. The cure in this case involves acknowledging the sins and vowing to improve one's behaviour. In the case of spiritual causes, disease-bearing spirits strike unexpectedly causing a variety of symptoms in their victims. Their invasion is unrelated to the individual's behaviour, who is therefore considered blameless and worthy of sympathetic help from others. In the case of ancestral shades causes, a pregnancy complication is ascribed to spirits of the ancestors whom they have offended and diagnosis takes place in a divinatory séance.

Results

Socio-demographic characteristics of the respondents

A total of 42 female respondents were interviewed, of whom 14 were pregnant and 28 were post-natal (Table 1). Half of the respondents had acquired primary education. All respondents were age 18 years and above and more than 26 respondents were between 20 and 29 years of age. Many respondents ($n = 30$) were married and almost all worked in the informal economy as subsistence farmers, homemakers or small entrepreneurs. Only 13 of the respondents were first-time mothers and the other 29 had 2–8 children. For the recent pregnancy, three respondents did not seek any ANC from the health facility. For those who attended ANC at the health facility, only three did so in the first trimester while the majority started after 6 months of pregnancy.

Table 1 Demographic characteristics of the respondents

Characteristic	Categories	Number of cases ($N = 42$)
Maternal status	Ante-natal	14
	Post-natal	28
Parity	First Pregnancy/child	13
	1–3	15
	4–6	11
	7–8	3
Gestational age at the first ANC visit	Never visited	3
	2 months	3
	4 months	3
	5 months	6
	6 months	16
	≥ 7 months	11
Age of respondents (years)	≤ 19	4
	20–24	16
	25–29	10
	30–34	7
	≥ 35	5
Marital status	Never married	8
	Currently married	30
	Separated	2
	Widowed	2
Educational level	Primary Education	21
	Secondary Education	16
	Tertiary Education	5
Occupation	Student/pupil	4
	Business	7
	Farming	26
	Formal employment	1
	Other	4
Sub-ethnic groups	Nandi	31
	Keiyo	4
	Marakwet	5
	Terik	1
	Kipsigis	1

Perceptions of and responses to adverse pregnancy outcomes

Several perceived causes of pregnancy complications and the remedies adopted were identified and classified into four major categories based on Helman's [15] classification of lay-illness aetiologies model as illustrated in Fig. 1. Further, sub-categories and themes that emerged were established and are presented in Table 2.

Table 2 Interpretation of pregnancy complications and remedies

Category (Cause)	Subcategory (Sub-cause)	Theme (perceived causes)	N = 42 (%)	Theme (perceived remedies)
Individual causes	Physical activities	Doing heavy duties	25(60%)	Avoid doing heavy duties
		Having sexual intercourse during pregnancy	10(24%)	Abstain from sexual intercourse during pregnancy
		Idling	9(21%)	Do light duties
		Standing or peeping at the door/ window way	6(14%)	Either walk out quickly or stay
		Running or walking long distances	5(12%)	Avoid running and long walks
		Oversleeping	4(10%)	Avoid over sleeping
		Boarding a motorbike	2(5%)	Avoid using motor bikes
		Sitting and sleeping style	2(5%)	Sit with legs straight, Sleep on the side, not on back
		Dress code	2(5%)	Avoid dressing accessories around the body including necklace, belts or clothes with bands around the waist
	Diet	Eating restricted food (eggs, avocado, meat, oily food, fresh milk, cold ugali cold water, alcohol and cigarettes)	41(98%)	Avoid restricted food
		Not eating recommended food and herbal medicine (traditional vegetables, milk, liver, ugali)	41(98%)	Eat recommended food Use herbal medicine
Natural Causes	Sickness and hereditary complications	Severe cramps during menses	8(19%)	Seek herbal treatment
		Wrong foetal presentation	3(7%)	Seek TBA care to turn the foetus
		Malaria	2(5%)	Take preventive herbal remedies Only take prescribed drugs
		Amount of hair and sex of the foetus	2(5%)	Seek TBA advice/treatment
		Yellow fever	1(2%)	Seek herbal treatment
Social world	Getting in contact with dangerous people	Contact with a woman who had an abortion, or whose child died recently, or who had a wrong foetal presentation during birth, multiple births or who develops severe cramps during menses, or who have evil eyes	10(24%)	Reduce movements Avoid going to public places Use protective herbs
	Social relations	Quarrelling with/abusing someone	5(12%)	Maintain peaceful relations Confession and repentance
		Made to cry or stressed	2(5%)	Avoid emotional events
Super natural causes	Evil spirits	Eating meat of a "misfortune animal"	16(38%)	Avoid eating "evil meat"
		Killing an animal	12(29%)	Avoid killing any animal
		An animal crossing your way or meeting two snakes on your way	3(7%)	End the journey whenever one meets world animal, mostly a snake, on the way
	Gods	Laughing at a deformed person	8(19%)	Do not lough at a deformed person
	Ancestral spirits	Viewing or burying a dead person	11 (26%)	Avoid burials Do not view a dead body
		A relative committed evil actions towards the ancestor	4 (10%)	Conduct a reconciliation ritual

Individual causes

Individual cause is one of the factors that strongly emerged in this study. Under this category, pregnancy complications are seen as evidence of the pregnant woman's carelessness and as a result she should feel guilty about her incorrect practices during her pregnancy. These are particularly related to physical activities and diet.

Physical activities

One of the restricted activities that strongly emerged in the study, as reported by 60% of the respondents, is that a pregnant woman should be exempted from performing "heavy duties". Heavy duties that were commonly forbidden according to the respondents refer to activities that involve bending for long hours, carrying heavy loads, fetching water from an open well, "scooping soil" (digging), carrying soil and smearing mud houses. Other activities reported include: hand washing many clothes, splitting firewood, collecting water from the river using a heavy container (e.g. 20 kg), or carrying a heavy load of firewood. Heavy duties are believed to cause lower back pain that may cause a miscarriage, pre-term birth and excessive bleeding after birth or low birth weight. Splitting firewood is also believed to make the baby's fontanelle abnormally large, which is dangerous because it is believed to cause its death.

Heavy duties like digging, splitting firewood should be avoided because it drains all the energy from the lower back making it ache and become weak. This is dangerous....it can make the baby come out [abortion].

To avoid lower back pains that cause a miscarriage, it is perceived that a pregnant woman should not only avoid heavy activities, but also seek herbal treatment. The herbs are believed to strengthen the lower back and thus minimise back pains during pregnancy and after the birth.

When a woman is pregnant, she should not overwork herself with housework or digging. This is why some of them come to me complaining of back pains. I give them pain relief herbs and I normally tell them to completely avoid overworking themselves. (Herbalist 2)

Some respondents felt that fetching water from an open well is risky; a woman might lose her balance and fall into the well. Collecting water from the well is discouraged in the first 4 months of pregnancy, because at this stage, pregnancy is still considered immature hence fragile and easy to abort. Thus, such activity can be undertaken after a pregnancy is 5 months or more. A pregnant woman may also carry a light load (10 kg or less) that she can easily lift without being assisted.

Sometimes there are women when giving birth, legs of the baby come out first instead of the head or those who experience severe cramps during menses. Such a woman should not assist you in lifting the load to your head or back when you are pregnant. You will also give birth like her or have an abortion.

A pregnant woman is also advised to abstain from having sexual intercourse, as reported by 24% of the respondents. However, the period of abstinence varied; to some, abstinence should begin the moment you realise you are pregnant, to others from 6 months onwards. The semen is believed to make the baby dirty, because it sticks on the baby's skin and scalp, creating a white substance. Thus, the baby must be washed with herbs for several days to clear it off. The "semen" is also believed to be dangerous for the foetus because it is thought to block the nasal passages and this could make breathing difficult and subsequently cause death. It is also thought that the "semen" can be swallowed by the foetus and remain stuck in the chest, causing a wheezing chest. The condition is believed to be more dangerous if the baby is a boy because males are considered less active in the uterus and cannot wash it off into the amniotic fluid. A woman who did not abstain from sex will be detected during birth because "she will be messy with semen" and nobody will be willing to assist her delivery, including the midwife. Instead, they will use plastic bags as gloves in assisting delivery, and the woman and her husband will be abused and ostracised.

.....ejaculations of the man are dangerous to the baby and messy, even those facilitating your birth might run away and leave you, they do not like looking at those things. They will be forced to use plastic bags to remove the baby and give you to wash it by yourself. They only assist you well if you give birth to a clean baby.

Some respondents, including one of the CHWs, reported that they use condoms during pregnancy to prevent the semen from reaching the baby.

On the other hand, a pregnant woman should not be idle (21%) and should not oversleep (10%) but perform light duties. Light duties include washing a few clothes, grazing cows, weeding a small plot, or taking a nature walk. It is believed that, when a woman is idle or asleep, the foetus also becomes idle, inactive and docile because it tends to sleep a lot. A docile foetus, according to the respondents, is not strong enough to assist the mother when she is pushing during delivery, resulting in prolonged labour. Similarly, if a pregnant woman is idling or sleeping a lot makes her muscles will be weak during labour and she will not find it easy to push out the baby.

I was told not to sleep too much but to be active in doing light duties like grazing animals and digging but not too much of it. It makes the baby play well and be positioned in the right part of the womb; otherwise I will have trouble during birth. The pain will extend for long.

Domestic duties like washing utensils, and when your body is okay you can go to the farm. It helps blood to flow very well, and the body to function well, but if you just stay idle it can even bring you diseases like high blood pressure and diabetes.

A pregnant woman, as reported by 14% of the respondents, should not peep through or stand in the doorway or window of a house. If she has a tendency to do this and return, during labour, the baby will also peep though the cervix, trying to come out, but instead return back into the uterus, thus prolonging labour. To avoid the chances of prolonged labour, a pregnant woman should decisively either stay inside or just walk out of the house and avoid standing in the doorway.

A pregnant woman should also avoid running or walking long distances, as reported by 12% of the respondents:

One should not run when pregnant, she can accidentally fall down causing the pregnancy to pain [contractions] *before term.*

Other restricted activities during pregnancy that were reported by less than 10% of the respondents include boarding a motorbike (the means of transport commonly used in rural areas), the dress code, sitting style and sleeping positions. High heels are considered dangerous because they might cause a woman to fall, and that could lead to pre-term contractions/miscarriage. Pregnant women should also avoid clothes with a band around the waist, such as skirts, trousers and belts. Bands around the waist are believed to make the umbilical cord twist around the baby during birth, which they believe may cause stillbirth. A pregnant woman should sit with her legs straight and apart. Sitting with her legs twisted or bent, they believe, will block the birth canal and result in obstructed labour.

Diet

Pregnancy complications were also thought to be caused by the wrong diet during pregnancy. Some foods, as reported by 98% of the respondents, were considered to jeopardise a pregnancy if consumed in excess, while others can endanger pregnancy if they are not eaten in sufficient quantity. Thus, a pregnant woman is required to eat sparingly and selectively. High-protein and energy-rich foods were believed to make the foetus grow big. A big foetus cannot be pushed out easily and will cause an obstruction, thus prolonging labour and possibly lead to caesarean section (CS). CS is believed to be a risky process in the sense that it halves the chances of mother or child survival, unlike an uncomplicated vaginal delivery. The big foetus also results in a prolonged labour and may cause tears by forcing itself out. Eggs, avocado, and oily food were commonly reported as needing to be avoided or restricted.

I was told not to eat strong food like eggs and avocado. The baby will grow big and later will give me problems when giving birth and I can even be operated.

Other foods of this kind that should be eaten sparingly include: meat, fresh milk, cooked bananas, and cold *ugali*. TBAs/herbalists prescribe herbs to regularise the size of the baby especially if it is judged to be too big.

Consumption of alcohol and cigarettes is restricted during pregnancy because it is believed to result in low birthweight and mentally retarded babies. Furthermore, when in labour, a pregnant woman should not drink cold water. It is believed to freeze contractions and thus lead to prolonged labour.

Some foods were believed to be good for pregnancy, hence encouraged to be eaten in plenty. According to most respondents, a pregnant woman is recommended to increase her blood volume and energy. A woman with less blood volume is considered not to have strength to push out the baby, will bleed to death during labour, and might require blood transfusion, which is believed to be risky. Therefore, lots of the foods that are believed to increase the amount of blood should be eaten for the entire period of pregnancy. These include indigenous vegetables (mostly leafy greens, including pigweed, black nightshade, spider plant, spinach, white vine spinach, pumpkin leaves and cowpea leaves), fruits, liver, animal blood, milk (especially when mixed with animal blood), red beans and their soup, meat, porridge made of finger millet flour, red soil or red stones and some traditional herbs.

When your blood is less, it will only help you to get a baby, thereafter; you will bleed until your body dries up and you die.

A pregnant woman is also required to be stronger during pregnancy. It is believed that a weak woman will not be able to push the baby out.

If you do not feed well on the pregnancy recommended food, you will not have strength for pushing out the baby during birth. You will be weak, you can even faint. They will demand an operation in order to remove the baby. With the operation you might die.

It is therefore recommended for her to eat "strong" energy-giving food during the pregnancy and minimise "less" energy food. *Ugali* and porridge were the commonly reported foods believed to be rich in energy. Others were milk, rice, sweet potatoes, Irish potatoes and herbs. However, rice and Irish potatoes are regarded as 'less energy-giving food' that should be eaten only once in a while.

Use of preventive herbs during pregnancy was reported by the majority of the respondents, mainly to prevent mother-to-child transmission. A TBA presented 10 different herbal medicines that are boiled together for pregnant women to drink, whether sick or not. Hence, a pregnant woman will be held responsible for any miscarriage if she refuses to take these preventive herbs.

Natural causes

Some aspects of the natural environment were also believed to cause pregnancy complications, though not reported by as many respondents as other aspects of Helman's model. The aspects of natural causes that emerged in this study were mainly infectious and hereditary diseases. Severe pre-pregnancy menstrual cramps (*chepsaliat*), as reported by 19%, are believed to cause miscarriage or pre-term contractions during the first months of pregnancy. Therefore, it is thought that girls who experience severe pre-pregnancy menstrual cramps are likely to abort within 4 months of conception if they do not seek herbal treatment before conceiving.

> *I had a miscarriage at two and a half months in my previous pregnancy, my grandmother told me it was caused by cramps. When I was a girl, I used to have severe menstrual cramps.*

Severe menstrual cramps, as explained by the herbalist, are inherited and are extended to pregnancy and are believed to pierce the capillaries supplying blood to the uterus resulting in "blood leakage" that supposedly causes spontaneous abortion mostly within the fourth month of pregnancy.

To avoid the chances of early miscarriage, girls who experience pre-pregnancy *chepsaliat* are highly recommended to seek herbal treatment before conception. However, if the woman notices unusual contractions or spots of blood and seeks immediate herbal attention, "the capillaries can be sealed" (spontaneous abortion can be controlled) as explained by a TBA/herbalist:

> *....If someone ignores the herbs and instead opts for hospital treatment before taking the herbs, she cannot control the bleeding even if I give her the herbs. That one is beyond repair, the herbs cannot help her. Whoever ignores these herbs aborts.* (Herbalist 2)

If a pregnant woman falls sick, her illness is also believed to be transferable to the foetus causing foetal death (miscarriage or perinatal death). The reported diseases were malaria and yellow fever. As a result, maternal sickness or the possibility of mother-to-child transmission should be prevented by periodically drinking herbs or be treated using mild herbal medicine. Hospital medicines are acceptable but believed to be 'too strong' and may cause spontaneous abortion, hence herbs were preferred.

> *When I miscarried my previous pregnancy, the TBA told me a different causal reason from my grand mum.... The cause she told me was yellow fever. When I conceived this second pregnancy, she gave me preventive herbs. I started taking from the time my pregnancy was 1 month old. I used to take them daily for 5 days per month until I finished 3 months then she terminated the dose.*

Other natural causes were associated with the foetus itself. For instance, the sex of the foetus and its amount of hair were considered a determining factor of the mother's feelings and physical status during pregnancy. Female foetuses are believed to give the mother nausea, lack of appetite, feeling sickly and make her thin and moody, whereas male foetuses are believed to make the mother crave certain types of food, increased appetite, look healthy, strong and jovial. Abundant foetal hair is associated with heartburn to the mother. It is believed that the long hair stretches to the throat causing the irritation.

Numbness of one leg, which complicates movement during pregnancy, is thought to be caused by the abnormal presentation of the foetus and this is believed to cause complicated delivery. TBAs are believed to have inherited skills to massage the uterus and correctly reposition the foetus, hence relieving discomfort to the mother and making birth easier.

Social causes

The social-based explanations that emerged strongly from the study, as reported by 24% of the respondents, is that a pregnant woman should not contact "dangerous people".

Pregnancy complications were believed to be contagious. For instance, a woman who had ever had an abortion or whose child died recently is considered to be contagious, and if she is in contact with a pregnant woman or her shadow falls on the body of a pregnant woman, it is believed to cause miscarriage, stillbirth, and perinatal death or make the woman sick. Other women believed to be dangerous and who should be avoided included those who had a breech or traverse presentation during birth or a multiple birth, or who experience severe menstrual cramps. This can cause pre-term contractions that might cause spontaneous abortion.

I was told not to meet someone whose child died or to get near her or the one who encountered an abortion. If she gets close to you, your baby might also come out [abortion] *or you can even fall sick.*

Some people are known to have evil eyes that can cause a miscarriage if they meet a pregnant woman. Therefore, a pregnant woman should stay away from such people. Some of these "dangerous" people are known, while others are not. Hence, the main way to reduce the chances of meeting them is to restrict movement outside the homestead, avoid walking along public roads, and going to crowded places such as market centres or other social gatherings.

I was just told when someone is pregnant like me now; I should avoid going where there are a lot of people.

Women are not allowed to visit to places when pregnant. They can meet evil people that can cause problems to the foetus. (Herbalist 1)

As a remedy, herbs are available in a roasted powder form, called *bosarok*, which is to be licked every morning. Pig oil can also be applied on the pregnant woman's face and tummy, especially when she is going on a journey, to counter evil eyes. Such herbs were commonly reported by respondents during the study.

When you wake up in the morning, the first thing you should do even before you wash your face is to lick the 'bosarok' [herbs]. *The timings and location of these women is not known. She might come to your house early in the morning to borrow tea leaves for breakfast. These herbs keep the baby safe in the stomach [womb]. If you use them as reserved, these spirits cannot attack the baby.*

Social relations

A pregnant woman should not exchange utterances or abusive words with anyone. This is because the opponent might "abuse her badly". The feared abuse mostly reported was "you will give birth but you will not hold that baby", referring to a stillbirth. If a pregnant woman is abused with these words, it is believed that this woman will have a stillbirth, or her baby will die shortly after birth. Moreover, the husband of a pregnant woman or any other close person should not do anything or utter words that might annoy or make her cry or emotionally stressed.

When pregnant, you should not quarrel or exchange words with anybody even if you find a person red handed backbiting you or doing something wrong to you. You simply stay silent and assume that nothing is wrong. If you start exchanging words, the person might abuse you badly and at the end you will give birth and your baby dies.

It is not good for a pregnant woman to cry. This is like moaning for her death or that of her unborn child. She might die or give birth to a dead baby.

Therefore, to avoid complications that may lead to a stillbirth or perinatal death, it is recommended to maintain peaceful relationships by avoiding quarrels. Similarly, a pregnant woman should not be abused or offended even if she transgresses anyone. Should she be abused or offended accidentally, the offending person should apologise immediately. If a pregnant woman had a dispute with someone, and this was not resolved, and she develops a complicated labour, the person concerned or who caused her stress will be sought to come and confess, in order to ease labour and facilitate birth. The offender will be held accountable for any calamity and this will cause the person emotions of shame and guilt. Therefore, a pregnant woman is expected to be respected by members of the community.

Supernatural causes

In this category, explanations of pregnancy complications were ascribed to supernatural causes, mostly spirits and to some extent ancestral spirits and gods.

Evil spirit of the dead

A pregnant woman is not supposed to eat meat of an animal carcass, as reported by 38% of the respondents. Such meat was believed to possess evil spirits that are transferable when eaten. The meat commonly reported to be avoided is an animal that was slaughtered because it suffered and died from pregnancy-related complications, such as placental retention, haemorrhage, an abortion or stillbirth. If eaten, it is believed that the "bad blood" that caused such complications is transferred, causing very similar complications to a pregnant woman who consumed it. Similarly, an animal that was slaughtered because it was sick, for unknown reasons, struck by lightning or by strangling itself with its umbilical cord, should not be consumed. The former is believed to cause maternal death whereas the latter will make the umbilical cord coil around the baby's neck resulting in stillbirth. Thus, a pregnant woman should be aware of the meat she eats. However, if she eats it without knowing its provenance, cleansing rituals must be performed to clear off the spirits of the bad blood.

In case there was a goat which died with kids in the stomach, that meat should not be eaten. Or a cow that died during labour, for example the calf came out but placenta retained she should not eat its meat. If she eats it, the placenta will also be retained during birth or she will die just like that animal.

On the other hand, as reported by 29% of the respondents, a pregnant woman or her husband should not kill any animal (wild nor domestic) or insects. Instead, they should get someone from the neighbourhood to do it for them. Otherwise it is believed that she will give birth to a baby with similar features of that animal. Unless they conduct rituals that involve giving the baby the name of that animal, the baby will retain those features to maturity, some of which are dangerous. The commonly mentioned animals were snakes, cats, dogs and chicken, and the killing was believed to cause disabilities such as blindness, lameness or even death.

I was told not to kill a snake; my baby will look like a snake... will have red eyes that look away from each other and unstable neck, just like a snake. They will call the baby 'Kiberen' continuously until the features disappear. The baby will also cry like a cat if you killed a cat or walk using toes like dog with a funny head if you killed a dog. (TBA 3)

Similarly, 26% of the respondents further reported that a pregnant woman is not allowed to view a dead body. The commonly reported forbidden act is viewing the body while inside the coffin or inside the grave. Traditionally, they were not allowed to even attend the funeral as reported by a key informant. If a person dies in the homestead, she moves away until the burial rituals are completed. The husband of a pregnant woman is not allowed to take part in digging the grave and burying of the dead. Many respondents could not understand why it is prohibited, yet they obeyed the custom. However, some respondents reported that a funeral is emotional and it worsens when viewing the body or burying the corpse. These emotions can make one faint and collapse which can cause damage to the uterus resulting in miscarriage e, stillbirth or maternal death.

Gods

Foetal deformity, as reported by 19% of the respondents, could arise if the pregnant woman makes fun of a person with a physical or mental disability. It is believed that this could result in God afflicting the infant with a similar disability.

Other beliefs ascribed to supernatural causes that emerged in the study were based on ancestral spirits, especially if a close relative of the pregnant woman's husband committed an evil act to a deceased member of the family and did not reconcile before he/she died. In this case, therefore, when a pregnant woman undergoes prolonged labour, male elders will be called to conduct reconciliation rituals at the graveyard of the deceased.

Discussion

This study examined the lay meanings ascribed to adverse pregnancy outcomes and the adopted treatment and remedies among the Kalenjin in rural Uasin-Gishu County in Kenya. A healthy pregnancy is perceived as a process that pregnant women are able to manipulate by observing behaviours, and taking remedies against natural, social and supernatural forces during pregnancy. The explanatory models of these local meanings are deliberate attempts to reduce and prevent pregnancy complications but are in many cases based on an understanding of disease transmission that differs from biomedical explanations. Some remedies are beneficial, others make no sense at all, while others to some extent can even be detrimental to maternal health as indicated below.

Restricting geographical mobility

In this study, pregnancy complications are attributed to evil people, so pregnant women are confined to the homestead to avoid contracting evil people and are encouraged to apply medicinal herbs to counter evil. Restrictions on geographical mobility reduce vulnerability to contracting infectious diseases. Pregnant women are at a higher risk and more susceptible to or more severely affected by infectious diseases because of the unique "immunological" condition caused by pregnancy. Infections contracted during pregnancy are in most cases associated with maternal death, stillbirth, spontaneous abortion and pre-term birth, hence this is a good practice that should be enhanced. However, the fears of meeting evil people can result in disruptive or non-use of public health facilities by avoiding going outside. Beliefs in witchcraft, poisoning or spiritual attacks are a major component of African cultures' explanatory model of pregnancy complications and illness and have been established as a major barrier to accessing health facilities for care [18, 19].

Use of herbal medicine

Preventive herbs are believed to protect pregnant woman from getting sick and from transmitting sickness to the foetus. Naturally, pregnancy is a state of immunological weakness, and therefore of increased susceptibility to infectious diseases. Improving the immune system is one of the most important ways of protecting the mother against the environmental infections and preventing damage to the foetus. Malaria In Pregnancy (MIP) is a major public health problem in areas of sub-Saharan Africa, including parts of Kenya, where malaria is endemic, and has important consequences for the birth outcome. Similarly, the risk of pre-term delivery and of miscarriage was found to be high in mothers with HIV and with MIP occurring within 2 weeks of delivery [20]. Use of minerals, plants, and animal products as medicines during pregnancy is a common practice in Kenya, especially among the Kalenjin, to treat pregnancy-related complications and symptoms [10, 21, 22]. Some herbal plants have been confirmed to have antibacterial, anti-inflammatory, antimicrobial and antimalarial properties [23]. However, the safety and efficacy of many of these medicinal herbs, especially during pregnancy, when the human body is vulnerable, still needs to be established.

Avoid sexual intercourse during pregnancy

Ante-natal sexual taboos, which prohibit couples from having sexual intercourse from the second trimester of pregnancy, were also established in the study. In African societies, abstinence from sexual intercourse during pregnancy and for some period after childbirth is a common phenomenon, and is believed to be associated with contamination that might be harmful to the unborn baby or the husband and that the mother is considered to be too fragile to have sex [19, 24, 25]. These women may not justify sexual abstinence during pregnancy in biomedical terms, but scientifically the latent function of this custom is to prevent the transmission of sexually transmitted infections (STIs) to a pregnant woman. STIs, including HIV/AIDS, among pregnant women are common in Kenya [26–28] and have been associated with a number of adverse pregnancy outcomes, such as spontaneous abortion, ectopic pregnancy, pre-term delivery, low birthweight, stillbirth, postpartum sepsis, and congenital infection [28], thus justifying the custom. However, encouraging sexual abstinence during pregnancy might result in men seeking extra-marital sex and might thereby increase the spread of STIs. Some pregnant women in this study opt to use condoms during sexual intercourse to overcome the complications, a practice that needs to be encouraged.

Minimise emotional stress

The belief that a pregnant woman is not supposed to experience emotional stress was also established in this study. Morris [24], in his study in south-eastern Madagascar, also established that prolonged labour and other delivery complications were viewed as resulting from an unsettled feud with someone, especially one's parents or partner, and this can be prevented by resolving feuds or obtaining benediction before or during delivery in order to prevent or resolve complications. A belief that quarrelling, fighting and emotional stress during pregnancy could lead to adverse pregnancy outcomes was also established in some communities in Ghana and Zambia [24, 27]. This is an adoptive practice that is supported by scientific explanations. It not only enhances social cohesion and harmony, but is also beneficial to the wellbeing of the mother and unborn baby. Studies have confirmed that gastritis, hypertensive disorders, pre-term labour, prematurity birth, low birthweight and perinatal death are significantly more frequent among emotionally stressed women [29, 30].

Avoid heavy duties and risky activities but do not stay idle

A number of activities were considered taboo during pregnancy because of their potentially harmful effect on pregnancy and the foetus. Heavy duties such as collecting water from an open well, splitting firewood, digging and bending for long hours as well as running and standing at the doorway are highly discouraged during pregnancy. Some of these activities endanger the pregnancy and others can cause physical injuries, in the case of a fall. Activity during pregnancy is recommended, but heavy duties should be avoided, and enough rest periods assured, especially in late pregnancy and among women with a high-risk profile [31]. Strenuous work, especially involving long hours of standing and walking, seem to have a negative influence on the growth of the foetus and increase the risk of pre-term delivery [31].

On the other hand, physical activities during pregnancy are encouraged. A pregnant woman is recommended to stay active by engaging in light duties. Bed rest during pregnancy decreases the risk of developing severe hypertension [32] and can improve foetal growth [32]. A belief in maintaining light duties during pregnancy was also established in Zambia [33] and Ghana [34]. Hence this belief and practice of avoiding heavy duties and engaging in light physical activities to exercise the body should be encouraged with scientific explanations.

Observing an appropriate diet

Pregnancy food precautions as a concern for a healthy pregnancy and birth outcome were established in this study. Pregnant women are restricted from consuming protein-rich food such as eggs, meat, and fresh milk for fear of CS arising from big babies. More than half of the respondents in this study reported that they were small-scale farmers and the reported farm produce were vegetables, milk and chicken. This means that eggs, milk and meat are the major sources of protein that are readily available and accessible in their environment are restricted. Protein deficiency is often associated with spontaneous abortion [35] hence there is need for health practitioners to raise awareness against this belief for the benefit of the pregnant women and their children. However, in case of cultural sensitivity against this practice, culturally acceptable high-protein foods should be encouraged. Pregnancy food taboos as a way of restricting the foetus from growing too big in order to facilitate an easy birth as found in this study was also established among other communities in Kenya, Ghana, Ethiopia and south-east Nigeria [36–41].

Consumption of the meat of an animal carcass is a taboo that is highly condemned as reported by 38% of the respondents. This is a good practice that needs to be encouraged because studies have confirmed that bacteria in animal carcasses can lead to human illness if consumed [42].

On the other hand, pregnant women were encouraged to eat certain foods that were believed to be important in increasing blood volume and facilitating easy labour and birth. Food believed to increase blood volume include traditional green leafy vegetables, liver, animal blood, fruits, milk, beans, and fish. Iron deficiency anaemia during pregnancy has long been implicated in miscarriage [43] and is the major contributor to post-partum haemorrhage (PPH), which is the single leading cause of maternal mortality and morbidity in low-income countries [44]. More than half of all maternal deaths occur within 24 h of delivery, mostly from excessive bleeding, thus, women's belief is justified and the foods believed to increase the "volume" of blood are truly rich in iron, hence the practice needs to be encouraged. A belief in the importance of iron-rich food in a successful pregnancy outcome was also established in Ghana [45] and Kenya [37, 38].

Pregnant women were also encouraged to consume foods believed to make a pregnant woman strong, because energy is associated with easy birth. Food believed to make a woman strong include *ugali* and porridge made from finger millet mixed with sorghum, and traditional vegetables, milk, traditional herbs and meat. Some of these foods are indeed energy-rich and studies have confirmed that the risk of spontaneous pre-term birth and low birthweight increases in women with limited weight gain [46], hence this practice needs to be encouraged. The importance of acquiring strength during pregnancy was also established in Ghana [45].

Remedies against supernatural attacks

In this study, pregnant women are restricted from killing any animal. The commonly reported animals that should not be killed because of supernatural reasons include dogs, cats, snakes, chicken and insects. These animals if agitated may produce chemical toxins through a bite or sting, which can kill as a defence against the attacker; hence it is a good practice to avoid them. According to Huntingford [47], among the Nandi, it is believed that the spirits of dead ancestors or relatives return to this world to visit their people and they normally travel in the bodies of snakes, moles, or rats, which they use as vehicles to carry them to and from the houses of the living. If a snake or these animals go to people's houses especially at night or to the pregnant woman's bed or house, they may not be killed, as it is believed that they personify the spirit of a deceased ancestor or relative, and that have been sent to indicate to the woman that her next child will be born safely. Instead milk is poured on the ground for it to drink, and then it is allowed to leave the house. If the animal is killed, it will be unable to get back to spirit-land without great difficulty and will be very angry with the offender, resulting in punishment from the spirit. Usually this punishment takes the form of death or illness in man or beast.

In the event that such animals are killed, a pregnant woman is expected to undergo cleansing rituals to end any calamity that is likely to follow her after exposure. The belief that killing of animals will lead into birth of visually impaired child was also established by Ogechi and Ruto among the Gusii and Nandi of Kenya and these were corrected by conducting a ritual [48]. Scientifically, it has been established that maintaining health through spiritual harmony and spiritual healing reduces anxiety, tension and stress associated with (or causing) illness if the patient has faith in the healer, thus increasing the chance for the prescribed therapy to be effective [49]. However, these spiritual healings may coexist or compete with biomedical treatment, thus negatively affecting access and use of health facilities.

Limitations and strengths of the study

This study focused only on pregnancy-related beliefs up to the point of birth. Post-pregnancy beliefs were beyond the scope of this study and hence need follow-up research. Further exploration of views is necessary to explain some of the Kalenjin perceptions and practices. We are also aware that the respondents who were interviewed were those who had sought care at health facilities. They might have different views from those who do not seek such care. Similarly, respondents were selected from rural Uasin Gishu County health facilities, and we do not know the extent to which respondents attending urban facilities might have different perceptions. However, this being an exploratory qualitative study provides a deeper understanding of the phenomenon on question.

Conclusion

This study aimed to gain insight into the socio-cultural perceptions of maternal morbidity, mortality and other complications associated with pregnancy and childbirth and to establish how these perceptions influence maternal health and care-seeking behaviours. This study has shown that traditional beliefs of health and illness continue to shape reproductive and maternal health practices among the Kalenjin women of Kenya. This is shown by the fact that many respondents attribute maternal health complications to taboos of pregnancy and childbirth, such as acceptable foods to eat, places women can and cannot go, activities in which women should or should not engage during pregnancy and the spirits of dead animals and ancestors. Participants also reported using traditional herbal medicine as a healing and preventive remedy during pregnancy and after birth. These cultural taboos and beliefs allow Kalenjin women to make sense of their maternal experiences, and to care for their health, hence shaping their care-seeking behaviours. Some of the cultural remedies adopted to prevent morbidity and mortality during pregnancy are cultural adaptive mechanisms that indirectly control the transmission of disease and improve maternal health and thus should not be considered to be exclusively folk or primitive. Such activities include: condemning the consumption of meat from a dead animal, avoiding heavy duties and going to crowded areas, maintaining good social relations and avoiding emotional events such as funerals. However, other cultural remedies such as restricting diet and geographical mobility, may pose risks to the pregnant woman's health and access to health facilities. The delay in deciding to seek maternal care is a result of women's failure to recognise symptoms and maternal health problems as potentially needing hospital care, and this failure stems from culturally informed perceptions of symptoms of maternal morbidity and pregnancy complications that differ significantly from biomedical implications.

Abbreviations

ANC: Antenatal care; ASALI: A sustainable approach to livelihood improvement; CHWs: Community health workers; CIS: Centre for International Studies; CS: Caesarean section; FGM: Female genital mutilation; KII: Key informant interviews; MCH: Maternal and child healthcare; MIP: Malaria in pregnancy; MMR: Maternal mortality rate; NACOSTI: National Commission for Science, Technology and Innovation; PNC: Post natal care; SEKU: South Eastern Kenya University; STD: Sexually transmitted diseases; STI: Sexually transmitted infection; TB: Tuberculosis; TBAs: Traditional birth attendants; VU: Vrije Universiteit Amsterdam

Acknowledgements

The authors wish to acknowledge the Uasin Gishu County Director of Health and the Health Officers in charge of the health facilities we visited, who were always willing to collaborate or assist us during field research. We also thank the key informants and the women, who willingly shared their childbirth practices, encounters and beliefs with the research team. I would also like to acknowledge Professor Jos van Roosmalen whose contributions enriched the content of this work.

Funding

The authors acknowledge the financial support from A Sustainable Approach to Livelihood Improvement (ASALI) Project. The Project is coordinated by Dr. Denyse Snelder of the Centre for International Students (CIS) at the VU University Amsterdam. ASALI is a joint collaboration project of Moi University Kenya, South Eastern Kenya University (SEKU) and VU University (Vrije Universteit) Amsterdam that is being implemented in Kenya. This financial support proved fundamental to the design of the study, the collection and analysis of data, and the writing of this manuscript.

Declarations

This article is our original work. The data used to write this article is part of broader research investigating the socio-cultural context of maternal nutrition and health in rural Uasin Gishu County in western Kenya. Hence parts of the results presented in this article (demographic characteristics of the respondents, some narratives, ethical clearance, and description of the study area) have been used to publish some work in other journals.

Authors' contributions

RMR, a doctoral candidate, is the main author. She contributed to the conception, study design, planning, data collection, analysis and interpretation and prepared a first draft of the paper. JEWB is the promoter and AKN the co-promoter of RR's PhD program. They both contributed to the study design and interpretation of results. All the authors critically revised the paper and approved the final manuscript for submission.

Authors' information

Roselyter Riang'a is an Assistant Lecturer in the Department of Sociology and Psychology, School of Arts and Social Sciences, Moi University, Kenya. She is also a PhD candidate of Maternal Nutrition and Health at Athena Institute for Research on Innovation and Communication, in the Faculty Science, at the VU University Amsterdam, Prof. Anne Nangulu is the director of quality assurance at the Commission for University Education (CUE) in Kenya and also a professor of economic history at Moi University, Kenya. Prof. Dr. Jacqueline Broerse is Professor of Innovation and Communication at the VU University, Amsterdam in the Health and Life Sciences. She is also the Research Director of the Faculty of Sciences, VU University, Amsterdam.

Competing interests

The authors declare that they have no financial or personal relationship(s) that may have inappropriately influenced them in writing this article. The financial grant for this study was only meant for the design of the study, the collection and analysis of data, and the writing of this manuscript.

Author details

[1]School of Arts and Social Sciences, Moi University, P.O. Box 3900-30100, Eldoret, Kenya. [2]Athena Institute, Faculty of Science, Vrije Universiteit Amsterdam, De Boelelaan 1085, 1081 HV Amsterdam, The Netherlands.
[3]Commission for University Education, Red Hill Road, off Limuru Road, Gigiri, PO Box 54999 – 00200, Nairobi, Kenya.

References

1. Adegoke AA, Van Den Broek N. Skilled birth attendance-lessons learnt. BJOG Int J Obstet Gynaecol. 2009;116:33–40.
2. Cheptum JJ, Oyore JP. Poor pregnancy outcomes in public health facilities in Kenya. Afr J Midwifery Womens. Health. 2012;6:185–90.
3. World Health Organization. Trends in maternal mortality: 1990 to 2015. Geneva: WHO Press; 2015.
4. Jebet J, Oyore JP. Poor pregnancy outcomes in public health facilities in Kenya; 2015. p. 4–10.
5. Magadi M, Diamond IAN, Madise N. Analysis of factors associated with maternal mortality in Kenyan hospitals. J Biosoc Sci. 2001;33:375–89.
6. World Health Organization. WHO Global Health Observatory (GHO) data global on maternal health indicators, 2017 update [internet]. Genever: World Health Organization; 2017. Available from: http://www.who.int/gho/maternal_health/en/

7. Kenya National Bureau of Statistics, ICF Macro. Kenya Demographic and Health Survey 2014. Rockville: ICF International; 2014.
8. Wanjira C, Mwangi M, Mathenge E, Mbugua G, Ng'ang'a Z. Delivery practices and associated factors among mothers seeking child welfare Services in Selected Health Facilities in Nyandarua South District, Kenya. BMC Public Health. 2011;11:360 Available from: http://www.biomedcentral.com/1471-2458/11/360.
9. van Eijk AM, Bles HM, Odhiambo F, Ayisi JG, Blokland IE, Rosen DH, et al. Use of antenatal services and delivery care among women in rural western Kenya: a community based survey. Reprod Health. 2006;3:2.
10. Kaingu CK, Oduma JA, Kanui TI. Practices of traditional birth attendants in Machakos District, Kenya. J Ethnopharmacol. 2011;137:495–502 Available from: http://ac.els-cdn.com/S0378874111004090/1-s2.0-S0378874111004090-main.pdf?_tid=41a99bf2-f8a7-11e4-b07d-00000aacb361&acdnat=1431435977_24d6321d00c99d0e264a9f6cda97caaa.
11. Kenya National Bureau of Statistics (KNBS); ORC Macro. Kenya Demographic and Health Survey 2008-09. Maryland: Calverton; 2010.
12. County Government of Uasin Gishu Department of Health Services. County health strategic and investment plan 2013-2018. Nairobi; 2013.
13. Miller E. Maternal health and knowledge and infant health outcomes in the Ariaal people of northern Kenya. Soc Sci Med. 2011;73:1266–1274. Available from: https://doi.org/10.1016/J.SOCSCIMED.2011.07.009
14. Montesanti SR. Cultural Perceptions of Maternal Illness among Khmer Women in Krong Kep, Cambodia. vis-à-vis Explor Anthropol. 2011;11:90–106 Available from: http://vav.library.utoronto.ca/index.php/vav/article/view/12664.
15. Helman CG. Cuture health and Illiness. 5th. Purdy JK and S, editor. London: Hodder Arnold; 2007.
16. Kothari CR. Research methodology: methods and techniques. New Delhi: New Age International (P) Limited; 2004.
17. Grinnel RM, Unrau YA. Social work research and evaluation: foundations of evidence based-evaluations. 8th ed. New York: Open University Press; 2007.
18. Mathole T, Lindmark G, Majoko F, Lecturer S, Ahlberg BM. A qualitative study of women ' s perspectives of antenatal care in a rural area of Zimbabwe; 2004. p. 122–32.
19. Ngomane S, Mulaudzi FM. Indigenous beliefs and practices that influence the delayed attendance of antenatal clinics by women in the Bohlabelo district in Limpopo, South Africa. Midwifery. 2012;28:30–8 Available from: http://www.sciencedirect.com/science/article/pii/S0266613810001816.
20. de Beaudrap P, Turyakira E, White LJ, Nabasumba C, Tumwebaze B, Muehlenbachs A, et al. Impact of malaria during pregnancy on pregnancy outcomes in a Ugandan prospective cohort with intensive malaria screening and prompt treatment; 2013. p. 1–11.
21. Hillary NC. Utilization of herbal medicine during pregnancy, labour and post-partum period among women at Embu provincial general hospital: Nairobi University, College of Humanities and Social Sciences, Sociology; 2013.
22. Mothupi MC. Use of herbal medicine during pregnancy among women with access to public healthcare in Nairobi, Kenya: a cross-sectional survey. BMC Complement Altern Med. 2014. Article Number 432. Date Publ. Novemb. 04, 2014. 2014;1–8.
23. Towns AM, Van Andel T. Wild plants, pregnancy, and the food-medicine continuum in the southern regions of Ghana and Benin. J Ethnopharmacol. 2016;179:375–82.
24. Morris JL, Short S, Robson L, Andriatsihosena MS. Maternal health practices, beliefs and traditions in Southeast Madagascar. Afr J Reprod Health. 2014;18:101–17.
25. Maimbolwa MC, Yamba B, Diwan V, Ransjö-Arvidson AB. Cultural childbirth practices and beliefs in Zambia. J Adv Nurs. 2003;43:263–74.
26. Fonck K, Kidula N, Jaoko W, Estambale B, Claeys P, Kirui P, et al. Validity of the vaginal discharge algorithm among pregnant and non-pregnant women in Nairobi, Kenya; 2000. p. 33–8.
27. Masha SC, Wahome E, Vaneechoutte M, Cools P, Crucitti T, Sanders EJ. High prevalence of curable sexually transmitted infections among pregnant women in a rural county hospital in Kilifi, Kenya. 2017;1–16. Available from: doi: https://doi.org/10.1371/journal.pone.0175166
28. Mullick S, Beksinska M, Mabey D. Sexually transmitted infections in pregnancy: prevalence, impact on pregnancy outcomes, and approach to treatment in developing countries. Trop Med. 2005;81:294–302.
29. Lukasse M, Helbig A, Eberhard-gran M. Antenatal Maternal Emotional Distress and Duration of Pregnancy; 2014. p. 9.
30. Tandu-umba B, Dedetemo DK, Mananga GL. Maternal stress and pregnancy outcomes *. Open J Obstet Gynecol. 2014;4:361–70.
31. Ahlborg JG. Physical work load and pregnancy outcome. J Occup Environ Med. 1995;37:941–4.
32. Crowther CA, Bouwmeester AM, Ashurst HM. Does admission to hospital for bed rest prevent disease progression or improve fetal outcome in pregnancy complicated by non-proteinuric hypertension? Obstet Gynaecol. 1992;99:13–7.
33. M'soka NC, Mabuza LH, Pretorius D. Cultural and health beliefs of pregnant women in Zambia regarding pregnancy and child birth. Curationis. 2015;38:1–7 Available from: http://www.curationis.org.za/index.php/curationis/article/view/1232.
34. Dako-Gyeke P, Aikins M, Aryeetey R, McCough L, Adongo PB. The influence of socio-cultural interpretations of pregnancy threats on health-seeking behavior among pregnant women in urban Accra, Ghana. BMC Pregnancy Childbirth. 2013;13:211.
35. Ebina Y, Ieko M, Naito S, Kobashi G, Deguchi M, Minakami H, Tatsuya Atsumi HY. O127. Low levels of plasma protein S, protein C and coagulation factor XII during early pregnancy and adverse pregnancy outcome. Pregnancy Hypertens An Int J Women's Cardiovasc Heal. 2015;5:239–40.
36. Ekwochi U, Osuorah CDI, Ndu IK, Ifediora C, Asinobi IN, Eke CB. Food taboos and myths in south eastern Nigeria: the belief and practice of mothers in the region. J Ethnobiol Ethnomed. 2016;12:17 Available from: http://www.ethnobiomed.com/content/12/1/7.
37. Riang'a RM, Broerse J, Nangulu AK. Food beliefs and practices among the Kalenjin pregnant women in rural Uasin Gishu County , Kenya. J Ethnobiol Ethnomed. 2017;13:29.
38. Riang'a RM, Nangulu AK, Broerse JEW. "When a woman is pregnant, her grave is open": health beliefs concerning dietary practices among pregnant Kalenjin women in rural Uasin Gishu County, Kenya. J Health Popul Nutr. 2017;36:53 Available from: https://jhpn.biomedcentral.com/articles/10.1186/s41043-017-0130-0.
39. Zepro NB. Food taboos and misconceptions among pregnant women of Shashemene District, Ethiopia, 2012. Scinence J Public Heal. 2015;3:410–6.
40. Arzoaquoi SK, Essuman EE, Gbagbo FY, Tenkorang EY, Soyiri I, Laar AK. Motivations for food prohibitions during pregnancy and their enforcement mechanisms in a rural Ghanaian district. J Ethnobiol Ethnomed. 2015;11:59 Available from: http://www.ethnobiomed.com/content/11/1/59.
41. Demissie T, Muroki N, Kogi-makau W. Food taboos among pregnant women in Hadiya zone. Ethiop J Heal Dev [Internet]. 1998;12:2–7 Available from: http://www.ethiopianreview.com/1995/Tsegaye_Demissie_Nelson_Muroki_Wamboi_Kogi_Makau_1995.pdf.
42. Crump JA, Griffin PM, Angulo FJ. Bacterial contamination of animal feed and its relationship to human foodborne illness. Clin Infect Dis. 2002;35:859–65.
43. Nair M, Choudhury MK, Choudhury SS, Kakoty SD, Sarma UC, Webster P, et al. Association between maternal anaemia and pregnancy outcomes: a cohort study in Assam, India. BMJ Glob Heal. 2016;1:e000026 Available from: http://gh.bmj.com/lookup/doi/10.1136/bmjgh-2015-000026.
44. Khan KS, Wojdyla D, Say L, Gulmezoglu AM, Van Look PF. WHO analysis of causes of maternal death: a systematic review. Lancet. 2006;367:1066–74.
45. Aikins A. Food beliefs and practices during pregnancy in Ghana: implications for maternal health interventions. Health Care Women Int. 2014;9332:954–72.
46. Lumbanraja S, Lutan D, Usman I. Maternal weight gain and correlation with birth weight infants. Procedia Soc Behav Sci. 2013;103:647–56 Available from: http://www.sciencedirect.com/science/article/pii/S1877042813038287.
47. Huntingford GWB. The Nandi of Kenya: tribal control in pastoral socirty. First. London: Routledge and Kegan Paul Ltd; 1953.
48. Ogechi NO, Ruto SJ. Portrayal of disability through personal names and proverbs in Kenya: evidence from Ekegusii and Nandi. Stichproben Wiener Zeitschrift für Krit Afrikastudien. 2002;3:63–82.
49. Stark L. Cleansing the wounds of war: an examination of traditional healing, psychosocial health and reintegration in Sierra Leone. Intervention. 2006;4:206–18.

Incidence of maternal near miss in the public health sector of Harare, Zimbabwe

Henry Chikadaya*, Mugove Gerald Madziyire and Stephen P. Munjanja

Abstract

Background: Maternal 'near miss' can be a proxy for maternal death and it describes women who nearly died due to obstetric complications. It measures life threatening pregnancy related complications and allows the assessment of the quality of obstetric care.

Methods: A prospective descriptive study was carried out from October 1 2016 to 31 December 2016, using the WHO criteria for maternal 'near miss' at the two tertiary public hospitals which receive referrals of all obstetric complications in Harare city, Zimbabwe. The objective was to calculate the ratio of maternal 'near miss' and associated factors. All pregnant women who developed life threatening complications classified as maternal near miss using the WHO criteria were recruited and followed up for six weeks from discharge, delivery or termination of pregnancy or up to the time of death.

Results: During this period there were 11,871 births. One hundred and twenty three (123) women developed severe maternal outcomes, 110 were maternal 'near miss' morbidity and 13 were maternal deaths. The maternal 'near miss' ratio was 9.3 per 1000 deliveries, the mortality index (MI) was 10.6% and the maternal mortality ratio was 110 per 100,000 deliveries. The major organ dysfunction among cases with severe maternal outcomes (SMO) was cardiovascular dysfunction (76.9%). The major causes of maternal near miss were obstetric haemorrhage (31.8%), hypertensive disorders (28.2%) and complications of miscarriages (20%). The intensive care unit (ICU) admission rate was 7.3 per 100 cases of SMO and 88.8% of maternal deaths occurred without ICU admission.

Conclusion: The MNM ratio was comparable to that in the region. Obstetric haemorrhage was a leading cause of severe maternal morbidity though with less mortality when compared to hypertensive disorders and abortion complications. Zimbabwe should adopt maternal near miss ratio as an indicator for evaluating its maternal health services.

Keywords: Maternal near miss, Maternal mortality, Severe maternal morbidity, Severe maternal outcome, Mortality indexs

Background

Maternal morbidity is part of a continuum from maternal good health to maternal mortality. In any setting, women who suffer severe maternal complications share many circumstantial and pathological factors related to their condition [1]. Some women die as a result of these complications, but a proportion of them narrowly escape death either by chance or due to the quality of care they receive [2]. Maternal deaths (MD) can be likened to the 'tip of an iceberg' with the base being maternal morbidity, in that more women survive pregnancy complications than the ones who die [3, 4]. The primary indicator of maternal health care and hence quality of obstetric care is Maternal Mortality Ratio (MMR) [5]. By monitoring only maternal deaths at institutions, very few lessons can be learnt to prevent further deaths. This is further compounded by the fact that in maternal death review meetings most of the patient's records are either missing or incompletely filled [6, 7]. Quality of obstetric care can be assessed using either outcome indicators like maternal mortality ratio, or MNM

* Correspondence: drhenrychikadaya@gmail.com
Department of Obstetrics and Gynaecology, University of Zimbabwe College of Health Sciences, Central Hospital, P O Box ST 14, Southerton, Harare, Zimbabwe

indicators or using process indicators such as the use of prophylactic antibiotics for the reduction of puerperal sepsis after caesarian section [1, 8].

In 2009, the WHO introduced the concept of 'maternal near miss'(MNM) for evaluating the quality of care for severe pregnancy complications [1]. A MNM is defined as a case of a woman who nearly died but survived a complication that has occurred during pregnancy, childbirth or within 42 days of termination of pregnancy [1]. Studying MNM is increasingly being recognized as a useful means to improve the quality of obstetric care, particularly in low and middle income countries [2]. It is estimated that for every woman who dies 20 or more survive severe maternal complications as a result of the pregnancy or delivery [9].

The underlying assumptions of WHO MNM concept are that all maternal deaths involve at least one life threatening condition or organ dysfunction and a substantial proportion of women with one or more of these life threatening conditions are those who have severe pregnancy-related complications or receive critical interventions like blood transfusion and ICU admission [1].

The WHO criteria for MNM are based on clinical, laboratory as well as management based proxies for organ or system dysfunction [1]. The WHO recommends that the maternal near miss approach should be considered in national plans for improving maternal health care [10]. Using near miss indicators has several advantages in that it offers a large number of cases that allows a more rapid and precise assessment of quality of care, it has greater acceptability by involved health workers and institutions since death has not occurred, and it offers an opportunity for interviewing the women themselves [11]. Maternal mortality is among the worst performing health indicators in developing countries [7]. The WHO near miss clinical based criteria when used in Tanzania taking into account available resources, had an improved sensitivity (99.5%) and specificity (100%) for detecting maternal deaths [12].

In Zimbabwe maternal mortality remains high, even in urban settings although women in rural areas are at a significantly higher risk of dying from pregnancy complications [13, 14]. The latest maternal mortality ratio in Zimbabwe is 651 per 100,000 live births [15]. The quality of obstetric care is a large driver of poor maternal outcomes. Recently, there has been some studies that sought to address this issue [9, 14, 16–18]. The maternal mortality ratio patterns established using these retrospective studies are often imprecise and make it difficult to monitor trends or progress regarding the targets of improving maternal care [5]. The burden of severe maternal morbidity is unknown in Zimbabwe including in the public health sector of Harare. We therefore sought to assess the burden of severe maternal morbidity by calculating the MNM ratio and describe factors associated with MNM in the public health sector of Harare city.

Methods

Aim

We aimed to establish the MNM ratio and factors associated with severe maternal morbidity in the public sector of Harare.

Research design

A prospective descriptive study was carried out. This was a quantitative design that concentrated in the collection of numerical data on the occurrences of severe maternal outcomes and associated factors.

Setting

The population of the city of Harare is 1.542 million. The public sector health facilities of Harare are composed of two hospitals, Harare Central Hospital and Parirenyatwa Hospital and 12 local authority clinics which offer maternity services. The two hospitals are the tertiary hospitals which also serve as the teaching units for the University of Zimbabwe. The 12 local authority clinics are located in residential areas. They provide antenatal care, vaginal deliveries and postnatal care to low risk women. If a high risk pregnancy is identified, or there is a need for a caesarean section, or an obstetric emergency arises, referral is made to either of the two hospitals for further care. Women registered for follow up in a particular unit are referred to as having booked their pregnancies. The two tertiary hospitals also receive referrals from rural provinces across Zimbabwe. Private care maternity services are provided by five smaller facilities mainly located near the central business district.

Participants

The participants were women who delivered or miscarried, or who had antenatal complications leading to a near miss condition according to WHO near miss criteria in the public health sector of Harare City during the period 1st October to 31st December 2016. We excluded women who had been referred from facilities outside Harare.

A target sample size of 96 was determined using a single proportion formula [19], and the incidence of MNM in a study done at Haydom Lutheran Hospital in Tanzania (23.6 per 1000 live births) which had the highest incidence in the region [20].

Data collection

Identification of cases was carried out through review of all the women admitted into the obstetrics and gynaecology units at the two tertiary hospitals. Data was collected from patient registers and case notes by the principal researcher and two research assistants. Once the patient was treated and in a stable condition, informed consent was sought. The managing clinicians were questioned in case of doubt or missing information. At the local clinics data was obtained on the total number of deliveries. Data was collected from the 1st of October to the 31st of December 2016.

The primary outcome measure was the MNM ratio in the public sector of Harare during the study period. Secondary outcome indicators such as the MMR, Severe Maternal Outcomes (SMO) ratio, and the Mortality Index (MI) were calculated. SMO – refers to a life threatening condition, i.e. organ dysfunction or death hence includes MNM and maternal deaths. SMO ratio (SMOR) is the number of MNM plus MD per 1000 LB. MNM ratio refers to the number of maternal near-miss cases per 1000 live births (MNMR = MNM/LB). These two indicators, SMO ratio and MNM ratio, give an estimate of the amount of care and resources that would be needed in an area or facility. Maternal near-miss mortality ratio (MNM: 1 MD) refers to the ratio between maternal near- miss cases and maternal deaths. Higher ratios indicate better care. MI refers to the number of maternal deaths divided by the sum of women with life-threatening conditions and maternal deaths expressed as a percentage [MI = MD/ (MNM + MD)]. The higher the index the more women with life-threatening conditions die (low quality of care), whereas the lower the index the fewer women with life-threatening conditions die (better quality of care).

Data was entered and cleaned using IBM SPSS statistics data editor version 20. Frequency tables and cross tabulations were produced for the demographic and clinical variables as well as for the underlying causes.

Ethical clearance was sought and obtained from: Harare Central Hospital Ethics Committee (HCHEC 240616/40); The Director, City of Harare Department of Health; The Joint Research Ethics Committee (JREC Ref: 222/16); Medical Research Council of Zimbabwe (MRCZ/B/1130).

Results

The total number of deliveries in the public sector of Harare was 11,871 during the study period. Most of the deliveries occurred at the local clinics [6475(54%)], while 27% (3185) and 19% (2211) were delivered at Harare and Parirenyatwa hospitals respectively. Of these, 123 women developed SMO of which 13 were maternal deaths and 110 were maternal near misses. The median age for severe maternal outcomes was 28 years. Median parity was two. Most of the women were married, educated up to secondary level and 60.8% were homemakers. Most (80%) were Christians (Table 1). The maternal near miss ratio was 9.3 per 1000 deliveries, 95% confidence interval (C I) of 7.6–11.0 per 1000 deliveries, with a mortality index of 10.6%. For every maternal death, there were 8.5 maternal near miss events. The maternal mortality ratio was 110/100000 live births, 95% C I of 50–170 deaths per 100,000 live births (Table 2). Of the women who developed severe maternal outcomes 66.7% (82) were referred from local clinics, while 24% (30), 8% (10) were booked at Harare and Parirenyatwa hospitals respectively. One woman came from home.

The major underlying causes of maternal near miss were obstetric hemorrhage (31.8%), hypertensive disorders (28.2%) and complications of miscarriages (20%) (Table 3). Among maternal deaths hypertensive disorders of pregnancy were the leading cause accounting for four (30.8%) of deaths, followed by medical disorders [3(23.1%)] and obstetric haemorrhage [3(23.1%)]. The major organ dysfunction among cases with severe maternal outcomes was cardiovascular dysfunction (76.9%),

Table 1 Demographic data of women with severe maternal outcomes (n = 123) at Harare and Parirenyatwa hospitals in October–December 2016

Characteristic	Parameter	Number	%
Age	Median (interquartile range)	28 (10)	
Parity	Median (interquartile range)	2 (2)	
Marital status	Married	117	90.1
	Single (never married)	9	6.9
	Divorced/separated	2	1.5
	Widowed	2	1.5
Level of education	Primary	12	9.2
	Secondary	114	87.7
	Tertiary	4	3.1
Occupation	Homemaker	79	60.8
	Unskilled	25	19.2
	Peasant farmer	1	0.8
	Semi- skilled	22	16.9
	Skilled	3	2.3
Religion	Christianity	104	80.0
	Traditional	2	1.5
	Apostolic	23	17.7

Table 2 Summary of deliveries and severe maternal outcomes and near miss indicators in women delivering at public health sector institutions of Harare in October–December 2016

Outcomes	Near-miss indicators
Total deliveries	11,871
Severe maternal outcomes (SMO) cases (number)	123
Maternal deaths (n)	13
Maternal near-miss cases (n)	110
Severe maternal outcome ratio (per 1000 deliveries)	10.4
Maternal near-miss ratio (per 1000 deliveries)	9.3CI 95%: (7.6–11.0)
Maternal mortality ratio (per 100,000 live births)	110 CI 95%: (50–170)
Maternal near-miss: mortality ratio	8.5:1
Mortality index	10.6%

Table 3 Underlying causes and organ dysfunction in SMO

Underlying causes	MNM (*n* = 110) N (%)	MD (*n* = 13) N (%)	MI (%)
Obstetric hemorrhage	35 (31.8)	2 (15.4)	5.4
Hypertensive disorders	31 (28.2)	4 (30.6)	11.4
Abortion related complications	22 (20)	3 (23.1)	12
Pregnancy-related infection	15 (13.6)	1 (7.7)	6.3
Ruptured ectopic pregnancy	11 (10)	0 (0)	0
Medical disorder	4 (3.6)	3 (23.1)	75
Parasuicide/suicide	1 (0.9)	1 (7.7)	50
Unanticipated complications of management	1 (0.9)	0 (0)	0
Organ Dysfunction			
Cardiovascular dysfunction	72 (65.5)	10 (76.9)	
Respiratory dysfunction	23 (20.9)	9 (69.2)	
Coagulation/hematologic dysfunction	12 (10.9)	3 (23.1)	
Renal dysfunction	4 (3.6)	2 (15.4)	
Hepatic dysfunction	3 (2.7)	0 (0)	
Uterine dysfunction/hysterectomy	2 (1.8)	0 (0)	

SMO severe maternal outcomes which refers to women with life-threatening conditions and maternal deaths, *MNM* maternal near miss cases, *MD* maternal death cases, *MI* mortality index calculated as number of maternal deaths divided by the sum of women with life-threatening conditions and maternal deaths expressed as a percentage [MI = MD/ (MNM + MD)]

Respiratory dysfunction (69.2), haematologic dysfunction (23.1%) and renal dysfunction (15.4%). There were 9 out of 123 cases of severe maternal outcomes admitted into ICU, giving an ICU admission rate of 7.3 cases per 100 cases of SMO and 88.8% of maternal deaths occurred without ICU admission.

Discussion

The MNM ratio was 9.3 per 1000 deliveries and the leading cause was obstetric hemorrhage. The MNM ratio was within the range of MNM ratios described by WHO of around 7.5 cases per 1000 deliveries [1]. In a systematic review by Tuncalp et al., the MNM ratio varies depending on the criteria used and is higher in low and medium income countries [21]. Our MNM ratio is higher when compared to the MNM ratio from a South African study, which reported 4.3 per 1000 [22], and lower to that from a study in Tanzania, (23.6 per 1000 live births) [20].. This could be explained firstly by the fact that in this study we used a broader definition of MNM which included complications of miscarriages and ectopic pregnancies unlike the criteria in the South African study, secondly because the Tanzanian study was hospital based.

The MMR in this study was 110 per 100,000 live births which is lower than the national level of 651 per 100,000 live births [15] and a notable decrease from 361 per 100,000 live births in 2010 in the same population [23]. This shows a continued downward trend likely due to increased resource allocation. Most (67%) patients who developed SMO had booked at local clinics i.e. were low risk women. This was similar to findings from the South African study that reported that a significant proportion of serious complications occur in women who are otherwise regarded as low risk [22] highlighting increased vigilance during antenatal clinic visits for apparently low risk women. The leading underlying causes of SMO in this study are similar to the top 5 causes of maternal mortality in Zimbabwe quoted in various studies [9, 17, 23]. This confirms that MNM can be a proxy for MM [1]. The overall MI was 10.6%. which is comparable to the one from a South African study (14%) [22]. The MI was lowest for obstetric haemorrhage (5.4) and high for hypertensive disorders (11.4), abortion complications (12.0) and medical disorders. This is likely because of improved management of obstetric haemorrhage as a result of availability of free blood and in service training in obstetric emergencies funded by aid organizations. However, hemorrhage is still a leading cause of MNM and there is need for continued health system strengthening so as not to lose gains made by wide spread in service training in the management of obstetric emergencies. The MI for medical disorders is distorted by a low number of cases as there were only 4 cases and 3 of them died. A multi-disciplinary approach is however needed when managing patients with medical conditions in pregnancy so as to recognize complications early. While in service training in obstetric emergencies cover all areas there is need to improve the management protocols for hypertensive disorders and post abortion complications. Most deaths as a result of miscarriages were occurring within hours of arrival which suggests the unsafe nature of abortions in the communities. Earlier studies have also reported a higher case fatality rate from hypertensive disorders and this was reported to be due to inadequate case management [23, 24].

The ICU admission rate among SMO is low and most deaths occurred without being admitted into ICU. There is greater demand for ICU at our tertiary hospitals from non-obstetric cases as well as referrals from rural provinces. There is need to have an ICU dedicated to the maternity units alone. There is also need to better equip hospital wards to have high dependency units with adequate human and material resources so as to improve patient outcome.

Strengths and weakness

Strengths

This study was prospective in nature with every case of severe maternal outcome providing a full complete account of events as outlined in the questionnaire and hence avoiding problems associated with missing records in retrospective studies. We used a validated standard data collection tool and criteria for near miss morbidity that had been used elsewhere in similar low resource settings [11, 12, 20, 22, 25]. Our study was population based which avoids erroneous figures associated with institutional based data due to concentration of complicated cases.

Weaknesses

Data collection was based at the two tertiary hospitals and we did not capture cases that crossed over to or were completely managed in the private sector. This number will be low however as there are only 5 private hospitals in Harare with a capacity to attend to obstetric complications and their combined delivery capacity is about 6544/year versus about 50,000 per year for the tertiary hospitals [23]. This was a cross sectional study done over a 3 month period and hence can miss morbidity or mortality patterns due to seasonal trends.

Conclusion

The MNM ratio of 9.3 per thousand deliveries was comparable to other reports in the region. The mortality index was 10.6%, which is high. Obstetric haemorrhage was a leading cause of severe maternal morbidity though with less mortality when compared to hypertensive disorders and abortion complications. Zimbabwe should adopt the maternal near miss ratio as an indicator for evaluating its maternal health services. There is need for a nationwide study on the incidence of MNM to rule out regional variability and to include facilities that offer comprehensive emergency obstetric care in the sample. Well-equipped maternity HDUs and ICUs should be established to reduce the MI from obstetric emergencies.

Abbreviations

HDU: High dependence unit; ICU: Intensive care unit; MD: Maternal deaths; MI: Mortality index; MMR: Maternal mortality ratio; MNM: Maternal near miss; SMO: Severe maternal outcomes; WHO: World Health Organization

Acknowledgements

I would like to acknowledge Munyaradzi Damson for statistical support.

Funding

No external funding was obtained for this study.

Authors' contributions

HC was primarily responsible for conceiving of the project, and HC, MGM and SM for carrying out data collection, analysis and drafting of the manuscript. All authors have read and approved the final manuscript.

Competing interests

The authors declare that they have no competing interests.

References

1. WHO. Evalauting the quality of care for severe pregnancy complications. In: The WHO near-miss approach for maternal health; 2011. Report No.: 978 92 4 150222 1.
2. Filippi V, Brugha R, Browne E, Gohou V, Bacci A, De Brouwere V, et al. Obstetric audit in resource-poor settings: lessons from a multi-country project auditing 'near miss' obstetrical emergencies. Health Policy Plan. 2004 Jan;19(1):57–66.
3. Kilpatrick SK, Ecker JL, Callaghan WM. Severe maternal morbidity: screening and review. Am J Obstet Gynecol. 2016;215(3):B17–22.
4. Geller SE, Cox SM, Callaghan WM, Berg CJ. Morbidity and mortality in pregnancy: laying the groundwork for safe motherhood. Womens Health Issues. 2006 Jul-Aug;16(4):176–88.
5. Munjanja SP. Joining the dots: a plea for precise estimates of the maternal mortality ratio in sub-Saharan Africa. BJOG. 2009;116(Suppl 1):7–10.
6. Magwali TL, Mataya R, Munjanja SP, Chirehwa M. An assessment of the maternal death notification system in Zimbabwe--2006. The Central African journal of medicine. 2011;57(1–4):8–11.
7. Say L, Souza JP, Pattinson RC. Maternal near miss--towards a standard tool for monitoring quality of maternal health care. Best practice & research. 2009;23(3):287–96.
8. Silva AL, Mendes Ada C, Miranda GM, Sa DA, Souza WV, Lyra TM. Evaluation of maternal and neonatal hospital care: quality index of completeness. Revista de saude publica. 2014;48(4):682–91 discussion 91.
9. Ministry of Health and Child Care. Maternal and perinatal mortality 2007. Harare Ministry of health and Chid care 2009.
10. Pattinson R, Say L, Souza JP, Broek N, Rooney C. WHO maternal death and near-miss classifications. Bull World Health Organ. 2009;87(10):734.
11. Kalra P, Kachhwaha CP. Obstetric near miss morbidity and maternal mortality in a tertiary Care Centre in Western Rajasthan. Indian J Public Health. 2014;58(3):199–201.
12. Nelissen E, Mduma E, Broerse J, Ersdal H, Evjen-Olsen B, van Roosmalen J, et al. Applicability of the WHO maternal near miss criteria in a low-resource setting. PLoS One. 2013;8(4):e61248.
13. Lawson GW, Keirse MJ. Reflections on the maternal mortality millennium goal. Birth. 2013;40(2):96–102.
14. UN-ZW. Maternal Mortality in Zimbabwe. Evidence, Costs and Implications Periodic Publications 2013;Paper 1(Issue Paper Series).
15. Zimbabwe National Statistics Agency and ICF International. Zimbabwe Demographic and Health Survey 2015: Key Indicators;2016.
16. Zishiri C, Shodu LK, Tshimanga M, Nyirongo L. Post natal maternal morbidity patterns in mothers delivering in Gweru City (midlands province). The Central African journal of medicine. 1999;45(9):234–9.
17. Majoko F, Chipato T, Iliff V. Trends in maternal mortality for the greater Harare maternity unit: 1976 to 1997. The Central African journal of medicine. 2001;47(8):199–203.
18. MOHCW. Zimbabwe National Integrated Health Facility Assessment Dec 2011- Jan 2012. In: Ministry of Health and child welfare Zimbabwe; 2012.
19. Dobson AJ. Calculating sample size. Transactions of the Menzies Foundation. 1984;7:75–9.
20. Nelissen EJ, Mduma E, Ersdal HL, Evjen-Olsen B, van Roosmalen JJ, Stekelenburg J. Maternal near miss and mortality in a rural referral hospital in northern Tanzania: a cross-sectional study. BMC pregnancy and childbirth. 2013;13:141.
21. Tuncalp O, Hindin MJ, Souza JP, Chou D, Say L. The prevalence of maternal near miss: a systematic review. BJOG. 2012;119(6):653–61.
22. Soma-Pillay P, Pattinson RC, Langa-Mlambo L, Nkosi BS, Macdonald AP. Maternal near miss and maternal death in the Pretoria academic complex, South Africa: a population-based study. South African medical journal = Suid-Afrikaanse tydskrif vir geneeskunde. 2015;105(7):578–63.
23. Manjeya F. Trends in maternal mortality for Greater Harare Maternity Unit. 2010–2014. Harare: University of Zimbabwe; 2014.
24. Majoko F, Mujaji C. Maternal outcome in eclampsia at Harare maternity hospital. The Central African journal of medicine. 2001;47(5):123–8.

Maternal dietary consumption of legumes, vegetables and fruit during pregnancy, does it protect against small for gestational age?

Juan Miguel Martínez-Galiano[1,2*], Carmen Amezcua-Prieto[2,3,4], Inmaculada Salcedo-Bellido[2,3,4], Guadalupe González-Mata[1], Aurora Bueno-Cavanillas[2,3,4] and Miguel Delgado-Rodríguez[1,2]

Abstract

Background: Different diets during pregnancy might have an impact on the health, reflected in the birthweight of newborns. The consumption of fruits and vegetables during pregnancy and the relationship with newborn health status have been studied by several authors. However, these studies have shown inconsistent results. Purpose: We assessed whether certain foods were related to the risk of small for gestational age (SGA).

Methods: A matched by age (± 2 years) and hospital 1:1 case-control study of 518 pairs of pregnant Spanish women in five hospitals was conducted. The cases were women with an SGA newborn at delivery (neonates weighting less than the 10th percentile, adjusted for gestational age at delivery and sex, were diagnosed as SGA). The control group comprised women giving birth to babies adequate for gestational age (AGA). Mothers who gave birth to babies large for gestational age (LGA) were excluded. Data were gathered concerning demographic characteristics, socioeconomic status, toxic habits and diet. A food frequency questionnaire (FFQ) comprising 137 items was completed by all participants. The intake of vegetables, legumes and fruits was categorized in quintiles (Q1–Q5). Crude values and and adjusted odds ratios (AORs) and 95% confidence intervals (CIs) were estimated using conditional logistic regression. The variables for adjustment were as follows: preeclampsia, education, smoking, weight gain per week during pregnancy, fish intake and previous preterm/low birthweight newborns.

Results: Total pulse intake showed an inverse association with the risk of SGA (trend $p = 0.02$). Women with an intake of fruits above 420 g/day (Q5), compared with women in Q1 (≤ 121 g/day) showed a decreased risk of SGA (AOR = 0.63, 95% CI = 0.40–0.98). The total consumption of vegetables was not associated with the risk of SGA. The intake of selenium was assessed: a protective association was observed for Q3–5; a daily intake above 60 μg was associated with a lower risk of SGA (AOR = 0.39, 95% CI: 0.22–0.69).

Conclusions: Fruits, pulses and selenium reduce the risk of SGA in Spanish women.

Keywords: Small for gestational age, Maternal diet, Fruits, Legumes, Vegetables, Selenium

* Correspondence: juanmimartinezg@hotmail.com
[1]Department of Health Sciences, University of Jaen, Campus de Las Lagunillas s n Edificio B3, 23071 Jaén, Spain
[2]CIBER de Epidemiología y Salud Pública (CIBERESP), Jaén, Spain
Full list of author information is available at the end of the article

Background

Small for gestational age (SGA) newborns are defined as those with a birthweight in the <10th percentile according to gestational age [1]. There are important adverse consequences for SGA newborns, including higher mortality and psychic, physical and social health problems in the short, medium and long term [2–8]. Between 5.3% and 23.7% of live newborns are SGA [2, 8–10].

Several risk factors for SGA have been identified. Among the non-dietary variables, the main factors are maternal education, income, smoking, body mass index (BMI), low weight gain during pregnancy, diseases during pregnancy (anaemia, preeclampsia, hypertension, infections, etc.), previous low birthweight and factors related to preterm delivery, inter alia [9–15]. In this regard, maternal diet may play an important role. Among others, it may have an "additional" role in various risks during pregnancy, such as gestational diabetes, maternal hypertension/preeclampsia, preterm birth and foetal growth restriction [16, 17].

The consumption of fruits and vegetables during pregnancy and the relationship with newborn health status has been studied by several authors [18–20]. Previous studies show inconsistent results. In the *INfancia and Medio Ambiente* (INfancy and Environment [INMA]) cohort study undertaken in Spain, incorporating 787 pregnant women with 11.5% SGA, a high intake of vegetables during pregnancy showed a lower incidence of SGA; no association was observed for fruit consumption [18]. In a cohort study in Denmark with 43,585 women) [19], the results contradicted those of the INMA cohort; that is, maternal consumption of fruit, but not vegetables, during pregnancy was associated with increased birthweight. A systematic review that did not include meta-analysis found no evidence that the intake of fruits and vegetables during pregnancy reduced the risk of having a SGA newborn [20].

The negative association of the consumption of fruits and vegetables with the risk of SGA can be explained by the high content of vitamins and micronutrients. Some studies have reported an inverse association of different vitamins (D, folic acid, etc.) and the risk of SGA [21, 22]. Several studies have analysed the relationship between selenium and newborn size, also with conflicting results [23–27]. Selenium has been implied to influence inflammation, oxidation and the proper functioning of the immunological system [28].

The intake of legumes is very common in Spain and other Mediterranean countries, as these are key elements of the Mediterranean diet. However, there are no published studies relating legume consumption to the risk of SGA. Given that previous studies correlating vegetable and fruit consumption with the risk of SGA present conflicting results, the aim of this study is to provide a fresh assessment of the effect of the intake of vegetables, legumes and fruits on the risk of SGA in a Southern European population.

Methods

The study population included women attending five hospitals in Eastern Andalusia (Spain): the University of Jaen Hospital (UJH), Ubeda Hospital (UB), the University of Granada Hospitals ([UGH] two centres) and Poniente Hospital (PH), serving 1.8 million people. Case and control groups were collected from 15 May 2012 to 15 July 2015.

Ethical approval was obtained from the Ethics Committees of the hospitals participating in the study: Comité de Ética de la Investigación del Complejo Hospitalario Universitario de Granada (Committee of Ethics of Investigation of the UGH), Comité de Ética de la Investigación del Hospital de Poniente (the Committee of Ethics of Investigation of the PH), Comité de Ética de la Investigación del Complejo Hospitalario Universitario de Jaén; (the Committee of Ethics of Investigation of the UJH) and Comité de Ética de la Investigación del Hospita de Úbeda (the Committee of Ethics of Investigation of the UB). Informed consent was obtained from the women participating in the study and we followed the protocols established by the respective health centres for accessing data from medical records to carry out this type of research with the purpose of publication/disclosure to the scientific community.

We estimated the appropriate sample size based on the results of a similar study [29]. To detect a significant ($p < 0.05$, odds ratio [OR] = 0.6) difference between extreme quintiles with a statistical power of 80%, we estimated that 447 pairs of cases and controls were required.

Cases

The eligibility criteria for cases were the delivery of a single live newborn diagnosed as small for gestational age (SGA) according to the tables developed for the Spanish population [30], without congenital malformations, during the study period and resident in the referral area of the hospital. Nineteen women declined participation. A total of 533 cases were selected: 79 (UJH), 369 (UGH), 46 (UB) and 39 (PH).

Controls

A pair of newborns matched by age at delivery (± 2 years) was selected within a week of inclusion of a case at the same hospital. Eligible women were those with a newborn of the appropriate gestational age meeting the same inclusion criteria for cases (residence in the referral area of the hospital and no malformations); women with large for gestational age (LGA) newborns were excluded. Sixty-five women declined participation.

Data collection

Data were gathered through personal interviews (conducted in the hospital by a specifically trained midwife within two days of delivery), clinical charts and prenatal care records. Information was obtained for the following variables: mother's vital data (age at pregnancy, race, pre-pregnancy body mass index [BMI], educational level, marital status, income level and occupation), obstetric history (parity and abortions), previous adverse perinatal outcomes, conditions during pregnancy (infections, preeclampsia, diabetes and other obstetric conditions), birth weight (weight in grams in the delivery room), prescribed and over-the-counter drugs, smoking during pregnancy and prenatal care (number of visits and date of first visit, weight gain during pregnancy). Social class was coded according to five main levels (ranging from I [the highest] to V [the lowest]) based on the classification of the Spanish Society of Epidemiology [31], which is close to that of the Black Report [32]. Utilization of prenatal care was measured using the Kessner Index [33].

Alcohol consumption during and before pregnancy was assessed using a structured questionnaire in which the number and types of drinks on weekdays, weekends (including Friday evenings), and holidays (including the eve) were recorded.

Dietary assessment

The baseline questionnaire (Additional file 1) included a semiquantitative food frequency questionnaire, previously validated in Spain, comprising 137 items and open-ended questions to obtain information on use of dietary supplements [34]. The questionnaire was based on typical portion sizes and provided 9 options for the frequency of intake in the previous year for each food item (ranging from "never" or "almost never" to "≥ 6 times/day"). A dietician updated the nutrient data bank using the latest available information included in the food composition tables for Spain [35, 36]. After computing total energy intake, a total of 15 matched pairs were excluded because of unreliable dietary assessment (total energy intake > 4000 Kcal/day), leaving 518 pairs for analysis.

Statistical analysis

Food and nutrient intake were adjusted for total energy intake using the residuals method and separate regression models were performed to obtain the residuals [37]. Energy-adjusted food and nutrient intake were categorized in quintiles. It is recommended that selenium intake in pregnancy be at least 60 μg/day [38] and this cut-off level was also applied in the analysis of this micronutrient. Odds ratios (ORs) and 95% confidence intervals (CIs) were estimated with conditional regression logistic models, with adjustments for potential confounders (adjusted ORs [aORs]): preeclampsia, education, smoking, weight gain per week during pregnancy, fish intake and previous preterm/low birthweight newborns. The addition of other variables (such as BMI) did not change the coefficients of the models appreciably (< 10% change). All p-values are 2-tailed. Statistical significance was set at $p < 0.05$. Analyses were performed in the Stata 14 program (College Station, TX).

Results

In all, 1036 women – 518 cases and 518 controls – participated in the study. The description of the study population is shown in Table 1. Maternal marital status influences the risk of SGA ($p = 0.036$). Well-known risk factors for SGA showed significant relationships in our study population, such as maternal smoking, previous low birth weight and/or preterm delivery, maternal BMI, low weight gain during pregnancy, preeclampsia and fish intake. The duration of gestation was shorter in the cases than in the controls and the frequency of Caesarean section was similar in both groups.

The relationship between legume intake and risk of SGA is shown in Table 2. In general, the highest levels of consumption are associated with a lower risk of SGA, although statistical significance is only achieved for kidney beans (aOR = 0.67, 95% CI: 0.48–0.94). The total amount of legumes was also analysed in quintiles. Significant p-values for the trend can be observed in both the crude and adjusted analyses: the higher the intake, the lower the risk.

Women with an intake of fruits > 420 g/day (Q5) compared with those with an intake ≤121 g/day (Q1) showed a decreased risk of SGA (aOR = 0.63, 95% CI = 0.40–0.98), although the trend was not significant (p for the trend = 0.136) (Table 3). Regarding the consumption of specific fruits, only melon (an intake of two or more times a week vs no consumption) yielded a significant relationship (aOR = 0.48, 95% CI = 0.29–0.78).

The consumption of dried fruits and nuts is displayed in Table 4. Total dried fruits showed a lower risk in Q5 (> 3.8 g/day) vs Q1 (< 0.1 g/day) in the crude analysis, although in multivariate analysis the association was borderline (aOR = 0.67, 95% CI: 0.42–1.05. Walnuts and other nuts did not exhibit any association with SGA.

No association was found between the total consumption of vegetables and the risk of SGA (Table 5). Regarding specific vegetables, significant associations were observed for asparagus, garlic and green beans, with borderline associations for eggplants, but not for

Table 1 Description of the study population

Variable	Cases	Controls	*P*-value
Marital status, n (%)			0.036
Single	37 (7.1)	42 (8.1)	
Stable couple	161 (31.1)	124 (23.9)	
Married	320 (61.8)	352 (68.0)	
Education level, n (%)			0.084
Primary	112 (21.6)	93 (17.9)	
High school, not ended	42 (8.1)	28 (5.4)	
High school	185 (35.7)	190 (36.7)	
University	179 (34.6)	207 (40.0)	
Previous preterm/low birthweight newborn (yes), n (%)	64 (12.4)	26 (5.0)	< 0.001
Kessner index (prenatal care), n (%)			0.737
Adequate	259 (50.0)	253 (48.8)	
Intermediate	185 (35.7)	182 (35.2)	
Inadequate	74 (14.3)	83 (16.0)	
Smoking during pregnancy, n (%)	149 (28.8)	80 (15.4)	< 0.001
Preeclampsia, n (%)	46 (8.9)	11 (2.1)	< 0.001
Weight gain throughout pregnancy (g/week), mean (SD)	278 (121)	310 (114)	< 0.001
Body mass index in the first trimester of pregnancy (Kg/m^2), mean (SD)	23.1 (4.5)	23.9 (4.1)	< 0.001
Alcohol intake (g/week), mean (SD)	4.2 (18.5)	3.1 (15.2)	0.312
Fish intake (g/day), mean (SD)	83.4 (48.4)	92.0 (57.0)	0.009
Gestational age (days), mean (SD)	271 (11)	276 (9)	< 0.001
Delivery by caesarean, n (%)	127 (24.2)	120 (23.2)	0.854

the remaining vegetables. Finally, the consumption of selenium was assessed (Table 6): a protective association was observed for Q3–5. Given that the recommended daily intake is 60 μg, we found that an intake above this level was associated with a lower risk of SGA (aOR = 0.39, 95% CI: 0.22–0.69).

Discussion

The aim of this report was to assess the effect of the intake of vegetables, legumes and fruits on the risk of SGA in a Southern European population. According to our results, the overall consumption of legumes shows an inverse association with the frequency of SGA. The same holds for fruit consumption > 420 g/day. No relationship between the general consumption of vegetables and fruits and SGA was observed, nor for consumption of nuts. A protective association was observed with selenium intake above the recommended levels.

The consumption of fruits in the diet of pregnant women was studied in a case-control study in New Zealand comprising 844 cases (SGA) and 870 controls; it was reported that the insufficient consumption of fruit (intake < 0.75 servings of fruits a day) during pregnancy increased the risk of SGA [39]. Similar conclusions were obtained from a Danish cohort study [19] and an Indian prospective descriptive study carried out over two years [40]. In contrast, in the Spanish INMA cohort study [18], no such relationship was observed. We found an association for Q5 (> 420 g/day), although no significant trend was apparent. This association may be due to the high content of vitamins in fruits [41].

We did not find any significant relationship with dried fruits and nuts. These foods have interesting components in terms of reducing the risk of cardiovascular diseases [42] and they also have a high content of selenium. However, the amount ingested by women in our study was rather small: for Q5 consumption of dried fruits was > 3.8 g/day and of walnuts was > 5 g/day; this latter case implies a single unit per day.

The lack of a relationship between total vegetable intake and SGA in our study agrees with the conclusions of a systematic review [20]. In contrast, several studies have found that vegetable intake increases foetal size. The first of these is the INMA study [18], which reported a beneficial effect on foetal growth attributed by the authors to the high content of antioxidants and folic acid in vegetables. Two other reports, from Denmark

Table 2 Frequency of intake of different legumes and risk of SGA

Frequency of intake	Casesn (%)	Controlsn (%)	OR (95% CI)	aOR[a] (95% CI)
Lentils				
Never	21 (4.1)	19 (3.7)	1 (ref.)	1 (ref.)
1–3 times per month	81 (15.6)	85 (16.4)	0.85 (0.43–1.68)	0.81 (0.38–1.71)
Once per week	406 (78.4)	396 (76.5)	0.91 (0.49–1.70)	0.81 (0.41–1.60)
> Once per week	10 (1.9)	18 (3.5)	0.50 (0.19–1.35)	0.41 (0.14–1.22)
Kidney beans				
Never	134 (25.9)	106 (20.5)	1 (ref.)	1 (ref.)
1–3 times per month	145 (28.0)	141 (27.2)	0.80 (0.57–1.14)	0.84 (0.57–1.23)
≥ Once+ per week	239 (46.1)	271 (52.3)	0.70 (0.51–0.95)	0.67 (0.48–0.94)
Chickpeas				
Never	52 (10.0)	46 (8.9)	1 (ref.)	1 (ref.)
1–3 times per month	129 (24.9)	140 (24.9)	0.81 (0.51–1.30)	0.79 (0.47–1.31)
≥ Once per week	337 (65.1)	332 (64.1)	0.89 (0.58–1.39)	0.83 (0.51–1.33)
Peas				
Never	170 (32.8)	152 (29.3)	1 (ref.)	1 (ref.)
1–3 times per month	184 (35.5)	188 (36.3)	0.86 (0.63–1.16)	0.84 (0.61–1.18)
Once per week	148 (28.6)	158 (30.5)	0.83 (0.60–1.14)	0.78 (0.55–1.10)
> Once per week	16 (3.1)	20 (3.9)	0.69 (0.34–1.41)	0.59 (0.27–1.28)
Legumes, g/day in quintiles				
Q1 (≤ 16.4 g/d)	112 (21.6)	104 (20.1)	1 (ref.)	1 (ref.)
Q2 (16.5–23.6)	115 (22.2)	104 (20.1)	1.04 (0.72–1.54)	1.07 (0.70–1.64)
Q3 (23.7–28.3)	115 (22.2)	103 (19.9)	1.05 (0.71–1.56)	1.16 (0.76–1.77)
Q4 (28.4–33.0)	97 (18.7)	104 (20.1)	0.89 (0.60–1.32)	0.88 (0.58–1.36)
Q5 (> 33.0)	79 (15.3)	103 (19.9)	0.72 (0.49–1.07)	0.68 (0.44–1.04)
P for trend			0.050	0.020

[a] Adjusted for preeclampsia, education, smoking, gain weight per week during pregnancy, fish intake and previous preterm/low birthweight newborn

[19] and India [40], noted the same results. These studies did not analyse specific types of vegetables and therefore it is not possible to compare our results for green beans, garlic and asparagus (in which protective associations with SGA risk were observed).

Insufficient consumption of selenium increases the frequency of pre-eclampsia, a clear risk factor for SGA [23]. An analysis on a subset (126 pregnant adolescent women) from a prospective observational study in London found low levels of selenium in women delivering an SGA newborn [24]. Sun et al., in a cross-sectional study carried out in 209 pregnant women from Eastern China, observed that an increase in selenium intake could reduce serum cadmium levels, improving foetal growth [25]. However, Horan et al., in a cohort analysis of 554 infants from the Randomised cOntrol trial of LOw glycaemic index diet to prevent macrosomia (ROLO) study (a randomized controlled trial conducted in Ireland of 800 secundigravid women with a previous macrosomic baby) showed that selenium was inversely related with the womb perimeter of newborns [26]. Also, in a Spanish study with a rather small sample size ($n = 197$ women), without data on SGA, no association was observed between selenium intake and newborn size [27].

Legumes, mainly lentils and chickpeas, have a high selenium content. In general, the content of selenium in most vegetables is low. The exception is garlic, which has 23 times the content of selenium of tomato or lettuce; also, green beans have almost three times the amount of selenium of other common vegetables [35, 36, 43]. In our results, both garlic and green beans reduced SGA risk. However, mushrooms, with a high selenium content, were unrelated to SGA risk in our population.

It would be very interesting to analyse whether diet can overcome the influence of obesity, malnutrition and other unfavourable conditions, such as low socioeconomic status and smoking. This can be addressed in future studies. Our sample had no statistical power

Table 3 Frequency of intake of different fruits and risk of SGA

Frequency of intake	Casesn (%)	Controls n (%)	OR (95% CI)	aOR[a] (95% CI)
Orange				
Never	50 (9.7)	36 (7.0)	1 (ref.)	1 (ref.)
vs. ≥ Once per day	85 (16.4)	91 (17.6)	0.67 (0.40–1.13)	0.68 (0.38–1.21)
Banana				
Never	78 (15.1)	70 (13.5)	1 (ref.)	1 (ref.)
vs. ≥ 5 times per week	33 (1.4)	47 (9.1)	0.64 (0.37–1.11)	0.60 (0.32–1.11)
Apple				
Never	60 (11.6)	51 (9.9)	1 (ref.)	1 (ref.)
vs. ≥ 5 times per week	46 (7.7)	46 (8.9)	0.74 (0.42–1.30)	0.75 (0.41–1.39)
Strawberry				
Never	108 (20.9)	100 (19.3)	1 (ref.)	1 (ref.)
vs. ≥ 2 times per week	56 (10.8)	53 (10.2)	0.97 (0.61–1.53)	0.88 (0.54–1.45)
Cherry				
Never	140 (27.0)	123 (23.8)	1 (ref.)	1 (ref.)
vs. ≥ 2 times per week	39 (7.5)	49 (9.5)	0.69 (0.42–1.12)	0.63 (0.37–1.08)
Peach				
Never	111 (21.4)	94 (18.2)	1 (ref.)	1 (ref.)
vs. ≥ 2 times per week	66 (12.7)	78 (15.1)	0.72 (0.46–1.13)	0.79 (0.49–1.29)
Watermelon				
Never	82 (15.8)	69 (13.3)	1 (ref.)	1 (ref.)
vs. ≥ 5 times per week	31 (6.0)	34 (6.6)	0.74 (0.41–1.32)	0.64 (0.33–1.22)
Melon				
Never	108 (20.9)	80 (15.4)	1 (ref.)	1 (ref.)
vs. ≥ 2 times per week	59 (11.4)	82 (15.8)	0.53 (0.34–0.84)	0.48 (0.29–0.78)
Kiwi fruit				
Never	190 (36.7)	186 (35.9)	1 (ref.)	1 (ref.)
vs. ≥ 2 times per week	80 (15.4)	88 (17.0)	0.90 (0.62–1.29)	1.02 (0.68–1.52)
Grapes				
Never	190 (36.7	189 (36.5)	1 (ref.)	1 (ref.)
vs. ≥ 2 times per week	34 (6.6)	34 (6.6)	0.99 (0.60–1.66)	0.87 (0.50–1.50)
Fruit, g/day, quintiles				
Q1 (≤ 121 g/d)	129 (24.9)	104 (20.1)	1 (ref.)	1 (ref.)
Q2 (122–170)	109 (21.0)	104 (20.1)	0.84 (0.58–1.24)	0.87 (0.57–1.35)
Q3 (171–272)	100 (19.3)	103 (19.9)	0.76 (0.52–1.11)	0.73 (0.48–1.12)
Q4 (273–420)	98 (18.9)	104 (20.1)	0.74 (0.51–1.09)	0.73 (0.47–1.13)
Q5 (> 420)	82 (15.8)	103 (19.9)	0.63 (0.42–0.93)	0.63 (0.40–0.98)
P for trend			0.089	0.136

[a] Adjusted for preeclampsia, education, smoking, body mass index, gain weight per week during pregnancy, fish intake and previous preterm/low birthweight newborn

to allow reliable analysis of these important variables; in our sample, obesity (BMI ≥ 30) was 8% (41 women in controls and 43 in cases), none of the patients were diagnosed with malnutrition and smoking women with a low socioeconomic status only comprised 10% of the population ($n = 102$). Regardless, the benefits of a healthy diet (with an adequate consumption of fruits, vegetables and legumes) should be widespread in the population.

There were no problems recruiting participants. The response rate was very high, so selection bias was not unlikely. The food frequency questionnaire (FFQ)

Table 4 Frequency of intake of dried fruit and nuts and risk of SGA

Frequency of intake (quintiles, Q)	Casesn (%)	Controls n (%)	OR (95% CI)	aOR[a] (95% CI)
Dried fruit (g/day)				
Q1 (< 0.1)	126 (24.3)	104 (20.1)	1 (ref.)	1 (ref.)
Q2 (0.1–0.3)	113 (21.8)	104 (20.1)	0.89 (0.61–1.29)	0.88 (0.58–1.34)
Q3 (0.31–1.1)	105 (20.7)	103 (19.9)	0.83 (0.57–1.22)	0.89 (0.58–1.38)
Q4 (1.11–3.8)	91 (17.6)	104 (20.1)	0.70 (0.47–1.03)	0.70 (0.45–1.10)
Q5 (> 3.8)	83 (16.0)	103 (19.9)	0.63 (0.42–0.95)	0.67 (0.42–1.05)
P for trend			0.099	0.193
Walnuts (g/day)				
Q1 (< 0.3)	114 (22.0)	104 (20.1)	1 (ref.)	1 (ref.)
Q2 (0.3–1.4)	99 (19.1)	104 (20.1)	0.86 (0.58–1.27)	0.75 (0.49–1.14)
Q3 (1.41–2.6)	90 (17.4)	103 (19.9)	0.79 (0.54–1.17)	0.78 (0.51–1.21)
Q4 (2.61–5.0)	114 (22.0)	104 (20.1)	1.01 (0.69–1.46)	1.02 (0.68–1.53)
Q5 (> 5.0)	101 (19.5)	103 (19.9)	0.89 (0.60–1.31)	0.83 (0.55–1.27)
P for trend			0.873	0.517
Other nuts[b] (g/day)				
Q1 (< 0.8)	104 (20.8)	104 (20.1)	1 (ref.)	1 (ref.)
Q2 (0.8–2.0)	83 (16.0)	104 (20.1)	0.79 (0.52–1.17)	0.80 (0.51–1.24)
Q3 (2.01–3.4)	114 (22.0)	103 (19.9)	1.09 (0.74–1.60)	1.07 (0.70–1.64)
Q4 (3.41–5.5)	96 (18.5)	104 (20.1)	0.91 (0.62–1.35)	0.91 (0.59–1.40)
Q5 (> 5.5)	121 (23.4)	103 (19.9)	1.16 (0.80–1.66)	1.21 (0.81–1.81)
P for trend			0.188	0.234

[a]Adjusted for preeclampsia, education, smoking, body mass index, gain weight per week during pregnancy, fish intake and previous preterm/low birthweight newborn
[b]Almond, peanut, pistachio, etc.

had been validated and used previously with Spanish women [44, 45]. Mothers of normal newborns were density matched to cases to avoid the influence of season on the responses for certain types of foods. Also, women were matched by age to decrease generational effects on their food habits: younger women show a trend to have a more westernized diet than older ones, who adhere more to the Mediterranean diet [46].

In case-control studies certain problems of anamnestic bias cannot completely be ruled out, as women are aware of the newborn condition and this could influence their answers. During prenatal care no advice is given on taking specific foods, apart from avoiding raw meat and fish and reducing consumption of big fish (presumably with a higher content of mercury and other heavy metals). We asked women about any change in diet during pregnancy: 48.8% of cases reported increased vegetable intake vs. 46.7% of controls; the figures for fruit were 59.9% vs. 58.3 and 23.2% and 22.2% for legumes in cases and controls respectively. The percentages of change are roughly similar (although slightly higher in cases) between cases and controls and thus we believe that in the case of misclassification bias, it is most likely to be non-differential.

Confounding bias can also not be completely dismissed. Differences in weight gain, smoking and other variables were controlled for in multivariate analysis. This is a limitation inherent to most observational studies. Known risk factors for SGA help to explain only 30–40% of all cases, indicating that there is still much to be known about the epidemiology of this condition. We have also tried to control this bias by collecting data on the well-known risk factors for SGA and adjusting for them in the multivariable models.

Regarding specific legumes, a significant negative association was found with kidney beans; with other legumes, protective ORs were observed in the highest categories of intake, although none of them reached significance. When total legume intake was assessed, a significant negative trend was observed: the higher the intake, the lower the SGA risk. We have failed to identify any other report in which the intake of legumes is related to SGA or low birthweight and thus we cannot compare our results to other work.

Table 5 Frequency of intake of different vegetables and risk of SGA

Frequency of intake	Cases n (%)	Controls n (%)	OR (95% CI)	aOR[a] (95% CI)
Swiss chard				
Never	128 (24.7)	110 (21.2)	1 (ref.)	1 (ref.)
vs. ≥ 2 times per week	79 (15.3)	72 (13.9)	0.91 (0.60–1.39)	0.88 (0.55–1.39)
Cabbage				
Never	234 (45.2)	220 (42.5)	1 (ref.)	1 (ref.)
vs. ≥ 2 times per week	44 (8.5)	41 (7.9)	1.01 (0.63–1.58)	0.94 (0.57–1.55)
Lettuce				
Never	40 (7.7)	33 (6.4)	1 (ref.)	1 (ref.)
vs. ≥ 5 times per week	141 (27.2)	122 (23.6)	0.94 (0.56–1.60)	0.83 (0.46–1.51)
Tomato				
Never	50 (9.7)	40 (7.7)	1 (ref.)	1 (ref.)
vs. ≥ 5 times per week ek	193 (37.3)	177 (34.2)	0.86 (0.53–1.40)	1.02 (0.60–1.75)
Carrot				
Never	97 (18.7)	68 (13.1)	1 (ref.)	1 (ref.)
vs. ≥ 5 times per week	74 (14.3)	60 (11.6)	0.88 (0.56–1.39)	0.90 (0.55–1.48)
Green bean				
Never	124 (23.9)	90 (17.4)	1 (ref.)	1 (ref.)
vs. ever	398 (76.1)	428 (82.6)	0.66 (0.49–0.90)	0.55 (0.38–0.90)
Eggplants				
Never	71 (13.7)	57 (11.0)	1 (ref.)	1 (ref.)
vs. ≥ 2 times per week	70 (13.5)	87 (16.8)	0.63 (0.38–1.02)	0.59 (0.34–1.01)
Pepper				
Never	102 (19.7)	93 (18.0)	1 (ref.)	1 (ref.)
vs. ≥ 2 times per week	96 (18.5)	105 (20.3)	0.83 (0.56–1.24)	0.77 (0.50–1.20)
Asparagus				
Never	191 (36.9)	163 (31.5)	1 (ref.)	1 (ref.)
vs. ≥ 2 times per week	36 (7.0)	48 (9.3)	0.64 (0.39–1.03)	0.53 (0.31–0.89)
Cold vegetable soup (Spanish 'gazpacho')				
Never	196 (37.8)	169 (32.6)	1 (ref.)	1 (ref.)
vs. ≥ 2 times per week	44 (8.5)	41 (7.9)	0.91 (0.58–1.46)	0.75 (0.45–1.24)
Onion				
Never	78 (15.1)	73 (14.1)	1 (ref.)	1 (ref.)
vs. ≥ 5 times per week	159 (30.7)	117 (22.6)	1.32 (0.89–1.96)	1.26 (0.81–1.97)
Garlic				
Never	104 (20.1)	75 (14.5)	1 (ref.)	1 (ref.)
vs. ever	414 (79.9)	443 (75.5)	0.68 (0.49–0.94)	0.67 (0.46–0.97)
Mushrooms				
Never	139 (26.8)	126 (24.3)	1 (ref.)	1 (ref.)
vs. ≥ 2 times per week	36 (7.0)	32 (6.2)	1.01 (0.59–1.74)	0.90 (0.48–1.67)
Total amount of vegetables (g/day), quintiles				
Q1 (≤ 228.9)	122 (23.6)	104 (20.1)	1 (ref.)	1 (ref.)
Q2 (229.0–329.1)	89 (17.2)	104 (20.1)	0.72 (0.49–1.07)	0.75 (0.48–1.15)
Q3 (329.2–432.5)	90 (17.4)	103 (19.9)	0.72 (0.49–1.08)	0.75 (0.48–1.15)
Q4 (432.6–573.0)	96 (18.5)	104 (20.1)	0.77 (0.53–1.13)	0.80 (0.53–1.22)
Q5 (> 573.0)	121 (23.4)	103 (19.9)	0.99 (0.69–1.44)	0.91 (0.60–1.39)
P for trend			0.177	0.401

[a] Adjusted for preeclampsia, education, smoking, gain weight per week during pregnancy, fish intake and previous preterm/low birthweight newborn

Table 6 Association between selenium (µg/day) and risk of SGA

Quintiles	Casesn (%)	Controls n (%)	OR (95% CI)	aOR[a] (95% CI)
Selenium (µg/day)				
Q1 (≤ 72.25)	132 (25.5)	104 (20.1)	1 (ref.)	1 (ref.)
Q2 (72.26–84.49)	110 (21.4)	104 (20.1)	0.83 (0.57–1.20)	0.73 (0.44–1.22)
Q3 (84.50–96.20)	86 (16.6)	103 (19.9)	0.63 (0.42–0.95)	0.46 (0.27–0.80)
Q4 (96.21–110.63)	94 (18.2)	104 (20.1)	0.71 (0.49–1.03)	0.58 (0.36–0.94)
Q5 (> 110.63)	96 (18.5)	103 (19.9)	0.72 (0.49–1.07)	0.53 (0.32–0.87)
P for trend			0.581	0.594
< 60	65 (12.6)	32 (6.2)	1 (ref.)	1 (ref.)
≥ 60	453 (87.4)	486 (93.8)	0.47 (0.30–0.73)	0.39 (0.22–0.69)

[a] Adjusted for preeclampsia, education, smoking, body mass index, gain weight per week during pregnancy and previous preterm/low birthweight newborn

Conclusion

In conclusion, the intake of legumes and fruits seems to reduce the risk of SGA in Spanish women. Several vegetables containing selenium also reduced the incidence of SGA in our population. Nevertheless, the available information is scarce and more studies are needed on this subject.

Abbreviations

AGA: Adequate for gestational age; aOR: Adjusted odds ratio; BMI: Body mass index; CIs: Confidence intervals; FFQ: Food frequency questionnaire; INMA: "INfancia and Medio Ambiente" (INMA, INfancy and Environment); LGA: Large for gestational age; OR: Odds ratio; PH: Poniente Hospital; Q1: Quintile 1; Q2: Quintile 2; Q3: Quintile 3; Q4: Quintile 4; Q5: Quintile 5; ROLO: Randomised cOntrol trial of LOw glycaemic index diet to prevent macrosomia; SGA: small for gestational age; UGH: University of Granada Hospital; UH: Ubeda Hospital; UJH: University of Jaen Hospital

Acknowledgements

Women participating in the study and interviewers.

Funding

This work was supported by a grant from the National Institute of Health Carlos III [PI11/02199].

Authors' contributions

MDR and JMMG conceived the study; MDR, JMMG, ABC, CAP, GGM and ISB designed the study; MDR, JMMG and ABC analysed the data. CAP, GGM, ISB and JMMG coordinated data collection. The first draft of the paper was written by MDR and JMMG. All the authors discussed, made contributions to the article and approved the final version.

Ethics approval and consent to participate

Ethical approval was obtained from the Ethics Committees of the hospitals participating in the study: Comité de Ética de la Investigación del Complejo Hospitalario Universitario de Granada (Committee of Ethics of Investigation of the UGH), Comité de Ética de la Investigación del Hospital de Poniente (the Committee of Ethics of Investigation of the PH), Comité de Ética de la Investigación del Complejo Hospitalario Universitario de Jaén; (the Committee of Ethics of Investigation of the UJH) and Comité de Ética de la Investigación del Hospita de Úbeda (the Committee of Ethics of Investigation of the UB). The informed consent was verbally obtained because no interventions were performed on the study. It was to answer a survey's questions. It was more pragmatic to obtain a verbal consent. The different Ethics Committes authorized and were aware about verbally consent use on the study. Informed consent was obtained from the women participating in the study and we followed the protocols established by the respective health centres for accessing data from medical records to carry out this type of research with the purpose of publication/disclosure to the scientific community.

Competing interests

The authors declare that they have no competing interests.

Author details

[1]Department of Health Sciences, University of Jaen, Campus de Las Lagunillas s n Edificio B3, 23071 Jaén, Spain. [2]CIBER de Epidemiología y Salud Pública (CIBERESP), Jaén, Spain. [3]Department of Preventive Medicine and Public Health, University of Granada, Granada, Spain. [4]Biosanitary Research Institute Granada (IBS-Granada), Granada, Spain.

References

1. American College of Obstetricians and Gynecologists. ACOG practice bulletin no. 134: fetal growth restriction. Obstet Gynecol. 2013;121:1122–33.
2. Kozuki N, Katz J, Christian P, Lee ACC, Liu L, Silveira MF, et al. Comparison of US birth weight references and the international fetal and newborn growth consortium for the 21st century standard. JAMA Pediatr. 2015;169(7):e151438.
3. Yi KH, Yi YY, Hwang IT. Behavioral and intelligence outcome in 8- to 16-year-old born small for gestational age. Korean J Pediatr. 2016; 59(10):414–20.
4. Steiner N, Wainstock T, Sheiner E, Segal I, Landau D, Waslfisch A. Small for gestational age as an independent risk factor for long-term pediatric gastrointestinal morbidity of the offspring. J Matern Fetal Neonatal Med. 2017;4:1–5.
5. Chauhan SP, Rice MM, Grobman WA, Bailit J, Reddy UM, Wapner RJ, et al. MSCE, for the Eunice Kennedy Shriver National Institute of Child Health and Human Development (NICHD) maternal-fetal medicine units (MFMU) network. Neonatal morbidity of small- and large-for-gestational-age neonates born at term in uncomplicated pregnancies. Obstet Gynecol. 2017;130(3):511–9.
6. Mendez-Figueroa H, Truong VT, Pedroza C, Khan AM, Chauhan SP. Small-for-gestational-age infants among uncomplicated pregnancies at term: a secondary analysis of 9 maternal-fetal medicine units network studies. Am J Obstet Gynecol. 2016;215(5):628.e1–7.
7. Lee AC, Kozuki N, Cousens S, Setevens GA, Blencowe H, Silveira MF, et al. Estimates of burden and consequences of infants born small for gestational age in low and middle income countries with INTERGROWTH-21st standard: analysis of CHERG datasets. BMJ. 2017;358:j3677. https://doi.org/10.1136/bmj.j3677.
8. Black RE. Global prevalence of small for gestational age births. Nestle Nutr Inst Workshop Ser. 2015. https://doi.org/10.1159/000365790.

9. Gaudineau A. Prevalence, risk factors, maternal and fetal morbidity and mortality of intrauterine growth restriction and small-for-gestational age. J Gynecol Obstet Biol Reprod (Paris). 2013;42(8):895–910.
10. Chiavaroli V, Castorani V, Guidone P, Derraik JG, Liberati M, Chiarelli F, et al. Incidence of infants born small- and large-for-gestational-age in an Italian cohort over a 20-year period and associated risk factors. Ital J Pediatr. 2016;26(42):42.
11. Bushnik T, Yang S, Kaufman JS, Kramer MS, Wilkins R. Socioeconomic disparities in small-for-gestational-age birth and preterm birth. Health Rep. 2017;28(11):3–10.
12. Fisher SC, Van Zutphen AR, Romitti PA, Browne ML. National Birth Defects Prevention Study. Maternal hypertension, antihypertensive medication use, and small for gestational age births in the National Birth Defects Prevention Study, 1997–2011. Matern Child Health J. 2018;22(2):237–46.
13. Margerison Zilko CE, Rehkopf D, Abrams B. Association of maternal gestational weight gain with short- and long-term maternal and child health outcomes. Am J Obstet Gynecol. 2010;202(6):574.e1–8.
14 Usynina AA, Grjibovski AM, Odland JØ, Krettek A. Social correlates of term small for gestational age babies in a Russian Arctic setting. Int J Circumpolar Health. 2016;75:32883. https://doi.org/10.3402/ijch.v75.32883 eCollection 2016.
15. McCowan L, Horgan RP. Risk factors for small for gestational age infants. Best Pract Res Clin Obstet Gynaecol. 2009;23(6):779–93.
16. Parlapani E, Agakidis C, Karagiozoglou-Lampoudi T, Sarafidis K, Agakidou E, Athanasiadis A, et al. The Mediterranean diet adherence by pregnant women delivering prematurely: association with size at birth and complications of prematurity. J Matern Fetal Neonatal Med. 13:1–8. https://doi.org/10.1080/14767058.2017.1399120.
17. Bain E, Crane M, Tieu J, Han S, Crowther CA, Middleton P. Diet and exercise interventions for preventing gestational diabetes mellitus. Cochrane Database Syst Rev. 2015;4:CD010443. https://doi.org/10.1002/14651858.CD010443.pub2.
18. Ramón R, Ballester F, Iñiguez C, Rebagliato M, Murcia M, Esplugues A, et al. Vegetable but not fruit intake during pregnancy is associated with newborn anthropometric measures. J Nutr. 2009;139(3):561–7.
19. Mikkelsen TB, Osler M, Orozova-Bekkevold I, Knudsen VK, Olsen SF. Association between fruit and vegetable consumption and birth weight: a prospective study among 43,585 Danish women. Scand J Public Health. 2006;34(6):616–22.
20. Murphy MM, Stettler N, Smith KM, Reiss R. Associations of consumption of fruits and vegetables during pregnancy with infant birth weight or small for gestational age births: a systematic review of the literature. Int J Womens Health. 2014;6:899–912. https://doi.org/10.2147/IJWH.S67130 eCollection 2014.
21. Catov J, Bodnar LM, Ness RB, Markovic N, Roberts JM. Association of periconceptional multivitamin use and risk of preterm or small-for-gestational-age births. Am J Epidemiol. 2007;166(3):296–303.
22. Chen Y, Zhu B, Wu X, Li S, Tao F. Association between maternal vitamin D deficiency and small for gestational age: evidence from a meta-analysis of prospective cohort studies. BMJ Open. 2017;7(8):e016404. https://doi.org/10.1136/bmjopen-2017-016404.
23. Ghaemi SZ, Forouhari S, Dabbaghmanesh MH, Sayadi M, Bakhshayeshkaram M, Vaziri F, et al. A prospective study of selenium concentration and risk of. Preeclampsia in pregnant Iranian women: a nested case-control study. Biol Trace Elem Res. 2013;152(2):174–9.
24. Mistry HD, Kurlak LO, Young SD, Briley AL, Pipkin FB, Baker PN, et al. Maternal selenium, copper and zinc concentrations in pregnancy associated with. Small-for-gestational-age infants. Matern Child Nutr. 2014;10(3):327–34.
25. Sun H, Chen W, Wang D, Jin Y, Chen X, Xu Y. The effects of prenatal exposure to low-level cadmium, lead and selenium on birth outcomes. Chemosphere. 2014;108:33–9.
26. Horan MK, McGowan CA, Gibney ER, Donnelly JM, FM MA. The association between maternal dietary micronutrient intake and neonatal. Anthropometry-secondary analysis from the ROLO study. Nutr J. 2015;14:105.
27. Zaragoza-Noguera R. Influence of the diet of the pregnant woman on fetal growth, Doctoral thesis. Murcia: University of Murcia; 2017.
28. Rayman MP. Selenium and human health. Lancet. 2012;379(9822):1256–68. https://doi.org/10.1016/S0140-6736(11)61452-9.
29. Ricci E, Chiaffarino F, Cipriani S, et al. Diet in pregnancy and risk of small for gestational age birth: results from a retrospective case control study in Italy. Matern Child Nutr. 2010;6:297–305.
30. Delgado-Beltrán P, Melchor-Marcos JC, Rodríguez-Alarcón J, Linares-Uribe A, Fernández-Llebrez del Rey L, Barbazán-Cortés MJ, et al. The fetal development curves of newborn infants in the hospital de cruces (Vizcaya). I. Weight. An Esp Pediatr. 1996;44(1):50–4
31. Álvarez-Dardet C, Alonso J, Domingo A, Regidor E. La Medición de la Clase Social en Ciencias de la Salud, Informe de un Grupo de Trabajo de la Sociedad Española de Epidemiología. Madrid: SG Editores; 1995.
32. Townsend P, Davidson N. Inequalities in health, the Black report. Hammonsworth: Penguin; 1982.
33. Kessner DM, Singer J, Kalk CE. Infant death: an analysis by maternal risk and health care. Contrasts in health status. Washington: Institute of Medicine, National Academy of Sciences; 1973.
34. Fernández-Ballart JD, Piñol JL, Zazpe I, et al. Relative validity of a semi-. Quantitative food-frequency questionnaire in an elderly Mediterranean population of. Spain. Br J Nutr. 2010;103:1808.
35. Mataix VJ. Tabla de composición de alimentos españoles (Spanish food composition tables). Granada: Universidad de Granada; 2003.
36. Moreiras O, Carbajal A, Cabrera L, Cuadrado C. Tablas de composición de alimentos (Spanish food composition tables). Madrid: Pirámide; 2003.
37. Willett WC. Nutritional epidemiology. New York: Oxford University Press; 1998.
38. Institute of Medicine (US) Committee to Review Dietary Reference Intakes for Vitamin D and Calcium, Ross AC, Taylor CL, Yaktine AL, et al. Recommended dietary allowances and adequate intakes, elements. Washington: National Academies Press (US); 2011.
39. Mitchell EA, Robinson E, Clark PM, Becroft DM, Glavish N, Pattison NS, et al. Maternal birth size is not associated with maternal intake and status of folate during the second trimester nutritional risk factors for small for gestational age babies in a developed country: a case-control study. Arch Dis Child Fetal Neonatal Ed. 2004;89(5):F431–5.
40. Rao S, Yajnik CS, Kanade A, Fall CH, Margetts BM, Jackson AA, et al. Intake of micronutrient-rich foods in rural Indian mothers is associated with the size of their babies at birth: Pune maternal nutrition study. J Nutr. 2001;131(4):1217–24.
41. Salcedo-Bellido I, Martínez-Galiano JM, Olmedo-Requena R, Mozas-Moreno J, Bueno-Cavanillas A, Jimenez-Moleon JJ, et al. Association between vitamin intake during pregnancy and risk of small for gestional age. Nutrients. 2017;9(12):1277.
42. Martínez-González MA, Salas-Salvadó J, Estruch R, Corella D, Fitó M, Ros E, et al. Benefits of the Mediterranean diet: insights from the PREDIMED study. Prog Cardiovasc Dis. 2015;58(1):50–60.
43. Asociación EuroFIR AISBL. Spanish Database of Food Composition. http://www.bedca.net/ Accessed 26 Jan 2018.
44. De la Fuente-Arrillaga C, Ruiz ZV, Bes-Rastrollo M, Sampson L, Martinez-González MA. Reproducibility of an FFQ validated in Spain. Public Health Nutr. 2010;13(9):1364–72. https://doi.org/10.1017/S1368980009993065.
45. Olmedo-Requena R, Amezcua-Prieto C, de Dios L-D-CJ, Lewis-Mikhael AM, Mozas-Moreno J, Bueno-Cavanillas A, et al. Association between low dairy intake during pregnancy and risk of small-for-gestational-age infants. Matern Child Health J. 2016;20(6):1296–304.
46. Bibiloni MM, González M, Julibert A, Llompart I, Pons A, Tur JA. Ten-year trends (1999–2010) of adherence to the Mediterranean diet among the Balearic Islands' adult population. Nutrients. 2017;9(7):749.

16

A focus group study of women's views and experiences of maternity care as delivered collaboratively by midwives and health visitors in England

Maria Raisa Jessica V. Aquino[1*], Ellinor K. Olander[2] and Rosamund M. Bryar[2]

Abstract

Background: Research suggests that collaboratively delivered maternity care can positively impact health outcomes. However, women's perspectives on models of care involving interprofessional collaboration between midwives and health visitors are not well understood. Accounts of women's maternity care experiences are key to improving maternity services. This study considered women's views and experiences of maternity care as collaboratively provided by midwives and health visitors in England.

Methods: A qualitative focus group study with an exercise exploring women's ideal maternity care pathway was conducted. Three focus groups were conducted in London, England between June and August 2017 with women who had had a child within 18 months prior to the study. The participants ($n = 12$) were recruited from two Children's Centres in London, England. Data were analysed using thematic analysis.

Results: Four themes were identified: 'Women's experiences of maternity care from midwives and health visitors', 'Midwife-health visitor communication', 'Midwife-health visitor collaboration for tailored care', and 'Women's ideal maternity care pathway'. Regarding women's experiences of interprofessional collaboration between midwives and health visitors, this was rarely encountered, but welcomed by women. Women's observations of limited tailored care and co-ordination led to several suggestions to improve maternity care, including secure, shared medical recordkeeping systems, clarity on midwives' and health visitors' roles, as well as increased communication.

Conclusions: Maternity care that is collaboratively delivered by midwives and health visitors, from the perspectives of the women in this study, is not routinely provided. However, women recognise the potential benefits of midwife-health visitor collaboration. Future research should explore service configurations that support integrated maternity care pathways, and evaluate the impact of midwife-health visitor collaboration on health and service outcomes.

Keywords: Maternal health, Interprofessional collaboration, Women's experiences, Qualitative enquiry, Thematic analysis, Pregnancy, Postnatal, Midwife, Health visitor

* Correspondence: ra532@medschl.cam.ac.uk
[1]Primary Care Unit, Department of Public Health and Primary Care, University of Cambridge, Cambridge, UK
Full list of author information is available at the end of the article

Background

Interprofessional collaboration is widely promoted across health services, including maternal and child health services, both in the UK [1, 2] and internationally [3]. According to the World Health Organization, interprofessional collaboration occurs when different healthcare professionals work together to improve care [4]. The mounting evidence concerning the importance of one's early childhood to the rest of the lifespan puts interprofessional collaboration high on government agendas as a strategy for addressing women's and their families' unmet needs and improving outcomes [3, 5–7].

In the UK, midwives and health visitors (specialist community public health nurses) are key maternity care providers. These groups share overlapping professional remits both antenatally and postnatally and are encouraged to work together [8]. Specifically, Public Health England and Department of Health (UK) partnership pathway outlines this working relationship such that midwives and health visitors should be communicating with each other during and after pregnancy regarding the health and wellbeing of mother and baby [8]. Our recent systematic review of the international evidence on interprofessional collaboration between midwives and health visitors showed that collaboration in practice varied, and is influenced by interlinked structural (e.g. geographical distance, limited resources) and individual factors (e.g. communication, support for colleagues) [9].

Previous research suggests that collaborative maternity care models can have a positive impact on health outcomes [10], including breastfeeding [7], mental health and smoking cessation [11]. Conversely, poor interprofessional collaboration is associated with negative maternity care experiences, and can result in failures in care [12]. It is therefore important to identify women's experiences of midwife-health visitor collaboration, and explore how they envisage maternity services to be developed.

Women's involvement in the exploration of interprofessional collaboration care models in maternity is limited (e.g. [13, 14]), despite being service users [15]. Sandall and colleagues [12] have suggested that further research on women's experiences of continuity of care models, which include various health professionals working together, is needed. A recent systematic review of continuity of care with doctors demonstrated that greater continuity of care (defined as repeated contact between a patient and a doctor) was associated with lower mortality [16]. Continuity of care is also encouraged in maternity care guidance set out by the National Health Service (NHS) in England [17].

Critical realism [18–20] is a philosophical approach that allows for the understanding of the layers shaping individuals' experience and reality, and the links between these [21]. This asserts that reality is comprised of three levels: the empirical, the actual, and the real [19, 20]. In the context of midwife-health visitor collaboration, the *empirical* level concerns the directly observable, perceived and experienced. For example, a woman observes a midwife and a health visitor communicating about her care. Midwives' and health visitors' professional competencies as applied to care provision represent the *actual* level; these influence the empirical, and are not always observable [20]. At the deepest level – the *real* – are the generative mechanisms causing the observable events. For example, relational factors such as mutual trust for each other [22] and healthcare professionals' limited control of financial or structural constraints imposed by the healthcare system [14]. Therefore, women's experiences of collaborative care as provided by midwives and health visitors are key to better understanding their care needs and service provision more generally. This study aimed to explore women's (i) experiences of maternity care as collaboratively provided by midwives and health visitors, and (ii) their perspectives of how their maternity care can best be provided by these healthcare professionals together.

Methods

Study design and setting

This study applied a qualitative, cross-sectional design, to elicit women's views and experiences of midwife-health visitor collaboration. Focus groups were selected as they are an accessible, flexible method for generating data on a selected topic [23], and capitalise on group interaction [24]. Midwife-health visitor collaboration may be difficult to discuss for some women, due to limited experiences of this; thus, focus groups are appropriate because participants can comment on each other's views and experiences, ask each other questions and seek clarification [23, 24]. Therefore, there is an immediate opportunity to compare and contrast experiences [24]. Data collection took place in a Children's Centre in London, England.

Participant recruitment

To be eligible to participate in this study, mothers needed to be over 18 years of age, have a child less than 18 months old, read and speak English and provide written consent to participate. Participant recruitment was approached through face-to-face contact with women in Children's Centres, word of mouth, and social media (i.e. Twitter), enabling wide dissemination of study information.

A specifically developed topic guide was used (Additional file 1), informed by our systematic review of midwife-health visitor collaboration [9] and the research aims. As aligned with a critical realist approach, we presented a summary of the existing literature and sought women's views of midwife-health visitor collaboration, and encouraged them to speak and discuss the topic freely and flexibly [20, 21]. Broadly, this covered: Experiences of women's maternity care as provided by midwives and health visitors, opinions of health visitor antenatal contact, and women's envisaged ideal maternity care pathway as collaboratively provided by midwives and health visitors.

Data collection

In order to capture as diverse a population as reasonably possible, 74 Children's Centres and other community-based groups in and around London were approached by email with a follow up email 1 week later. Of these, 10 centres responded (13.5%) to the email contact, with three agreeing to participate. Due to logistical constraints (e.g. Children's Centre closures, lack of availability of co-moderator), face-to-face recruitment focussed on two Children's Centres.

Following ethical approval from the Centre for Maternal and Child Health Research, School of Health Sciences (ref.: MCH/PR/PhD/17–18/01) in June 2017, recruitment commenced. Two members of the research team (RA, RB) were present at the focus group discussions. One acted as moderator (RA), and the other as assistant moderator (RB) responsible for note-taking. To accommodate women's babies, baby bouncers and a soft play area was organised. All focus groups were audio-recorded following written informed consent of all participants.

The focus groups started with introductions, followed by sharing of experiences of meeting midwives and health visitors, and care women received. Participants were also invited to discuss their opinions on midwife-health visitor collaboration. Then, as a group, participants were invited to consider the maternity care pathway, and draw out their ideal collaborative maternity care model. Previous research has demonstrated that visual approaches can enhance discussion by representing relationships between the topics discussed, thereby increasing one's understanding of a situation [25]. The aim of this exercise was to identify the most important aspects of maternity care that needed to be delivered collaboratively by midwives and health visitors. Including a visual approach to the focus group offered the opportunity to explore not only what women valued in relation to midwife-health visitor collaboration, but also construct their shared understanding of this beyond their individual experiences – a cornerstone of critical realism [20, 26]. Finally, participants were thanked for their participation in the study and offered a £10 voucher as a token of appreciation.

Analysis

Audio-recordings were transcribed verbatim by a professional transcription agency and checked for accuracy by RA. Thematic analysis was applied to the data corpus in order to identify repeated patterns (i.e. themes) within the data, following several phases of analysis [27, 26]. Critical realism seeks to develop an understanding of reality through active engagement with existing knowledge and experience; as such, a combination of inductive and deductive thematic analysis was used [27], allowing for the developed themes to be guided by the data, the research aims, and the existing literature [9].

The first author led data analysis using QSR NVivo 11.4.1 [28]. The first steps were data driven [27], specifically: Familiarisation, or the reading and rereading of transcripts and generation of initial codes to identify noteworthy topics. Then, this was combined with a deductive approach: Codes were based on the research aims, and used as a template to organise the data into themes. This phase of the analysis was an iterative process and involved exploring the relationships between the themes and subthemes, and the research aims. A member of the research team (RB) reviewed the themes derived from the analysis, which involved assessing whether the codes within the themes were appropriate, and discussing these with the first author. Finally, a member of the research team (EO) read the themes (and codes within these) agreed upon by the two researchers (RA, RB) to ascertain whether these themes were representative of the data and made recommendations for defining and naming the final set of themes. One of the researchers (RB) is a midwife and health visitor, and two are health psychology researchers (RA, EO). The participants were not aware of the researchers' clinical and academic backgrounds.

The data obtained from the group exercise concerning women's descriptions of their ideal maternity care pathway were summarised narratively using notes on flipcharts and transcriptions (see Figs. 1, 2, and 3), and then compared and contrasted.

Results

Sample characteristics

Twenty-two women expressed interest in the study by providing their contact details. Twelve women participated (54.5%) across three focus groups. Reasons for dropout included ill health and schedule clashes. All bar one of the women had given birth to all their children in London. The remaining participant had given birth in London and another country outside of the UK. Participant characteristics are summarised in Table 1.

Themes

Data analysis resulted in four themes, these are presented below (see Table 2 for a summary).

Theme 1: Women's experiences of maternity care from midwives and health visitors

This theme represents women's relationships with midwives and health visitors, and their experiences of care as collaboratively provided by these healthcare professionals. Women's accounts comprised of both positive and negative

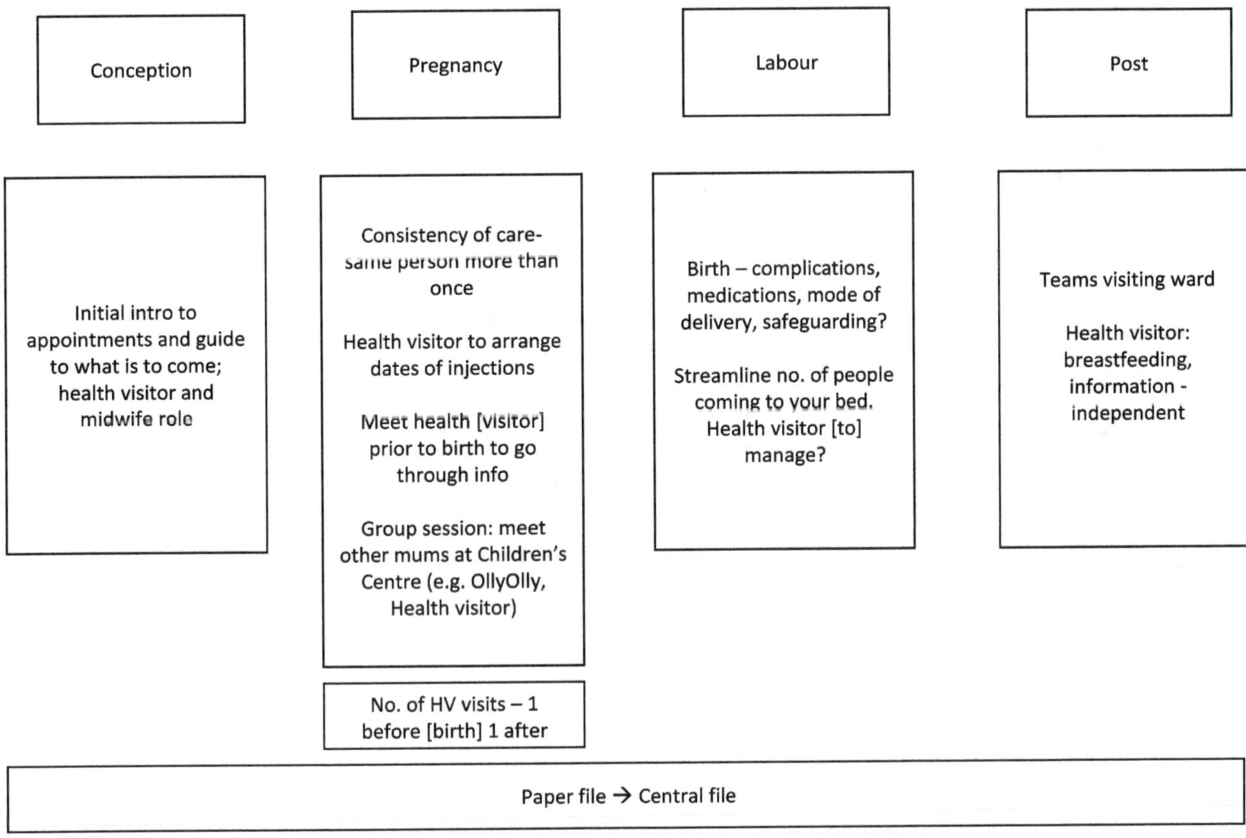

Fig. 1 Focus group 1 transcribed group exercise notes outlining their ideal maternity care pathway

experiences of care, which related to their expectations of care from midwives and health visitors. Positive experiences were characterised by helpful midwives and health visitors, who provided them with extensive support. Women linked this to healthcare professionals' experience and manner of communicating with them:

> *I really liked our health visitor, she was really interested, she was very, she seemed professional at what she was doing, caring, like you said, I felt like she really sort of saw you as an individual not just like tick the box type of thing, and so that was really nice.*
>
> Focus group (FG) 2, P7

Some women reported having less positive experiences from both healthcare professionals, such as pressure to breastfeed with limited support on how to achieve this. Women observed a lack of engagement from health visitors, particularly when going through routine questions:

> *So she [a health visitor] just went through loads of forms and just circled stuff, you know, that I had to remember and then that was it really and then she went, but yeah, it was, it was a bit of a waste of time, really. [...] There wasn't much point to the visit.*
>
> FG 1, P2

Although the majority of the participants reported not having any contact with their health visitors antenatally, those that did shared that this contact was positive, individualised and supportive:

> *So I met my health visitor, contacted me when I was pregnant and met me [...] and we just had an introduction [...]. And I thought it was quite helpful actually, because it was quite nice that we've already got to know her then, and then she said that she would be my health visitor and be the person who'll come and see us once the baby got home and she did.*
>
> FG2, P10

Moreover, women expressed a desire to meet health visitors in pregnancy to establish rapport, process the information that is given to them, and ask questions about areas of care that they are concerned about (e.g. parent groups, immunisations):

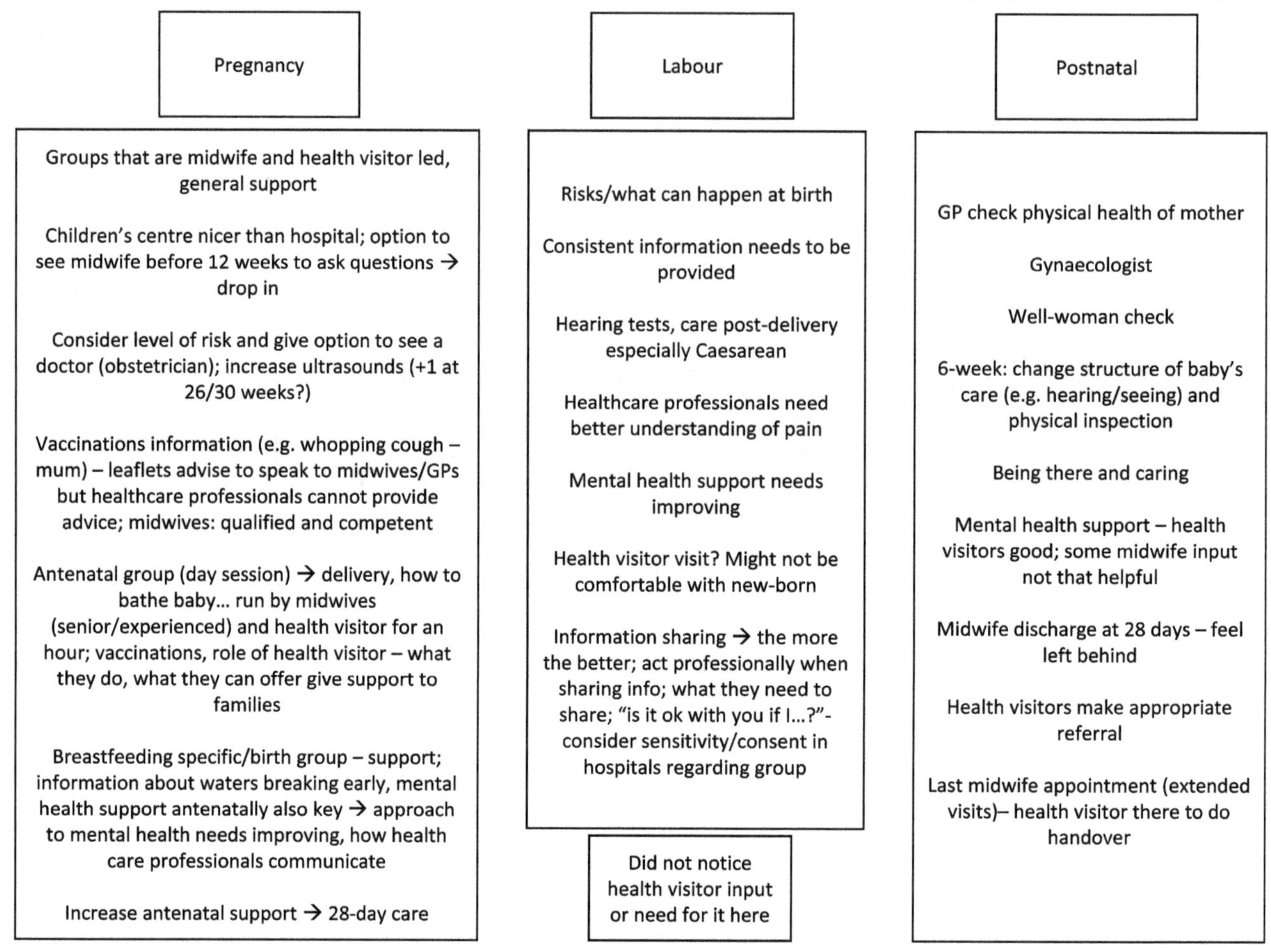

Fig. 2 Focus group 2 transcribed group exercise notes outlining ideal maternity care pathway

P1: *[...] if they could introduce themselves to you before you have the baby, but ...*

P3: *Yes, I definitely agree that to have the session that I had at home, to have had that prior to birth would have been much more helpful, because it [New Birth Visit] was literally leaflet after leaflet after leaflet, and then I keep meaning to go through it and you know, it takes a while to get round, [...] some downtime so even prior, just before the birth, I would have found it more beneficial, just information overload I think at a really quite manic time.*

FG 1

Theme 2: Midwife-health visitor communication

Regarding midwife-health visitor communication, women reported that this appeared to take place largely via their Red Book[1] [29] or notes, and observed evident fragmentation between midwives and health visitors:

> *Mine were definitely completely fragmented, because on the days that [...], but perhaps that was to do with the miscommunication initially with the addresses, but I would get a call from the health visitor on the day the midwife was coming, saying she was coming and I'd have to say no, I've already seen the midwife today, so there was definitely no communication between the teams in my experience.*
>
> FG 1, P3

Although women reported limited communication between midwives and health visitors taking place, they noticed that midwives had an awareness of health visitors being responsible for seeing women at home postnatally: *"No, no, but the midwives did check if the health visitor was coming, so yeah, so I think there was some connection, but yeah that's it really"* (FG 1, P1).

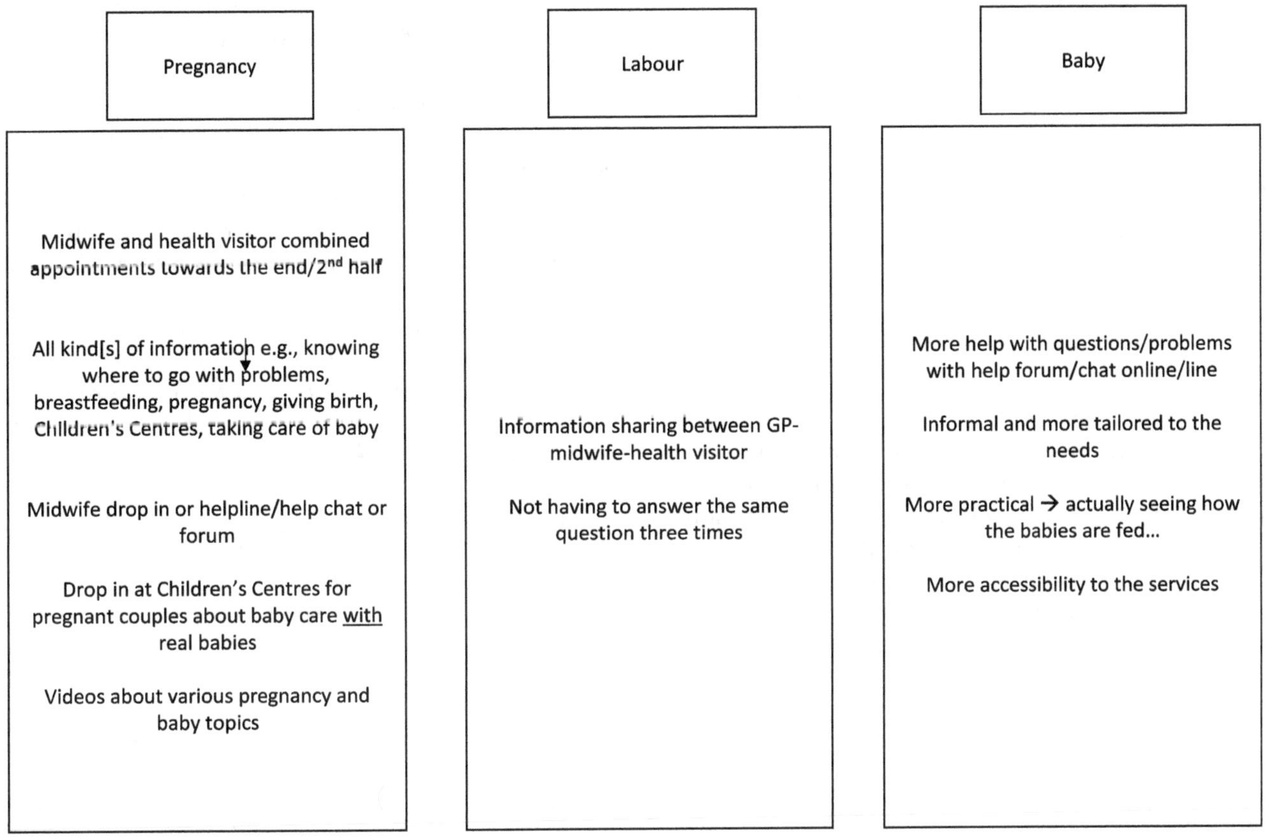

Fig. 3 Focus group 3 transcribed exercise notes outlining ideal maternity care pathway

In addition, women in this study reported valuing continuity of care, and of carer. Women shared experiences of seeing various health professionals throughout their pregnancy and after the birth, reflecting a lack of continuity of carer. This was associated with variations in the level and quality of care that the women receive as well as conflicting advice:

> *...they [midwives and health visitors] all came to my house on the same day, after they got back they must have talked and I asked them one question about what kind [...] oil to put on the baby because she was quite bad and they couldn't agree. So they then had a disagreement about what the midwife was recommend this and the health visitor would recommend this, and they kind of knew that they would give different recommendations but, so they were talking amongst themselves and then I was like, oh I'll just ask someone else.*
>
> FG 3, P10

Table 1 Participant characteristics

Age range (mean)	30–44 years (34.67 years)
Ethnicity	
White English/British	3
White Other	5
Asian/Asian Other	2
Mixed (White and Black African/French; White and Black Caribbean)	2
Range of number of children	1–2 children
Age range of youngest child (mean)	1.75–8 months (5.06 months)

However, participants acknowledged that whilst it would be ideal to have a single healthcare professional providing maternity care (i.e., one named midwife and one named health visitor) this might not be feasible.

Theme 3: Midwife-health visitor collaboration for tailored care

This theme represents maternity care areas where midwife-health visitor collaboration could be beneficial. Participants focussed on information that they received from midwives and health visitors, and the co-ordination of their care.

Women expressed concerns regarding the inconsistent information they received and suggested that centralised

Table 2 Summary of themes linked to research aims

Research aim	Theme
To explore women's experiences of maternity care as collaboratively provided by midwives and health visitors	Women's experiences of maternity care from midwives and health visitors
To explore women's perspectives of how their maternity care can best be provided by these healthcare professionals together.	Midwife-health visitor communication
	Midwife-health visitor collaboration for tailored care
	Women's ideal maternity care pathway

records accessible to midwives and health visitors could be useful. All participants agreed it was important for midwives and health visitors to be aware of their health status and relevant medical information, to counter unnecessarily narrating their needs repeatedly. This aligns with women's suggestions on how maternity care should be co-ordinated; in particular, through midwife-health visitor led antenatal group classes, and joint midwife-health visitor appointments. They considered group classes apt for learning about pregnancy and parenting from midwives and health visitors, along with other parents-to-be:

> P2: *Even if they [midwives and health visitors] did a group session within the area, so you, it's a chance to meet other mums going through the same thing before giving birth.*
>
> *[...]*
>
> P4: *Yeah, that's true because things like what immunisations they need could be said.*
>
> P2: *Yeah. And that gives a chance for mums to share any concerns and stuff at the same time and they're all at the same stage of their pregnancy, so that's nice.*
>
> FG1

Participants acknowledged that there could be greater clarity around the health visitor's role in order to maximise women's engagement with them. This was especially important for women who immigrated to the UK. Women expressed interest in learning about what health visitors can offer, and midwives could help to facilitate this:

> *[...] for me it would have been nice to meet them during their [midwives'] session and have them deliver something for 20 min or maybe on their role, what they do, da, da, da, da, that might be quite nice.*
>
> FG 2, P5

Women suggested that joint appointments/visits could enable transfer of care particularly in the postnatal period: *"So maybe it would be helpful if they have a last midwife appointment, the health visitor would be there then to do a handover"* (FG 2, P7). In addition, participants identified Children's Centres as potentially useful venues for meeting midwives and health visitors, along with other parents and/or parents-to-be, to do group activities and seek support and/or expert advice:

> *Yes, actually being introduced to the children's centre, I think lots of mums don't actually get automatically told about children's centres and playgroups and things like that, and actually it can be a real life saver in those first few weeks.*
>
> FG 1, P1

Theme 4: Women's ideal maternity care pathway

Drawing from the women's accounts and visual data (see Figs. 1, 2 and 3) from the group exercise, this theme sets out participants' suggestions for improving maternity care from pregnancy up to the postpartum period. It has been divided into pregnancy, labour/birth and postpartum care.

Table 3 summarises the common suggestions made by women across the three focus groups.

Pregnancy In pregnancy, all three groups agreed that a midwife and health visitor-led group session would be beneficial to guide parents-to-be about what is to come, and could be less labour intensive for midwives and health visitors. Regarding this session's content, women wanted to be better informed about their maternity care pathway particularly the appointments they would be invited to, the health professionals leading each of these, and their respective role remits:

> P5: *Yeah, I didn't really know what they [health visitors] do really.*
>
> P7: *I thought this was a general check that they do and I could imagine that for, they're also maybe checking for everyone so that they can catch on families where things are difficult, but they are there to help, maybe. I thought that was part of their role, just to make, inform a little bit about, there's a pathway of vaccinations to some general bits, but also to check if the baby is fine, where maybe families are difficult, that's what I sort of thought was their role as well, just to check on everyone but if there's some trouble that they could pick it up and help.*
>
> FG 2

Table 3 Aggregated suggestions for improving the maternity care pathway as collaboratively provided by midwives and health visitors

Pregnancy	Labour/birth	Postnatal
• Midwife-health visitor combined session/appointment	•Information sharing between midwives and health visitors	•Increased postnatal support
Content: Introduction session, guidance regarding what is to come, opportunity to ask questions	Ensure that information shared is consistent or accurate	Make appropriate referrals
Format: Group or combined midwife-health visitor appointment	Obtain consent in a respectful way	Increase mental health, and breastfeeding support
Where: Group sessions could be at Children's Centres		
When: Towards end/ second half of pregnancy		

Women reported preferring a group setting, to meet other parents-to-be, and hear about questions or concerns other than their own. Sessions could be offered towards the end of pregnancy or in the second half of the pregnancy, to give women a chance to reflect on the information they are given:

P4: *I think so, but maybe not too early on, because, I don't know about everyone else but when I was first pregnant especially I was just so wrapped up in the pregnancy I found it really hard to imagine actually having a baby and it felt faraway still, so maybe towards the end of the pregnancy when you're like, OK, I do actually have to look beyond.*

P1: *And also I think towards the end of your pregnancy, you, like you were saying, you had a bit more time, some, not everyone, but some people have, will have a bit of, will stop work a bit before the baby's due, and actually I think it would be quite nice if they did do a session in the children's centre.*

FG 1

Labour/birth There was consensus across the groups that birth-related and other relevant information (e.g. safeguarding issues) should be shared by healthcare professionals; midwives and health visitors having good knowledge of women's history demonstrates connectedness between them. Participants were confident that the healthcare professionals involved in their care would share only pertinent information about women/families relevant to their welfare. At the same time, some women recognised that this could be more challenging for women who might present with vulnerabilities. Reflecting on personal experiences, however, the majority were comfortable with midwives and health visitors sharing information about them:

[...] I do, personally, I'm happy with that information being shared between health visitor and midwife, I think it's quite helpful and [...] if the health visitor knows that you've had a C section, you've had a particularly traumatic birth, then they can be a bit more sensitive, I think that's quite useful.

FG 1, P1

Women were enthusiastic about centralised files that healthcare professionals could access in order to share accurate information with each other, and provide women with adequate, individualised support and advice:

P9: *[...] if there could be something, like I said tongue tie it is in their system, I know it's categorising and listing again, but if we make it a bit more focussed and individualised rather than give you general knowledge, then perhaps that is something that midwives and health visitors could easily share.*

FG 3

One participant (FG 1) had experience of meeting various healthcare professionals who had shared access to her information, which she appreciated.

Postpartum care Participants' key recommendation for postpartum care was increased support from midwives and health visitors. The groups had a variety of suggestions including having the opportunity for informal discussions with healthcare professionals (e.g. drop-ins), midwives and health visitors ensuring appropriate referrals, and providing adequate breastfeeding and mental health support:

P7: *I think what could be quite useful is if there was groups in general, maybe led by midwives or health visitors, during pregnancy, and afterwards for mums to just go to, so not just for breastfeeding, but say, you know you're not feeling well afterwards.*

P6: *Yeah*

[...]

P5: *Like a support group almost.*

FG2

Extended midwife and health visitor involvement was important for making women feel cared for and supported, with their specific needs addressed.

Discussion

This study explored women's experiences of midwife-health visitor collaboration, as well as their ideal maternity care pathway. The main findings are: 1) women's experiences of maternity care as delivered by midwives and health visitors are varied, 2) women perceived the communication between midwives and health visitors as limited, fragmented, and associated with conflicting advice, and 3) collaboration throughout the maternity pathway could be beneficial particularly in relation to information-giving and care co-ordination. Each of these will be discussed sequentially.

First, concerning midwife-health visitor collaboration, the findings showed that women's experiences were a mixture of positive and negative ones, supporting previous research [30, 31]. For example, a national survey of women's maternity care in the UK (N= >4500) found that over 75% of the respondents had positive care experiences [32]. Women in this study reported valuing their relationships with midwives and health visitors who are supportive (e.g. showing interest in mother and baby) and active listeners. Interestingly, despite the women living in the same geographical area with similar service providers, women still reported varied experiences of care particularly in relation to contacts with health visitors in pregnancy. One possible explanation is the decline of the health visiting workforce in England by 10% (9491 vs. 8588 Full-Time Equivalent) in the 12-month period between June 2016–2017 [33]. In addition, there has been a 16.88% reduction of antenatal contacts carried out nationally in Quarter 2 of 2017 (60,853 contacts) compared to Quarter 2 of 2016 (73,213 contacts) [34]. A critical realist approach would also suggest that factors at the real level (e.g. healthcare workforce structure) are influencing the *empirical* level given the diversity in women's reported experiences [18–21].

Second, women reported observing service fragmentation, evidenced by scant communication between midwives and health visitors. This reflects findings from the National Maternity Review, where women emphasised that good communication and information sharing amongst health professionals is essential [35]. However, participants also acknowledged that women's needs differ, which could partially explain why they reported limited midwife-health visitor communication. Research has shown that shared goals (e.g. smoking cessation targets) enhanced relationships between healthcare professionals including midwives and health visitors, which could be directly observed by women who are in contact with such services [36]. Women reported continuity of care, and of carer as important. This has been shown to be linked with lower mortality in terms of continuity with doctors [16] and needs to be explored in the context midwifery and health visiting. Whilst NHS England [17] also highlights the value of continuity of care, and of carer, this is focussed on midwifery care.

Finally, women contributed strategies for improving current maternity care provisions, aligned with the National Maternity Review [35] and Public Health England and Department of Health (UK) midwife-health visitor partnership pathway [8], specifically focussed on interprofessional collaboration. These included service changes, most notably an increased offering of group-based antenatal care collaboratively delivered by midwives and health visitors within community-based services. Existing maternity care pathways set out in line with policies such as the *Healthy Child Programme* [1] recommend group-based antenatal classes delivered in community or healthcare settings to enhance social support. Accordingly, women in this study considered such classes as a valuable resource, and a channel through for obtaining social support. However, there is evidence to suggest that health visitor involvement in antenatal classes is lacking [36]. Thus, currently available classes [36] do not meet these women's suggestion of classes jointly provided by midwives and health visitors and needs to be considered. Successful collaborative working in maternal health have been characterised by the provision of opportunities for health professionals to interact with each other and have shared activities [32], which was also reported to be influential by midwives and health visitors. Taken together, the evidence highlights the potential value of group antenatal classes for women, midwives, and health visitors alike.

The participants also made recommendations for improving mental health and breastfeeding support. Both are core requirements of delivering the *Healthy Child Programme* [1]. Redshaw and Henderson's [32] research showed that the majority of the women they surveyed (N= >4500, 82%) reported having been asked about their mental health, mostly by midwives, in pregnancy. Similarly, 90% of those surveyed were asked about their mental health postnatally, with 63% of these women reported having received support [32]. It was not clear, however, which health professionals were involved in offering postnatal mental health support. It has been shown that group-based breastfeeding support interventions provided jointly by midwives and health visitors can improve breastfeeding, particularly when relationships between these healthcare professionals are strong [7]. One plausible explanation for the participants' desire for increased breastfeeding and mental health support is the nature of their personal circumstances. For example, some participants reported having limited proximal familial/social support. However, this finding needs to be interpreted with caution in keeping with a critical realist approach because women will have different constructions and interpretations of reality shaped by the resources and/or support available to them (*actual* level), as well as their views on the kind of care that healthcare professionals ought to provide (*real* level). Despite these differences which the participants were aware of, they still had shared experiences and needs, suggesting that these layers only provide a partial understanding of the complex nature of reality [20, 21].

Finally, women suggested that their care pathway could be made clearer to them. This is in line with previous research, where women have stressed the value of being better informed about what they could expect from perinatal care such as the frequency of appointments and the purpose of these [30]. Generally, it is known that communication is paramount to high-quality maternity care, both from women's/families' and health professionals' perspectives [35]. Communication was also reported as playing a pivotal role in enabling midwife-health visitor interprofessional collaboration [9], and identified by women as a key issue in maternal and child health [36]. Specifically, participants were confident in healthcare professionals' ability to communicate information in an appropriate manner. They stressed that obtaining their consent for health professionals to share information with each other needs to be done in a respectful way. From a critical realist standpoint, this finding suggests that women lack an awareness of the barriers to communication experienced by midwives and health visitors, which are beyond these individuals' direct/observed experiences. Specifically, these healthcare professionals do not presently have shared information systems [35], despite the evidence suggesting that such systems can facilitate collaborative working between these healthcare professionals [9, 10].

Strengths and limitations of the study

A key strength of this study lies in the manner in which women's views were elicited – through semi-structured interview questions, and women-led, open group discussion to visualise their ideal maternity care pathway [24]. This format allowed women to explore their experiences together, and comment on each other's views and experiences. The diversity of the views obtained from the participants is a further strength of this study. In addition, as is recommended in focus group literature [23], the groups maintained a level of homogeneity in that they were all based in the same geographical area, with some women attending the same General Practice (GP) surgery. Furthermore, the participants were similar in terms of the number of children they had and gave birth in similar settings.

However, the participants were a self-selected sample, and evidently proactive about their maternity care (e.g. accessing Children's centres that they advocated for). Additionally, there were pre-existing relationships between a few of the participants (i.e. some were known to each other) which could have influenced how they responded to the questions. However, all the women appeared comfortable in the group setting, and still openly discussed their experiences with the rest of the group.

Clinical practice and research implications

The present study contributes to the body of knowledge by validating past research [35, 36], and enhances our understanding of maternity care collaboratively provided by midwives and health visitors from the recipients' perspective. The findings indicate that it is paramount that women are listened to, offered consistent services, and provided unbiased information and advice by midwives **and** health visitors. In addition, women's care pathways need to be made clear to them at the outset, including information about the health professionals who may be involved in their care, and these professionals' roles. In terms of midwife-health visitor interprofessional collaboration, the participants showed an awareness of the issues previously raised by these healthcare professionals [10, 37–39] such as poor communication and limited access to shared information, thereby supporting the evidence on the identified barriers and enablers to collaborative working [9]. Whilst the recommendations presented here (e.g. group-based antenatal and postnatal appointments/drop-ins, centralised records) may not necessarily apply to nor be desired by all women, the findings highlight the importance of providing individualised care delivered collaboratively by midwives and health visitors. Thus, it is crucial that women's voices are heard and considered when providing care [12, 35], ultimately promoting informed choice.

Considerations for future research include exploring specific service changes for improving maternity care pathways such as the feasibility of group-based antenatal classes jointly provided by midwives and health visitors, and evaluating the impact of midwife-health visitor communication on health (e.g. rates of postnatal depression, mortality) and service outcomes (e.g. referral management). Maternity care models and guidance developed should include health visitor input if services are to achieve midwife-health visitor collaboration throughout the care pathway. In addition, future research should include other stakeholders such as policymakers and service commissioners to obtain a better understanding of how midwifery and health visiting services could be redesigned to support collaborative working.

Conclusions

This study explored women's views and experiences of collaboratively provided maternity care by midwives and health visitors. Women reported limited midwife-health visitor collaboration; however, they acknowledged the potential value of collaborative working between these groups. Reflecting upon their experiences of care, women were able to identify the issues that they perceived could benefit from collaborative working, such as the provision of inconsistent or inaccurate advice, as well as fragmentation between services. Moreover, the participants offered potential solutions to these, such as the provision of group-based midwife-health visitor antenatal appointments. Women also highlighted positive experiences of the care that they received, such as having helpful midwives and health visitors. Women's recommended strategies regarding how midwife-health visitor interprofessional collaborative practice could be improved demonstrate the necessity of their input in service development efforts.

Endnotes

[1]Red books, or Personal Child Health Records are standardised records of a child's development provided to parents.

Abbreviations

GP: General Practice; NHS: National Health Service

Acknowledgements

We wish to thank Gareth Prosser and Clara Babechuk for their contributions to the recruitment phase of this study.

Funding

This study was part of a PhD studentship funded by the School of Health Sciences, City, University of London. The Research Sustainability Fund at the School of Health Sciences, City, University of London paid for Open Access fees. City, University of London was not involved in the design, data collection, analysis or interpretation of data, in the writing of the manuscript or in the decision to submit the manuscript for publication. Additional funding to support the conduct of this study was obtained from the Psychology Postgraduate Affairs Group (PsyPAG). PsyPAG was not involved in the design, data collection, analysis or interpretation of data, in the writing of the manuscript or in the decision to submit the manuscript for publication.

Authors' contributions

RA led the design of the study protocol, with all other authors (RB, EO) contributing to its development. RA led the application for ethical approval with guidance from RB and EO. RA led recruitment, data collection, analysis and write-up of the study. RB contributed to data collection, analysis, and write-up of the study. EO contributed to data analysis and write-up of the study. All authors have read and approve of the final version of this manuscript.

Competing interests

RA and RB have no competing interests to declare. EO is a member of the editorial board (Associate Editor) of this journal.

Author details

[1]Primary Care Unit, Department of Public Health and Primary Care, University of Cambridge, Cambridge, UK. [2]Centre for Maternal and Child Health Research, School of Health Sciences, City, University of London, London, UK.

References

1. Department of Health. The healthy child Programme: pregnancy and the first five years of life. London: Department of Health; 2009.
2. Chief Nursing Officers of England, Northern Ireland, Scotland and Wales. Midwifery 2020: Delivering expectations. London: Author; 2010.
3. National Health and Medical Research Council. National Guidance on Collaborative Maternity Care. Available from: https://catalogue.nla.gov.au/Record/5055605. Accessed 7 July 2018.
4. World Health Organization. Framework for action on interprofessional education & collaborative practice. WHO, Geneva. 2010
5. Marmot M, Allen J, Goldblatt P, Boyce T, McNeish D, Grady M, Geddes I. Fair society, healthy lives: the Marmot review: The Marmot review; 2010.
6. Public Health England. Health matters: giving every child the best start in life. Available from: https://www.gov.uk/government/publications/health-matters-giving-every-child-the-best-start-in-life/health-matters-giving-every-child-the-best-start-in-life. Accessed 7 July 2018.
7. Hoddinott P, Pill R, Chalmers M. Health professionals, implementation and outcomes: reflections on a complex intervention to improve breastfeeding rates in primary care. Fam Pract. 2007;24(1):84–91.
8. Public Health England. Health Visiting Programme: Pathway to support professional practice and deliver new service offer: Health visiting and midwifery partnership – pregnancy and early weeks. Available from: https://assets.publishing.service.gov.uk/government/uploads/system/uploads/attachment_data/file/465344/2903819_PHE_Midwifery_accessible.pdf. Accessed 7 July 2018.
9. Aquino MRJ, Olander EK, Needle J, Bryar R. Midwives' and health visitors' collaborative relationships: a systematic review of qualitative and quantitative studies. Int J Nurs Stud. 2016;62:193–206.
10. Psaila K, Schmied V, Fowler C, Kruske S. Interprofessional collaboration at transition of care: perspectives of child and family health nurses and midwives. J Clin Nurs. 2014;24:160–72.
11. Schmied V, Mills A, Kruske S, Kemp L, Fowler C, Homer C. The nature and impact of collaboration and integrated service delivery for pregnant women, children and families. J Clin Nurs. 2010;19(23–24):3516–26.
12. Sandall J, Coxon K, Mackintosh N, Rayment-Jones H, Locock L, Page L. Relationships: the pathway to safe, high-quality maternity care. Report from the Sheila Kitzinger symposium at Green Templeton College October 2015. Oxford: Green Templeton College; 2016.
13. Penny RA, Windsor C. Collaboration: a critical exploration of the care continuum. Nurs Inq. 2017;24(2):e12164.
14. Munro S, Kornelsen J, Grzybowski S. Models of maternity care in rural environments: barriers and attributes of interprofessional collaboration with midwives. Midwifery. 2013;29(6):646–52.
15. Sword W, Heaman MI, Brooks S, Tough S, Janssen PA, Young D, Kingston D, Helewa ME, Akhtar-Danesh N, Hutton E. Women's and care providers' perspectives of quality prenatal care: a qualitative descriptive study. BMC Pregnancy Childbirth. 2012;12(1):29.
16. Pereira Gray DJ, Sidaway-Lee K, White E, Thorne A, Evans PH. Continuity of care with doctors—a matter of life and death? A systematic review of continuity of care and mortality. BMJ Open. 2018;8(6):e021161.
17. NHS England. Implementing Better Births: Continuity of Carer. Available from: https://www.england.nhs.uk/publication/implementing-better-births-continuity-of-carer/. Accessed 8 July 2018.

18. Bhaskar R. A realist theory of science. 2nd ed. London: Verso; 1997.
19. Clark AM, Lissel SL, Davis C. Complex critical realism: tenets and application in nursing research. Adv Nurs Sci. 2008;31(4):E67–79.
20. Walsh D, Evans K. Critical realism: an important theoretical perspective for midwifery research. Midwifery. 2014;30(1):1–6.
21. Fletcher AJ. Applying critical realism in qualitative research: methodology meets method. Int J Soc Res Methodol. 2017;20(2):181–94.
22. D'Amour D, Goulet L, Pineault R, Labadie JF, Remondin M. Comparative study of interorganizational collaboration in four health regions and its impact: the case of perinatal services. Research Report; 2004.
23. Barbour R. Doing focus groups: Sage; 2008.
24. Morgan DL: Focus groups as qualitative research, 16: Sage publications; 1997.
25. Jacobs CD, Heracleous LT. Constructing shared understanding: the role of embodied metaphors in organization development. J Appl Behav Sci. 2006; 42(2):207–26.
26. Braun V, Carke V. Using thematic analysis in psychology. Qual Res Psychol. 2006;3(2):77–101.
27. Fereday J, Muir-Cochrane E. Demonstrating rigor using thematic analysis : a hybrid approach of inductive and deductive coding and theme development. Int J Qual Methods. 2006;5:80–92.
28. International QSR: QSR NVivo for Mac 11.4.1. 2014.
29. Royal College of Paediatrics and Child Health. Personal child health record. Available from: https://www.rcpch.ac.uk/resources/personal-child-health-record-pchr. Accessed 7 July 2018.
30. Care Quality Commission. National findings from the 2013 survey of women's experiences of maternity care [Internet]. Care Quality Commission [cited 2018 July 7]. Available from: https://www.cqc.org.uk/sites/default/files/20180130_mat17_statisticalrelease.pdf.
31. Raine R, Cartwright M, Richens Y, Mahamed Z, Smith D. A qualitative study of women's experiences of communication in antenatal care: identifying areas for action. Matern Child Health J. 2010;14(4):590–9.
32. Redshaw M, Henderson J. Safely delivered: A national survey of women's experience of maternity care 2014 [Internet]. National Perinatal Epidemiology Unit [cited 2018 July 7]. Available from: https://www.npeu.ox.ac.uk/downloads/files/reports/Safely%20delivered%20NMS%202014.pdf.
33. NHS Workforce statistics. February 2018. Available from: https://digital.nhs.uk/data-and-information/publications/statistical/nhs-workforce-statistics/nhs-workforce-statistics%2D%2D-february-2018. Accessed 7 July 2018.
34. Statistical commentary. Health visitor service delivery metrics, quarter 2, 2017 to 2018. Available from: https://www.gov.uk/government/publications/health-visitor-service-delivery-metrics-2017-to-2018/statistical-commentary-health-visitor-service-delivery-metrics-quarter-2-2017-to-2018. Accessed 7 July 2018.
35. National Maternity Review. Better births: Improving outcomes of maternity services in England. A five year forward view for maternity care. Available from: https://www.england.nhs.uk/wp-content/uploads/2016/02/national-maternity-review-report.pdf. Accessed 7 July 2018.
36. Donetto S, Malone M, Hughes J, Morrow E, Cowley S, Maben J. Health visiting: The voice of service users. Available from: https://www.kcl.ac.uk/nursing/research/nnru/publications/Reports/Voice-of-service-user-report-July-2013-FINAL.pdf. Accessed 7 July 2018.
37. Cheyne H, McCourt C, Semple K. Mother knows best: developing a consumer led, evidence informed, research agenda for maternity care. Midwifery. 2013;29(6):705–12.
38. Draper J, Farmer S, Field S. The working relationship between the health visitor and community midwife. Health Visitor. 1984;57(12):366–8.
39. Psaila K, Schmied V, Fowler C, Kruske S. Discontinuities between maternity and child and family health services: health professional's perceptions. BMC Health Serv Res. 2014;14:4–4.

17

Male involvement in the maternal health care system: implication towards decreasing the high burden of maternal mortality

Amanual Getnet Mersha

Abstract

Background: One of the essential components of antenatal care (ANC) is birth preparedness and complication readiness (BP/CR). Strengthening BP/CR measures is one of the principal strategies to reduce maternal mortality and morbidity. The current study aimed at determining the level of men's knowledge about obstetric danger signs, and their involvement in BP/CR among community of Northwest Ethiopia.

Method: A cross-sectional community based survey was conducted in Northwest Ethiopia from May 2016 to July 2016. Data was analyzed by the Statistical Package for the Social Sciences software Version 21.0 for Windows. Participants' socio-demographic characteristics, knowledge of obstetric danger signs, and level of involvement in BP/CR were described using frequencies and percentages. Bivariate and multivariable logistic regressions were employed to explore the associated factors and *P*-value of 0.05 was used as a cut-off point to declare significant association.

Result: From 856 men who were invited for the study, 824 men agreed for the interview giving a response rate of 96.2%. Half of the men stated one danger sign that may occur during pregnancy 407(49.4%); one third during delivery 271(32.9%); and 213(25.8%) during postpartum period. Among all participants, 256(31.1%) had not made any preparations; 363(44.1%) made one step; 116(14.1%) made two steps; 82(9.9%) made three steps; 5(0.6%) made four steps; 2(0.24%) made five steps; and no one made all the birth preparation steps during the birth of their last child. BP/CR was significantly association with knowledge of at least one danger sign during pregnancy (AOR = 3.3, 95% CI: 3.1, 3.9); during delivery (AOR = 2.2, 95% CI: 1.1, 2.8); and post partum period (AOR = 1.8, 95% CI: 1.1, 2.4). Furthermore, BP/CR was found to be positively associated with being married, completing college education, escorting wife to antenatal care, and urban residence.

Conclusions: Men's level of knowledge about obstetric danger signs, and their involvement in BP/CR was found to be very poor. Considering the importance of male involvement in the maternal health care, it is recommended to advocate policies and strategies that can improve awareness of men and enhance their engagement in the maternal care.

Keywords: Ethiopia, Birth preparedness, Complication readiness

Correspondence: amanuelget16@gmail.com
Department of Gynecology and Obstetrics, School of Medicine, College of Medicine and Health Sciences, University of Gondar, P.O. Box: 196, Gondar, Ethiopia

Background

Globally, an estimated number of 303,000 maternal deaths occur annually from causes related to pregnancy and childbirth. Around 99% of these deaths occur in developing countries and sub-Saharan African accounts for almost half of the maternal deaths (44%) [1, 2]. Maternal death may occur from complications that may occur while a woman is pregnant, during labor or after delivery. Preparing for birth and related complications ahead of time markedly reduce the number of women dying from such preventable causes [3].

One of the essential components of antenatal care (ANC) is birth preparedness and complication readiness (BP/CR). Birth preparedness and complication readiness (BP/CR) includes detection of danger signs, a plan for a birth attendant, a plan for the place of delivery, preparing potential blood donor and saving money for transport or other [4]. Some of the obstetric complications such as hemorrhage are difficult to precisely predict which mother will develop the complications, therefore every pregnant woman and spouse should make the necessary birth plans [5]. After the International Conference on Population and Development (ICPD) and 4th World Conference on Women held at Cairo [6] and Beijing [7] respectively, men's involvement in maternal health care system is being advocated. Studies had shown the helpful impact of male participation in maternal health in developing countries by improving maternal access to antenatal and postnatal services [8, 9].

The 2015 World Health Organization (WHO) recommendation on maternal and newborn health promotion interventions included active involvement of men during pregnancy, child birth and post partum period as an effective intervention to improve maternal as well as newborn health outcomes. However, male involvement is recommended provided only that women's autonomy in making their own decisions is respected [8].

A systematic review that included 13 studies aimed at assessing the effect of male partner involvement in low and middle income countries as an intervention to improve maternal health outcomes was published in 2018. The review demonstrated that male engagement as an intervention improves antenatal care utilization, postpartum care utilization, delivery at health facilities, child birth by a skilled attendant, and birth preparation and complication readiness [9].

Social norms, beliefs and values affect the types and extent of support that a pregnant woman can receive from her husband or other family members. For instance, a study conducted in Bangladesh showed low level of facility delivery service utilization among women whose husbands believed childbirth is a natural physiologic process that does not require a medical care; and women whose husbands were pressurized by other family members about appropriate place of delivery [10].

In societies where social norms, beliefs and values weaken women's rights, men have social as well as economical supremacy over their partners. Hence, in such patriarchal societies men make a decision regarding sexual affairs, family size, women's access to economic resources and health care service utilization. Achieving sustainable development goals (SDGs) requires alleviating gender based inequalities as well as improving male partner participation in the maternal health care system [11]. Male involvement should be continuously monitored so that it will not worsen gender inequality and affect women's reproductive rights [8].

A study conducted in Oromia regional state of Ethiopia showed that 89% of males were involved in deciding home as their spouses place of deliver [12]. In Patriarchal societies social norms, values and low attitude towards empowering women affects a women's level of maternal health service utilization. Hence, a careful engagement of male partners in the maternal health service in such communities may be an effective strategy to improve maternal health service utilization and reduce maternal morbidity as well as mortality. It is essential to assess men's current level of awareness and involvement in the maternal health care system in order to plan an effective intervention strategy to improve their involvement. Therefore, the current study aimed at assessing men's level of knowledge concerning obstetric danger signs, their level of birth preparedness and complication readiness (BP/CR) in Northwest Ethiopia.

Methods

Study design and setting

A cross-sectional descriptive community survey was conducted in North Gondar Zone, Northwest Ethiopia from May 3, 2016 to July 5, 2016. This zone has 19 districts; the zone has a total population of 2,903,165, of this 14.1% being urban residents.

Sample size and sampling technique

The sample size was calculated by using single population proportion formula by taking 5% desired precision, 95% confidence interval, assuming 42% men awareness of danger signs [21], design effect of 2 for cluster sampling and 10% non response rate, which results in sample size of 710. A multi stage cluster sampling procedure was employed to select four districts out of 19 districts of North Gondar zone. Firstly four districts, three rural districts and one urban district were randomly selected. All households within the catchment areas having men whose wife had given birth within the last 2 years were invited to interview. A total of 856 men were invited to participate in the study.

Data collection and management

A self administered questionnaire was adopted for our setting from Johns Hopkins Program for International Education in Gynecology and Obstetrics (JHPIEGO) [13]. The questionnaire has three sections: The first section is regarding socio demographic characteristics of the participants. The second section assesses participant's knowledge of obstetric danger signs during pregnancy, labor and post partum periods. The final section assesses birth preparedness and complication readiness among participants during the birth of their last baby. The data collection process had taken 2 months (from May 3, 2016 to July 5, 2016). Data was collected by five properly trained research assistants with previous experiences in survey data collection. So as to maintain the quality of the data the researcher reviewed collected data daily and sent feedbacks to the data collectors continuously. BP/CR practice was considered "well prepared" for BP/CR when at least three of the following six practices were reported to have been made in the birth of the last baby: prepared birth kit, identified a skilled attendant, saved money, knew where to go in case of emergency, contacted a blood donor in advance and prepared transportation in advance. Men who reported less than half of the above stated steps were considered to be less prepared. If at least three steps were reported as having been made, the respondent was labeled as well prepared. The three out six was chosen because previous studies have used 50% and above to determine who was well prepared [14]. The questionnaire, originally written in English, was translated to local language (Amharic) and back to English in order to ensure that the translated version gives the proper meaning. The content validity of the questionnaire was confirmed by local experts, including reproductive health experts. (Additional file 1) The questionnaire was pretested on 5% of the sample size prior to the real data collection, which was excluded from the final study. Considering the high burden of puerperal sepsis in this community, which is common in the first 10 days of postpartum period and accounts for 13% of maternal deaths in Ethiopia [15], The time frame of first 2 days in the questionnaire used by Johns Hopkins Program for International Education in Gynecology and Obstetrics (JHPIEGO) was amended to cover maternal health problems in the first 10 days of the post partum period. Once data were collected, each questionnaire was checked for completeness.

Operational definitions

Male partner

Male who has/had a spouse by means of formal marriage or informal union.

Birth preparedness and complication readiness (BP/CR)

Is a process of planning for normal birth and anticipating the actions needed in cases of an emergency.

Level of birth preparedness and complication readiness (BP/CR)

The steps made to have a normal birth outcome during the previous child birth.

Well prepared for birth

If at least three of the following steps have been made in the childbirth process of the last baby: prepared birth kit, identified a skilled attendant, saved money, knew where to go in cases of emergency, contacted a blood donor in advance and prepared transportation in advance.

Statistical analysis

The final data collection tool was checked for completeness, and responses were entered into and analyzed by the Statistical Package for the Social Sciences software Version 21.0 for Windows. Participants' socio-demographic characteristics, knowledge of obstetric danger signs, and level of BP/CR were described using frequencies and percentages in tables. Bivariate logistic regression was conducted to explore factors associated with BP/CR and factors that were found to have a p value of less than 0.2 were entered in to multivariable logistic regression. To declare significant association P-value 0.05 was used as a cut-off point and results expressed by using odds ratio (OR) with 95% confidence interval (CI).

Ethical considerations

This study was approved by the Institutional review board of University of Gondar. Informed written consent was obtained from each participant before starting the interview and participants were also told their right to stop the interview at anytime. The participants were also told that participation is based on their willingness. The obtained information was kept anonymous and recorded in such a way that the respondent could never be known.

Results

Socio-demographic characteristics of participants and their spouses

From 856 men who were invited for participation, 824 men agreed to the interview giving a response rate of 96.2%. A total of 721(87.5%) of the participants were found to be married and half of them have 3–4 children 403(48.9%). One third of the respondents 288(34.9%) did not go to school or did not complete their primary education. Participants from the rural areas accounts for the majority of respondents 637(77.3%). Participants who had escorted their wives to ANC follow up in previous pregnancy accounted for 334(40.5%) of the total participants and a quarter 201(24.4%) of the participants' spouses had delivered in a health facility. A total of 118(14.3%) participants' spouses had obstetric complication in their last pregnancy. (Table 1).

Knowledge of obstetric danger signs

Half of the participants had stated at least one danger sign during pregnancy 407(49.4%); 271(32.9%) of the participants stated at least one danger sign during delivery 271(32.9%) and fewer, 213(25.8%), of the participants stated at least one danger sign during the postpartum period. The commonest mentioned danger sign during pregnancy was high fever 105(12.7%) and excessive vaginal bleeding accounts for the majority of responses during childbirth as well as during the post partum period. 85(10.3%) participants mentioned prolonged labor as a danger sign. There were also other signs mentioned which were not stated in the table such as anemia, dizziness, palpitation that accounted for 10.1% during pregnancy, 3.2% during delivery and 2.7% during postpartum period. (Table 2).

Table 1 Socio-demographic characteristics of men and spouse's obstetric characteristics

Characteristic	N (%)
Age	
18–24	154(18.7%)
25–34	198(24%)
35–44	353(42.8%)
> 44	119(14.4%)
Marital status	
Single/divorced/widowed	103(12.5%)
Married	721(87.5%)
Number of children	
1–2	173(21%)
3–4	403(48.9%)
More than 4	248(30.1%)
Education	
No education	150(18.2%)
Primary Incomplete	138(16.7%)
Primary Complete	311(37.7%)
Secondary	124(15%)
College and above	101(12.3%)
Residence	
Rural	637(77.3%)
Urban	187(22.7%)
Escorted wife to ANC previous pregnancy	
Yes	334(40.5%)
No	490(59.5%)
Obstetric complication in previous pregnancy	
Yes	118(14.3%)
No	706(85.7%)
Place of delivery previous pregnancy	
Home	623(75.6%)
Health facility	201(24.4%)

Level of BP/CR in spouses' previous pregnancy

As illustrated in table three, the most common preparations made during the birth of their last child were getting birth kit 309(37.5%) followed by saving money 218(26.5%). (Table 3) Furthermore, 91(11%) of the participants had arranged transportation, 25(3%) had identified which health facility to visit in case of emergency, 67(8.1%) had identified a skilled birth attendant, 3(0.4%) prepared possible blood donor during the birth of their last baby. Two hundred and fifty six men

Table 2 Men's knowledge of danger signs during pregnancy, labor and postpartum

Obstetric danger sign	N (%)
During Pregnancy	
High fever	105(12.7%)
Severe abdominal pain	97(11.8%)
Excessive vaginal bleeding	94(11.4%)
Abnormal body movements	61(7.4%)
Severe headache	70(8.5%)
Swollen hands/face	59(7.2%)
Loss of consciousness	33(4%)
Blurred vision	13(1.6%)
Knowledge of at least one sign	407(49.4%)
During Childbirth	
Excessive vaginal bleeding	102(12.4%)
Abnormal body movements	54(6.5%)
Retained placenta	37(4.5%)
High fever	98(11.9%)
Prolonged labor	85(10.3%)
Severe headache	64(7.8%)
Loss of consciousness	29(3.5%)
Knowledge of at least one sign	271(32.9%)
During postpartum	
Excessive vaginal bleeding	105(12.7%)
High fever	99(12%)
Abnormal body movements	56(6.8%)
Loss of consciousness	31(3.8%)
Foul smelling discharge	74(8.9%)
Severe headache	78(9.5%)
Knowledge at least one sign	213(25.8%)

Multiple responses possible

Table 3 BP/CR among men in previous pregnancy

BP/CR	N (%)
Identified birth kit	309(37.5%)
Saved money	218(26.5%)
Identified transport	91(11%)
Identified a blood donor in advance	3(0.4%)
Identified where to go for emergency	25(3%)
Identified skilled attendant	67(8.1%)
Made at least 3 steps	82(9.9%)

Multiple responses possible

(31.1%) had not done any preparations; 363(44.1%) had made one of the six birth preparing steps assessed; 116(14.1%) made two preparations; 82(9.9%) made three preparations; 5(0.6%) made four preparations; 2(0.24%) had made five preparations; furthermore, no one made all the six preparations assessed in the current study. (Fig. 1).

Factors associated with BP/CR

Place of residency, current marital status, escorting wife to antenatal care in previous pregnancy, number of children, level of education, knowledge of at least one danger sign during pregnancy, knowledge of at least one danger sign during delivery and knowledge of at least one danger sign during the postpartum period were associated with BP/CR in the bivariate logistic regression analysis. Further analysis by using multivariable logistic regression demonstrates that completing college education have a significant positive association with the steps taken for birth preparation and complication readiness (AOR = 3.2, 95% CI: 2.8, 4.6). Being married, escorting wife to antenatal care, and urban residence were also found to be significantly associated with the steps taken for birth preparation and complication readiness. Furthermore, the steps made towards birth preparation and complication readiness were found to have significant associations with knowledge of at least one danger sign during pregnancy (AOR = 3.3, 95% CI: 3.1, 3.9), during delivery (AOR = 2.2, 95% CI: 1.1, 2.8) and post partum period (AOR = 1.8, 95% CI: 1.1, 2.4). (Table 4).

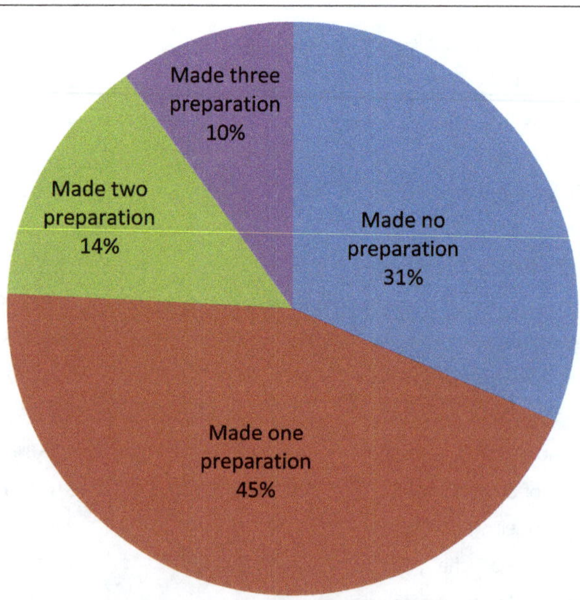

Fig. 1 Number of Preparations Made By Participants

Discussion

As part of a comprehensive antenatal care provision a pregnant woman and her family should be provided with detailed information about pregnancy, child birth, and obstetric danger signs that may occur in the process of child birth [4]. Antenatal care creates a good opportunity for the service providers to develop a birth plan with a women and her spouse. Involving men on the maternal health care system improves health service utilization, decrease rate of maternal depression, raise maternal self-esteem, and decreased possibility of childbirth complications [16–20].

Male residents in Northwest Ethiopia were found to have inadequate awareness regarding obstetric danger signs. This could be due to the low percentage of participants who had accompanied their spouses to antenatal care during previous pregnancy (40.5%) and low percentage of facility delivery rate (24.4%). It could also be due to deficiencies in community health education programs in the country. The findings of this research are similar with a study conducted in Southern Ethiopia which reported that only 42.2% of men were found to be aware of the obstetric danger signs [21]. Similarly, other studies conducted in different countries also reported men's inadequate knowledge concerning the obstetric danger signs. However, our findings are in contrast with one study that assessed Kenyan men's awareness of obstetric danger signs in which the median knowledge score was reported to be 9 out of 10 selected danger signs. This discrepancy may relate to differences in study method; in the Kenyan study men were asked to say yes or no after 10 danger signs were read to them by the interviewer [22].

Although majority of maternal morbidities and mortalities occur in the immediate postpartum period [23], men in this community were able to state fewer possible danger signs in the postpartum period as compared to other periods (ante partum and delivery). This may be due to low level of postnatal care utilization (20.2%) in communities of Northwest Ethiopia [24] and/or the cultural practice in rural parts of Ethiopia that postpartum women spend their postpartum period with their mothers. This result is in line with a study conducted in

Table 4 Association between selected socio-demographic characteristics, obstetric characteristics, knowledge of danger signs and BP/CR

Characteristic	Prepared N (%)	Less prepared N (%)	Bivariate Analysis Unadjusted OR (95%CI)	Multivariable Analysis AOR (95%CI)
Age				
18–24	12(7.8%)	142(92.2%)	1	
25–34	15(7.6%)	183(92.4%)	0.4 (0.3–1.2)	
35–44	43(12.2%)	310(87.8%)	1.7 (0.6–6.2)	
> 44	12(10.1%)	107(89.9%)	0.5 (0.2–2.8)	
Number of children				
1–2	18(10.4%)	155(89.6%)	1	
3–4	39(9.7%)	364(90.3%)	0.4 (0.2–5.4)	
More than 4	25(10.1%)	223(89.9%)	1.4 (1.3–2.1)	
Education				
No education	9(6%)	141(94%)	1	
Primary Incomplete	11(7.9%)	127(92.1%)	1.5 (0.3–6.2)	
Primary complete	20(6.4%)	291(93.6%)	1.7 (0.8–3.9)	
Secondary	17(13.7%)	107(86.3%)	1.3 (1.2–2.5)	
College and above	25(24.7%)	76(75.3%)	3.8 (2.9–5.1)	3.2(2.8–4.6)*
Marital status				
Married	78(10.8%)	643(89.2%)	3.1 (2.8–3.6)	2.3(1.6–3.5)*
Single/divorced/widowed	4(3.8%)	99(96.2%)	1	
Residence				
Urban	46(24.6%)	141(75.4%)	5.8 (4.3–6.3)	4.2(2.9–5.6)*
Rural	36(5.7%)	601(94.3%)	1	
Escorted Wife to ANC in the previous pregnancy				
Yes	43(12.9%)	291(87.1%)	2.7 (1.8–3.2)	1.7(1.6–2.9)*
No	39 (8%)	451 (92%)	1	
Knowledge of at least one danger sign during pregnancy				
Yes	61(15)	346(85)	3.1 (2.5–3.4)	3.3(3.1–3.9)*
No	21(5.1)	396(94.9)	1	
Knowledge of at least one danger sign during labor				
Yes	39(14.4)	232(85.6)	3.7 (2.3–3.8)	2.2(1.1–2.8)*
No	43(7.8)	510(92.2)	1	
Knowledge of at least one danger sign postpartum				
Yes	37(17.4%)	176(82.6%)	2.6 (1.5–2.7)	1.8(1.1–2.4)*
No	45(7.4%)	566(92.6%)	1	

*p value< 0.05, in the table the number "1" indicates the reference variable

rural Tanzania that reported higher numbers of danger signs stated in the ante partum period [14].

We found discrepancies between men's knowledge and the common causes of maternal complications. The most common obstetric danger signs men reported in relation to pregnancy were high fever (12.7%), severe abdominal pain (11.8%), and vaginal bleeding (11.4%). The finding of this study is in agreement with a study conducted in Southern Ethiopia that reported vaginal bleeding and severe abdominal pain as the most stated danger sign that may occur in the ante partum period [21]. In a Tanzanian study high fever, abdominal pain and vaginal bleeding were also commonly mentioned danger signs in the ante partum period [14]. A review conducted in 2014 reported that among all maternal deaths in Ethiopia obstructed labor and sepsis accounts for 29 and 13% respectively [15]. In a study conducted in Southwest Ethiopia, the incidence of obstructed labor was reported to be 12.2% [25]. However, prolonged labor as a danger sign during delivery was mentioned only by

10.3% of participants. Only 12% of participants mentioned fever as a danger sign in the postpartum period. Hence, awareness creation interventions are recommended in order to reduce major causes of maternal mortality and morbidity in this community.

Men's involvement in birth preparedness and complication readiness in this community was found to be scarce. Only 82(9.9%) participants reported making at least three of the six assessed steps during the birth of their last baby. A southern Ethiopian study also reported a low level (9.4%) of male involvement in BP/CR issues [21]. Moreover, the finding of this study is also in line with studies from other countries like Tanzania and Uganda [14, 26]. The low level of involvement in BP/CR may be explained by the low antenatal service utilization in this area, the poor quality of the service, mostly husbands did not accompany their wives during antenatal visit and even if they come there are also failures from the service providers to invite husbands to join the counseling process [26–29].

Higher level of education, being married, escorting wife to antenatal care, urban residence were found to have positive significant association with birth preparation and complication readiness. This may be due to the fact that those who have higher level of education have good level of understanding of the complications and importance of having a birth plan. In addition to that urban dwellers will access information as well as birth kits easily as compared to rural dwellers. Most of the educated ones have urban residency which can also explain the low level of birth preparation and complication readiness among rural residents. Escorting wife to antenatal care will increase exposure with health professionals that may improve the probability of being prepared for complications and childbirth. These factors were also found to be associated with men's involvement in BP/CR in studies conducted among other African countries like Tanzania and Uganda [30–32].

In the current study men's level of involvement in BP/CR was found to have a significant association with knowledge of obstetric danger signs during pregnancy, labor and postpartum. This may be due to the fact that knowledge of danger signs leads to greater anticipation and preparation to lessen effects of pregnancy and childbirth complications by reducing the first two delays (delay in decision making and delay in transportation) to tackle obstetric complications. The norms and values of the community towards women may have affected their interest of engaging in the maternal health issues. This finding is similar with a study conducted among male residents of southern Ethiopia which reported that awareness of danger signs doubles involvement [21].

Limitations and strengths of the study

As this is a cross sectional study, it is not possible to provide a causal relationship between being well-prepared and other variables. Moreover, the participants were required to remember things happened in the past 2 years so there is a possibility of recall bias. Although, all the necessary precautions were followed to maintain the quality of the data, it is not possible to avoid the effect of data collector's attitude on the quality of the data. These limitations mean that caution is required when generalizing the results to other settings. Despite these limitations our study demonstrates a lot of strengths. One of the strengths of this study was the large number of participate in the study and men's knowledge of danger signs and BP/CR were not assessed in this area previously.

Conclusions and recommendations

The current study demonstrated men's low level of knowledge concerning obstetrical danger signs as well as their involvement in birth preparedness and complication readiness in Northwest Ethiopia. This study also showed a strong association between BP/CR and men's level of awareness concerning obstetric danger signs. Additionally, BP/CR was also found to have a significant association with higher educational level, being married, escorting wife to antenatal care in their spouses' previous pregnancy, and being an urban resident. In patriarchal communities like Ethiopia so as to improve the maternal health service utilization, involving men in the maternal health care system without worsening the already existing gender inequalities is an essential strategy. Hence, it is recommended to advocate policies and strategies that can improve men's level of awareness and their engagement in the maternal care through health education and incentives. Community based awareness creation by utilizing mass media and campaigning is recommended. It is recommended to give special emphasis to improving utilization of postnatal care to improve the low level of knowledge in the post partum period, were most of maternal mortalities occur, as compared to the ante-partum and intra-partum period.

Abbreviations

ANC: Antenatal care; BP/CR: Birth preparedness and complication readiness

Acknowledgements

The author acknowledges the Support of University of Gondar, data analyst and data collectors. The author is very thankful for all the participants.

Funding

No financial support was gained to conduct this study.

Competing interests

The author declares that there are no competing interests.

References

1. Trends in maternal mortality. 1990 to 2015: estimates by WHO, UNICEF, UNFPA, World Bank Group and the United Nations Population Division. Geneva: World Health Organization. p. 2015.
2. Hogan MC, Foreman KJ, Naghavi M, Ahn SY, Wang M, Makela SM, et al. Maternal mortality for 181 countries, 1980-2008: a systematic analysis of progress towards millennium development goal 5. Lancet (London, England). 2010;375(9726):1609–23.
3. McPherson RA, Khadka N, Moore JM, Sharma M. Are birth-preparedness programmes effective? Results from a field trial in Siraha district, Nepal. J Health Popul Nutr. 2006;24(4):479–88.
4. Carroli G, Piaggio G, Khan-Neelofur D. WHO systematic review of randomised controlled trials of routine antenatal care. Lancet. 2001; 357(9268):1565–70. https://doi.org/10.1016/S0140-6736(00)04723-1.
5. Tura G, Afework MF, Yalew AW. The effect of birth preparedness and complication readiness on skilled care use: a prospective follow-up study in Southwest Ethiopia. Reprod Health. 2014;11:60.
6. Alison McIntosh C, L. Finkle J. The Cairo Conference on Population and Development: A New Paradigm? 1995. 223 p.
7. Larson EL.,"United Nations Fourth World Conference on Women: Action for Equality, Development, and Peace (Beijing, China: September 1995)",*Emory Int'l L Rev*,vol. 10, pp.1996. Accessed at http://www.un.org/womenwatch/daw/beijing/pdf/Beijing%20full%20report%20E.pdf.
8. Davis J, Luchters S and Holmes W. Men and maternal and newborn health: benefits, harms, challenges and potential strategies for engaging men. Melbourne: Centre for International Health, Burnet Institute; 2012 (http://www.comminit.com/hiv-aids/content/men-and-maternal-and-newborn-health-benefits-harms-challenges-and-potential-strategies-e. Accessed 12 Jan 2015).
9. Tokhi M, Comrie-Thomson L, Davis J, Portela A, Chersich M, Luchters S. Involving men to improve maternal and newborn health: a systematic review of the effectiveness of interventions. PLoS One. 2018;13(1):e0191620.
10. Story, et al. Husbands' involvement in delivery care utilization in rural Bangladesh: a qualitative study. BMC Pregnancy Childbirth. 2012;12:28. https://doi.org/10.1186/1471-2393-12-28.
11. Amnesty International. Women, Violence and health. London: Amnesty International; 2005. Accessed at https://www.amnestyusa.org/pdfs/mazeofinjustice.pdf.
12. Wassie L, Bekele A, Ismael A, Tariku N, Heran A, Getnet M, et al. Magnitude and factors that affect males' involvement in deciding partners' place of delivery in Tiyo District of Oromia region, Ethiopia. Ethiop J Heal Dev. 2014;28:1–43.
13. JHPIEGO (2004) Monitoring Birth Preparedness and Complication Readiness: Tools and Indicators for Maternal and Newborn Health. Baltimore: JHPIEGO;. Available: https://pdf.usaid.gov/pdf_docs/pnada619.pdf.
14. August F, Pembe AB, Mpembeni R, Axemo P, Darj E. Men's knowledge of obstetric danger signs, birth preparedness and complication readiness in rural Tanzania. PLoS One. 2015;10(5):e0125978.
15. Berhan Y, Berhan A. Causes of maternal mortality in Ethiopia: a significant decline in abortion related death. Ethiop J Health Sci. 2014;24(Suppl):15–28.
16. Schaffer MA, Lia-Hoagberg B. Effects of social support on prenatal care and health behaviors of low-income women. J Obstet Gynecol Neonatal Nurs. 1997;26:433–40.
17. Yargawa J, Leonardi-Bee J. Male involvement and maternal health outcomes: systematic review and meta-analysis. J Epidemiol Community Health. 2015;69(6):604–12.
18. Berhane Y. Male involvement in reproductive health. Ethiop J Health Dev. 2006;20(3):135–6.
19. Lewis G. Beyond the numbers: reviewing maternal deaths and complications to make pregnancy safer. Br Med Bull. 2003;67:27–37.
20. Koblinsky MA. Beyond maternal mortality--magnitude, interrelationship, and consequences of women's health, pregnancy-related complications and nutritional status on pregnancy outcomes. Int J Gynaecol Obstet. 1995; 48(Suppl):S21–32.
21. Debiso AT, Gello BM, Malaju MT. Factors Associated with Men’s Awareness of Danger Signs of Obstetric Complications and Its Effect on Men’s Involvement in Birth Preparedness Practice in Southern Ethiopia, 2014. Adv Public Health. 2015;2015:9.
22. Dunn A, Haque S, Innes M. Rural Kenyan men's awareness of danger signs of obstetric complications. Pan Afr Med J. 2011;10:39.
23. Khan KS, Wojdyla D, Say L, Gulmezoglu AM, Van Look PF. WHO analysis of causes of maternal death: a systematic review. Lancet. 2006;367:1066–74.
24. Workineh YG, Hailu DA. Factors Affecting Utilization of Postnatal Care Service in Amhara Region, Jabitena District, Ethiopia. Sci J Public Health. 2014;2(3):169–76. https://doi.org/10.11648/j.sjph.20140203.15.
25. Fantu S, Segni H, Alemseged F. Incidence, causes and outcome of obstructed labor in jimma university specialized hospital. Ethiop J Health Sci. 2010;20(3):145–51.
26. Kabakyenga JK, Ostergren PO, Turyakira E, Pettersson KO. Knowledge of obstetric danger signs and birth preparedness practices among women in rural Uganda. Reprod Health. 2011;8:33.
27. Sekoni OO, Owoaje ET. Male knowledge of danger signs of obstetric complications in an urban city in South west Nigeria. Annals of Ibadan postgraduate medicine. 2014;12(2):89–95.
28. Pembe AB, Urassa DP, Carlstedt A, Lindmark G, Nystrom L, Darj E. Rural Tanzanian women's awareness of danger signs of obstetric complications. BMC Pregnancy Childbirth. 2009;9:12.
29. Rashad WM, Essa R. Women's Awareness of Danger Signs of Obstetrics Complications; 2010. p. 1299–306.
30. Kakaire O, Kaye DK, Osinde MO. Male involvement in birth preparedness and complication readiness for emergency obstetric referrals in rural Uganda. Reprod Health. 2011;8(1):12.
31. Tweheyo R, Konde-Lule J, Tumwesigye NM, Sekandi JN. Male partner attendance of skilled antenatal care in peri-urban Gulu district, Northern Uganda. BMC Pregnancy Childbirth. 2010;10:53.
32. Redshaw M, Henderson J. Fathers' engagement in pregnancy and childbirth: evidence from a national survey. BMC Pregnancy Childbirth. 2013;13:70.

18

Assessing emergency obstetric and newborn care: can performance indicators capture health system weaknesses?

Andrea Solnes Miltenburg[1,2*], Richard Forget Kiritta[3], Thabea Benedicto Bishanga[4], Jos van Roosmalen[5,6] and Jelle Stekelenburg[7,8]

Abstract

Background: Regular monitoring and assessment of performance indicators for emergency obstetric and newborn care can help to identify priorities to improve health services for women and newborns. The aim of this study was to perform a district wide assessment of emergency obstetric and newborn care performance and identify ways for improvement.

Methods: Facility assessment of 13 dispensaries, four health centers and one district hospital in a rural district in Tanzania was performed in two data collection periods in 2014. Assessment included a facility walk-through to observe facility infrastructure and interviews with facility in-charges to assess available services, staff and supplies. In addition facility statistics were collected for the year 2013. Results were discussed with district representatives.

Results: Approximately 65% of expected births took place in health facilities and 22% of women with complications were treated in facilities expected to provide emergency care. None of the facilities was, however, able to perform at the expected level for emergency obstetric and newborn care since not all required signal functions could be provided. Inadequate availability of essential drugs such as uterotonics, antibiotics and anticonvulsants as well as lack of ability to perform vacuum extraction and blood transfusion limited performance.

Conclusions: Performance of emergency obstetric and newborn care in Magu District was not in accordance with expected guidelines and highly influenced by lack of available resources and an insufficiently functioning health care system. Improving assessment approaches, to look beyond the signal functions, can capture weaknesses in the system and will help to understand poor performance and identify locally applicable ways for improvement.

Keywords: Emergency obstetric and newborn care, Signal functions, Resource problems

Background

Emergency Obstetric and Newborn Care (EmONC) must be available and accessible to all women in order to avert maternal deaths and morbidities from the most frequent causes as haemorrhage, sepsis, eclampsia, obstructed labour and abortion complications. EmONC can also prevent fresh stillbirths and early neonatal deaths and morbidities [1].

The past decades Tanzania has given Reproductive Maternal Neonatal and Child Health (RMNCH) high priority which at policy level resulted in development of the 'One Plan – to accelerate reduction of maternal, newborn and child deaths between 2008 and 2015' [2, 3]. Implementation of policies, primarily the responsibility of regional and district councils, has received less attention, especially with regards to specific maternal and neonatal interventions [2, 4]. As a consequence insufficient progress has been made to reduce maternal and neonatal mortality, in particular in the Western and Lake Zone regions [2, 3].

There is no single intervention that works to achieve the desired reduction in maternal and neonatal mortality [5], as direct and underlying causes for poor maternal

* Correspondence: a.solnesmiltenburg@gmail.com
[1]Institute of Health and Society, Department of Community Medicine and Global Health, Faculty of Medicine, University of Oslo, Oslo, Norway
[2]Women Centered Care Project, a project of the African Woman Foundation, Magu, Mwanza Region, Tanzania
Full list of author information is available at the end of the article

health and mortality are complex [6]. Along the continuum of care from pre-conception to post-birth as well as from individual-, family-, community level up to facility and policy level, packages of interventions can have great impact if implemented well [7]. Skilled care at birth and access to EmONC is of vital importance especially for those 15% of pregnant women who are expected to experience life-threatening maternal and/or neonatal complications [8].

Over the years useful process indicators have been developed to evaluate availability, accessibility and quality of EmONC [9, 10]. Regular assessment and monitoring of EmONC indicators can help programme planners in the field of RMNCH to identify priorities and needs to strengthen health services for women and their newborns [10]. The aim of this study was to perform a district-wide assessment of EmONC performance, to identify gaps and propose ways for improvement.

Methods

Setting

Magu District is one of eight districts of Mwanza Region of Tanzania and is bordered to the north by Lake Victoria and to the west by the city of Mwanza, which is the second largest city in Tanzania. The estimated population in 2012 was 299,759 [11]. Magu district had 46 health facilities: one government district hospital, four government health centres, 30 government dispensaries, nine private dispensaries, one faith based dispensary and one parastatal dispensary. Out of all government health facilities 31 provided antenatal, delivery and postnatal care. In terms of ownership, facilities are funded and supported by the district council of which the Council Health Management Team (CHMT) is responsible for decision-making. Main actors in the provision of maternal health care are (assistant) medical officers, clinical officers, enrolled and registered nurses/midwives, as well as medical attendants.

Since 2012 the Woman Centered Care Project (WCCP), a project of the African Woman Foundation [12–14], has been performing baseline research activities in the district and formed a partnership with the Magu District Council with the aim to improve accessibility and availability of quality maternal health care. Although focus has mainly been on antenatal care services and community involvement, the project together with members of the CHMT discussed the need for an EmONC assessment as improvements in the health situation of women in the district can only be reached when the complete system functions well along the continuum of care.

Data collection

This study is based on two periods of data collection. A facility survey was performed at 13 dispensaries, one health centre and the district hospital in April-May 2014, including investigation of the availability of supplies and medicines to provide basic EmONC. Facilities were selected purposefully based on participation in the WCCP project locations. In December 2014 an EmONC assessment was performed including assessments at the district hospital and all four health centres in the district regarding their EmONC performance within the past three months. The research team interviewed (assistant) clinical officers or nurses in charge of the facilities. Facility visits included a walk-through to observe facility infrastructure, available services, staff and supplies. Maternal death review forms of 2013 were also reviewed. During the field visits and during meetings with different members of the CHMT and other stakeholders relevant observations were documented and discussed.

Data collection tools

For the facility survey in April-May a tool was developed based on the Johns Hopkins Program for International Education in Gynecology and Obstetrics (JHPIEGO) manual for monitoring birth preparedness and complication readiness [15]. The tool was digitalized using Magpi Data Collection Software [16]. Health facilities were visited to collect information on facility statistics for the year 2013, facility infrastructure, available services, equipment and supplies. The survey was conducted while facilities were awaiting their new batch of quarterly supplies. If supplies were told to be present but not able to be located or accessible during our visit, they were documented as absent. Non-functioning equipment was also recorded as not available.

For the EmONC assessment, the handbook 'Monitoring Emergency Obstetric Care' was used [10]. EmONC signal functions are the key medical interventions that are used to treat direct obstetric complications that cause the vast majority of maternal deaths around the globe. The seven functions of Basic EmONC are expected to be provided at health centre and dispensary level [3]. In referral district hospitals the nine functions of Comprehensive EmONC should be provided to save lives (see Table 1). For assessment of signal functions at dispensary level, focus was on availability of materials and supplies, rather than on performance in the last three months. Therefore signal function 4, manual removal of the placenta, was not included at dispensary level.

Data collection team

The data collection team consisted of members and volunteers of the WCCP, in collaboration with their partners. For the facility survey, a volunteer nurse-midwife from Australia performed facility visits together with ASM. The EmONC assessment was performed by co-authors JvR and JS, experts of the Working Party on International Safe Motherhood and Reproductive Health

Table 1 Signal functions for basic and comprehensive EmONC services

Basic EmONC services	Comprehensive EmONC services
1) Administer parenteral antibiotics	Perform signal functions 1–7, plus
2) Administer uterotonic drugs	8) Perform surgery (cesarean section)
3) Administer parenteral anticonvulsants	9) Perform blood transfusion
4) Manually remove the placenta	
5) Remove retained products	
6) Perform assisted vaginal delivery	
7) Perform basic neonatal resuscitation	

in the Netherlands, both consultant obstetricians with several years of working experience in Tanzania and other sub-Sahara African countries. Facilities were notified of the visit prior to arrival. For all facility visits representatives of the District Medical Officer accompanied the team and joined in the assessment. Interviews during the facility survey were conducted with the help of a translator, for the EmONC assessments interviews were done in Kiswahili, with occasional translation.

Data analysis

All data was entered in Microsoft Excel Version 15.0 to allow for calculation of frequency. To analyse the indicators, data collected from both the EmONC assessment and the facility survey at lower level facilities were used. Birth data was collected from registers (delivery register, admission register, operating theatre register, monthly reports) of the year 2013. If data was not accessible for the whole year, data was extrapolated from known parts of the year. To estimate the expected number of births in the district a Crude Birth Rate of 39 was used based on figures of the Demographic and Health Survey 2010, for mainland rural areas [17]. Research notes based on field visits were compared and discussed within the research team. A report of the facility survey was presented to the District Medical Officer and discussed with a Steering Committee on June 18th, 2014. The steering committee is overseeing project activities of the WCCP and comes together on a quarterly basis. Members included district and community representatives. After the EmONC assessment results were presented and discussed at a meeting of the CHMT during their annual planning meeting on December 6th, 2014.

Results

A total of 13 dispensaries, four health centres and one district hospital were included in the facility survey. In 2013, 2504 (21%) births took place in the district hospital and 2531 (22%) births in the four health centres. In dispensaries births ranged from 50 to 296 births per year, with a mean of 100 births. Assuming similar patterns in the facilities, which were not surveyed, births in dispensaries were estimated to cover a total of 2600 (22%) births. In total these facilities covered 7635 facility births, approximately 65% of the expected births.

None of the dispensaries complied with the guidelines to provide basic EmONC and were either not able to administer one or all of the essential drugs: anti-convulsants, uterotonics or antibiotics. None of the dispensaries had complete birth kits. Five facilities were able to locate all essential neonatal resuscitation equipment. An overview of availability of essential equipment and supplies is presented in Table 2.

Results with regards to the EmONC indicators are presented in Table 3. Three health centres did provide all signal functions for basic EmONC except administration of MgSO4 to prevent or treat eclampsia (supply problems) and performing assisted vaginal deliveries. One health centre appeared to have more problems; no manual vacuum aspirations were performed, parenteral antibiotics were not administered and newborn resuscitation was not performed. The district hospital was able to provide comprehensive EmONC but did not fully qualify due to non-availability of blood transfusions and no use of the available vacuum extractor in the past three months. Lack of blood was a contributing factor in at least three out of 22 maternal deaths and a frequent indication for referral to the regional hospital in Mwanza. Although a vacuum extractor was available and functioning, observations during the facility visit and lack of documentation on performance of vacuum extraction indicated it unlikely to be used.

Discussion

None of the facilities in Magu district was able to perform at the expected EmONC-level covering all signal functions. These findings are not surprising considering that the nation wide availability of basic and comprehensive EmONC facilities reduced between 2012 and 2015 [3, 18]. All facilities scored particularly poor on performance of assisted vaginal delivery. Poor clarity on who is qualified, lack of exposure and training and beliefs that higher cadres of health workers should perform such procedures contribute to almost district wide absence of performance of this signal function [1, 19]. Unavailability of facilities offering full basic and/or comprehensive EmONC is worrisome and contributes to poor outcomes, even after women have reached institutions. Previous studies in Tanzania reached similar conclusions [4, 19–22]. Negative in-facility experiences influence women's perceptions of care and might influence future care seeking, leading to

Table 2 Facility survey: availability of supplies[a] for EmOC in 2014

Audit items		District hospital ($N = 1$)	Health centre ($N = 1$)	Dispensaries ($N = 13$)
Basic equipment	Stethoscope	Yes	Yes	10/13
	BP machine	Yes	Yes	8/13
	Fetoscope	Yes	Yes	13/13
	Thermometer	Yes	Yes	9/13
	Urine dipstick	Yes	No	1/13
	Antiseptic	Yes	Yes	8/13
	Sterile gauze	Yes	No	3/13
	Syringes	Yes	Yes	13/13
	Suture material	Yes	Yes	12/13
	IV solutions	Yes	Yes	10/13
	IV giving set	Yes	No	10/13
	Urine catheters	Yes	No	2/13
Infection prevention	Clean/Utility gloves	Yes	Yes	9/13
	Sterile gloves	Yes	Yes	12/13
	Chlorine	Yes	Yes	8/13
	Buckets	Yes	Yes	9/13
	Ability to boil water	Yes	Yes	11/13
	Sharp containers	Yes	Yes	12/13
Childbirth equipment	Scissors	Yes	Yes	11/13
	Clamps	Yes	Yes	10/13
	Cord ties	Yes	No	8/13
	Ring forceps	Yes	Yes	5/13
	Needle holder	Yes	Yes	6/13
	Container for placenta	Yes	Yes	4/13
	Macintosh	Yes	Yes	10/13
	Protective wear	Yes	Yes	7/13
	Vacuum extractor	Yes	No	0/13
	Self inflating resuscitation bag	Yes	No	10/13
	Neonatal mask	No	No	7/13
	Suction equipment	Yes	No	6/13
MVA	MVA Set	Yes	Yes	3/13
Medication	Local anaesthetics	Yes	Yes	10/13
	Oxytocin/ergometrin	Yes	Yes	11/13
	Magnesium sulphate/Diazepam	Yes	No	6/13
	Ampiciline	Yes	Yes	1/13
	Erythromycin	Yes	No	6/13
	Gentamycin	Yes	No	5/13
	Paracetamol	Yes	No	4/13
	Misoprostol	Yes	Yes	1/13
	Nevarapine	Yes	Yes	9/13
Blood tests	Hb	Yes	Yes	0/13
	RPR	Yes	Yes	0/13
	Malaria	Yes	Yes	4/13
	HIV	Yes	Yes	2/13
	Blood grouping	Yes	No	0/13

[a]Supplies or materials were available if at least one item was available and functioning at the time of the audit

Table 3 Indicators, results and interpretations of EmONC indicators

	Indicator	Description[a]	Acceptable level	Results	Interpretations
1	Availability of emergency obstetric care: basic and comprehensive care facilities	The availability of EmONC services is measured by the number of facilities that perform the complete set of signal functions in relation to the size of the population. When staff has carried out the seven signal functions of basic EmONC in the 3-month period before the assessment, the facility is considered to be a fully functioning basic facility. The facility is classified as functioning at the comprehensive level when it offers the seven signal functions plus surgery (e.g. caesarean) and blood transfusion.	There are at least five emergency obstetric care facilities (including at least one comprehensive facility) for every 500 000 population	1 dispensary delivers 4 out of 6 (67%), 12 dispensaries deliver 3 or less out of 6 (≤50%) signal functions for BEmOC[b]; 3 health centres deliver 5 out of 7 (71%), 1 health centre delivers 2 out of 7 (29%) of the signal functions of BEmONC; the hospital delivers 7 out of 9 (78%) of the signal functions of comprehensive EmONC.	None of the health institutions in Magu District fulfilled the full package of expected level of EmONC
2	Geographical distribution of emergency obstetric care facilities	The geographical distribution of EmOC services is calculated in the same way as the first, but it takes into consideration the geographical distribution and accessibility of facilities. It can help program planners to gather information about equity in access to services at subnational level.	See above	The health centers and dispensaries are geographically equitably distributed over the district	The health centers and dispensaries are geographically equitably distributed over the district
3	Proportion of all births in emergency obstetric care facilities	The proportion of all births in an area that take place in EmOC health facilities (basic or comprehensive). The numerator is the number of women registered as having given birth in facilities classified as EmOC facilities. The denominator is an estimate of all the live births expected in the area, regardless of where the birth takes place.	At least 90% health facility births (Target based on Sharpened One Plan II)	Population 299,759; Crude Birth Rate (CBR) 39/1000; expected deliveries 11,690. Hospital births 2504 (21%); hospital + HCs 5035 (43%); all facilities 7635 (65%).	The majority of women give birth in facilities, which are expected to provide EmONC but remain underutilized by one third of the population.
4	Meeting the need for emergency obstetric care: proportion of women with major direct obstetric complications who are treated in such facilities	Met need' is an estimate of the proportion of all women with major direct obstetric complications who are treated in a health facility providing EmOC (basic or comprehensive). The numerator is the sum of all women treated for direct obstetric complications at emergency care facilities over a defined period, divided by the expected number of women who would have major obstetric complications, or 15% of expected births, during the same period in a specified area. The direct obstetric complications included in this indicator are: hemorrhage (antepartum and postpartum), prolonged and obstructed labour, postpartum sepsis, complications of abortion, severe pre-eclampsia and eclampsia, ectopic pregnancy and ruptured uterus.	100% of women estimated to have major direct obstetric complications are treated in emergency obstetric care facilities	Registered direct obstetric complications: 196; Caesarean sections (CS): 192 (assumption that CSs are done to treat or prevent direct obstetric complications) Expected number of direct obstetric complications: 11,690 × 0,15 = 1754 Met need = (192 + 196)/1754 × 100% = 22%	Health facilities are underutilized. 78% of women with complications are not seen in the facilities expected to provide EmONC services

Table 3 Indicators, results and interpretations of EmONC indicators *(Continued)*

5	Caesarean sections as a proportion of all births	The proportion of all deliveries by caesarean section in a geographical area is a measure of access to and use of a common obstetric intervention for averting maternal and neonatal deaths and for preventing complications such as obstetric fistula. The numerator is the number of caesarean sections performed in EmOC facilities for any indication during a specific period, and the denominator is the expected number of live births (in the whole catchment area, not just in institutions) during the same period.	The estimated proportion of births by caesarean section in the population is not less than 5% or more than 15%	All births: 11,690; Caesarean sections: 192. CS-percentage = 192/11,690 × 100% = 1.6% of all births Hospital-based CS percentage: 192/2504 × 100% = 7.7%	Health facilities are underutilized; many women who should have needed a CS did not get one, as a result of poor accessibility
6	Direct obstetric case fatality rate (CFR)	The direct obstetric case fatality rate is the proportion of women admitted to an EmOC facility with major direct obstetric complications, or who develop such complications after admission, and die before discharge.	<1%	Direct obstetric complications: 196 Maternal deaths: 22 (18 in the district hospital, 4 in the community) Direct obstetric CFR: 22/196 × 100% = 6%	Worries about quality of care in the facilities
7	Intrapartum and very early neonatal death rate	Indicator 7 is the proportion of births that result in a very early neonatal death or an intrapartum death (fresh stillbirth) in an EmOC facility. This new indicator has been proposed to shed light on the quality of intrapartum care for foetuses and newborns delivered at facilities. The numerator is the sum of intrapartum and very early neonatal deaths within the first 24 h of life occurring in the facility during a specific period. The denominator is the sum of all women who gave birth in the facility during the same period.	Standards to be determined	Fresh stillbirths (FSB) + very early neonatal deaths: 51 Hospital and health center births: 5035 Death rate: 51/5035 × 100% =1%	Low numbers of FSBs and early neonatal deaths are registered.
8	Proportion of maternal deaths due to indirect causes in emergency obstetric care facilities	The numerator of this indicator is all maternal deaths due to indirect causes in EmOC facilities during a specific period, and its denominator is all maternal deaths in the same facilities during the same period.	No standard can be set	Maternal deaths: 22; notification forms available: 16; maternal deaths classified: 15; indirect causes: 5 Proportion of indirect MD: 5/15 × 100% = 33%	Non-communicable diseases like malaria and HIV/AIDS are prevalent in the district, are important contributors to maternal mortality and are possibly inadequately prevented or treated during ANC.

[a]From the handbook 'Monitoring Emergency Obstetric Care' developed by AMDD, WHO, UNFPA and UNICEF, [10]
[b]Signal function 4 'Manual removal of placenta' was not assessed; therefore dispensaries were assessed based on 6 signal functions

an increase in delay to seek care and preference for home birth [6].

The average facility distribution of 31 facilities per 300.000 population shows there is adequate coverage and plotting the institutions on a map shows good geographical distribution of facilities. Our estimation that 65% of births took place in health facilities is encouraging, considering the national average of skilled birth attendance of 50% [17]. However, health facilities appear underutilized as only 22% of women with expected major obstetric complications were treated in facilities and 1.6% of births were caesarean sections, similar to findings in other sub-Saharan countries [23].

Although our assessment did not include the full range of Essential Newborn Care it is important to include the 'N' in EmONC when conducting such assessments. Newborns have been left out of the global agenda for decades but are now increasingly being acknowledged through initiatives such as the 'Every Newborn Action Plan' [24]. Since fresh stillbirth and early neonatal death are usually caused by complications during childbirth [25], the 'N' is a vital part of EmONC assessments. Our assessment found low numbers of fresh stillbirths and early neonatal deaths assuming severe underreporting. To our surprise we did not find any documentation of neonatal deaths outside the district hospital. Monthly reporting books do not request this information, other than number of stillbirths and number of children born with Apgar score below 7 after 5 min. Difficulties in distinguishing between fresh stillbirths versus early neonatal deaths and overall poor reporting of perinatal deaths were challenges found in other studies as well [26].

Maternal deaths have been relatively stable in the district over the past years ranging from 17 to 22 registered maternal deaths [27]. Of the registered deaths in 2013, 81% occurred in the district hospital. Review of notification forms raised concerns about the quality of care [28]. Of all maternal deaths, 33% were classified due to indirect causes and could have been prevented with adequate attendance and quality of antenatal care. These findings highlight the importance of ensuring quality of service delivery across the continuum of care.

Although the EmONC indicators are widely used to assess and monitor EmONC performance, their usefulness to understand and improve the level of performance is debated [4, 26]. Additional assessment methods, beyond reliance on routinely available data, are suggested to be necessary to get a complete picture of the challenges in providing EmONC [23]. Our study shows that assessing supply levels of facilities at a given moment in time can help in gaining a sense of their ability to perform at least 6 of the 7 signal functions. This is in particular useful for facilities with low level of activity (e.g dispensaries) where assessing performance of signal functions over the past three months would not give a realistic idea of their ability to tackle emergencies due to low numbers of births.

Also for the higher-level facilities, inadequate availability of essential medicines and supplies for EmONC affects their ability to perform all signal functions and is a common problem in Tanzania [4, 29, 30]. It is important to note that this does not mean facilities and their staff are not capable or skilled to provide EmONC services. On the contrary, highly skilled health workers can be demoralized due to continuous shortages affecting work motivation and consequently quality of care [31, 32]. Assessments of EmONC should therefore increase attention to supply chain problems, including available procurement and distribution systems and accountability mechanisms.

The assessment captured other weaknesses in the system contributing to poor availability, accessibility and quality of EmONC, which are not captured in the assessment of indicators alone. Poor utilization of the partograph to monitor birth process is a contributor to poor quality of monitoring labour progress and poor outcomes. Although monitoring and management of labour using partograph is part of the signal functions for routine care [9] we argue its use is significant for quality basic EmONC and should therefore not be left aside in EmONC assessments. Insufficient training and limited health worker knowledge contribute to poor use of the partograph [33], however health facility staff reported that unavailability of stationary or funds to print partograph was a major contributing factor for their lack of use.

Similarly, availability of an ambulance for emergency transport depends on families contributing for fuel and cesarean sections could not always be performed at the district hospital due to lack of functioning generator or lack of available anesthesia equipment or blood for transfusion. Such poor organization of services and human resources indicate weaknesses in the system which show how relatively small problems, such as lack of access to stationaries, can prevent access to life saving services [34]. Preventing maternal and perinatal mortality requires a functioning health system, including adequate quality of care in its EmONC facilities. EmONC assessments should therefore be supplemented by mixed methods designs, including qualitative studies, which allow for contextual understanding of findings [26, 35].

Limitations

Our findings should be interpreted with caution. Data collection in dispensaries was restricted to half of the available dispensaries and do, therefore, not necessarily give a complete picture of the district. However, our findings showing inadequate provision of basic EmONC services at all levels, make it very unlikely other lower level facilities are fully functioning EmONC facilities. Facility assessment in dispensaries was done prior to receiving new supplies, which should be taken into account. However re-assessment one year later after new supplies were provided did not show much improvement

Although our findings are typical for (maternal) health systems in poor rural districts in sub-Sahara Africa, our assessment was restricted to institutions in Magu District and the findings cannot be extrapolated to other districts. Neighbouring, Busega district, has no District Hospital and therefore women often rely on services of Magu District Hospital. This may have influenced the data explaining the relatively high percentage of facility births. Recall bias could have influenced data quality negatively, since we asked in-charges of health centres and district hospital about functioning of their facility in the past three months.

Data quality was limited at all levels of care. The research team observed many problems with documentation and reporting. All delivery books had missing information regarding outcome of birth and whether mother and child went home alive. Also many irregularities and inconsistencies were found between registries within facilities. At dispensary level there were no records of referral or adverse outcomes, despite staff informing us that these do occur. Poor documenting and reporting has been observed in other settings, and despite our knowledge of poor data quality, much of the decision-making is based on these poor numbers [36]. It is easy to assume there is underreporting of complications and poor outcomes, but at the same time many instances where staff do provide high quality of care also go undocumented.

Conclusions

Although availability of health facilities expected to deliver EmONC are adequate in Magu District, none of the facilities perform all signal functions of BEmONC or CEmONC. Performance of signal functions is dependent on sufficient availability of supplies and resources as well as adequately trained and qualified staff, which can be assessed in line with EmONC indicators. In addition robust data collection systems are required for reliable assessments. Improving assessment approaches to account for local realities and contextual constraints will help to strive for improvements over time. Based on the reported results recommendations were formulated and discussed together with the Council Health Management Team. Importance of implementation of the recommendations and follow up according to the quality cycle was emphasized.

Abbreviations

CHMT: Council Health Management Team; EMONC: Emergency Obstetrics and Neonatal Care; JHPIEGO: Johns Hopkins Program for International Education in Gynaecology and Obstetrics; RMNCH: Reproductive Maternal Neonatal and Child Health; WCCP: Woman Centered Care Project

Acknowledgements

We thank the District Medical Officer Dr Pembe, the District Nursing Officer Mr. Egdius Mtajwaha, the Hospital Matron Mrs. Joyce Sabora, the doctors in charge of the four health centres (Kabila, Nyanguge, Kahangara, Kisesa) and Naomi Maselle from the Woman Centered Care Project, for their cooperation and their kind assistance. The research team has appreciated the openness, helpfulness and trust of the DMO and his team to allow the research team to conduct this assessment.

Funding

During the time of writing of this manuscript ASM was supported by the Research Council of Norway through the Global Health and Vaccination Programme (GLOBVAC) for her PhD, project number 244674. The funding body had no role in the design of the study and collection, analysis, and interpretation of data, nor in writing of the manuscript.

Authors' contributions

The study was designed by ASM, JvR and JS. Data for the facility audit was collected by all authors. ASM, JvR and JS analysed and interpreted the data with assistance from TB and RK. ASM drafted the manuscript. All authors read and approved the final manuscript.

Competing interests

The authors declare that they have no competing interests.

Author details

[1]Institute of Health and Society, Department of Community Medicine and Global Health, Faculty of Medicine, University of Oslo, Oslo, Norway. [2]Women Centered Care Project, a project of the African Woman Foundation, Magu, Mwanza Region, Tanzania. [3]Department of Obstetrics and Gynaecology, Sekotoure Regional Referral Hospital, Mwanza, Mwanza Region, Tanzania. [4]Magu District Council, Magu, Mwanza Region, Tanzania. [5]Department of Obstetrics, Leiden University Medical Center, Leiden, The Netherlands. [6]Athena Institute, VU University, Amsterdam, The Netherlands. [7]Department of Obstetrics and Gynaecology, Leeuwarden Medical Centre, Henri Dunantweg 2, 8934 AD Leeuwarden, The Netherlands. [8]Department of Health Sciences, Community and Occupational Medicine, Global Health, University Medical Centre Groningen/University of Groningen, Antonius Deusinglaan 1, P.O. Box 1969700 AD Groningen, The Netherlands.

References

1. Ameh C, Msuya S, Hofman J, Raven J, Mathai M, van den Broek N. Status of emergency obstetric care in six developing countries five years before the MDG targets for maternal and newborn health. PLoS One. 2012;7(12):e49938.
2. Afnan-Holmes H, Magoma M, John T, Levira F, Msemo G, Armstrong CE, Martínez-Álvarez M, Kerber K, Kihinga C, Makuwani A, et al. Tanzania's countdown to 2015: an analysis of two decades of progress and gaps for reproductive, maternal, newborn, and child health, to inform priorities for post-2015. Lancet Glob Health. 2015;3(7):e396–409.
3. Ministry of Health and Social Welfare (MoHSW) Reproductive and Child Health Section. The national road map strategic plan to accelerate reduction of maternal, newborn and child deaths in Tanzania, 2008-2015. Dar es Salaam: Ministry of Health (MoH); 2008.
4. Olsen OE, Ndeki S, Norheim OF. Availability, distribution and use of emergency obstetric care in northern Tanzania. Health Policy Plan. 2005; 20(3):167–75.

5. Nyamtema AS, Urassa DP, van Roosmalen J. Maternal health interventions in resource limited countries: a systematic review of packages, impacts and factors for change. BMC Pregnancy Childbirth. 2011;11:30.
6. Thaddeus S, Maine D. Too far to walk: maternal mortality in context. Soc Sci Med. 1994;38(8):1091–110.
7. The Partnership for Maternal, Newborn & Child Health. A global review of the key interventions related to reproductive maternal and child health (RMNCH). Geneva: PMNCH; 2011.
8. Campbell OMR, Graham WJ. Strategies for reducing maternal mortality: getting on with what works. Lancet. 2006;368(9543):1284–99.
9. Gabrysch S, Civitelli G, Edmond KM, Mathai M, Ali M, Bhutta ZA, Campbell OM. New signal functions to measure the ability of health facilities to provide routine and emergency newborn care. PLoS Med. 2012;9(11):e1001340.
10. WHO, UNFPA, AMDD, UNICEF. Monitoring Emergency Obstetric Care: a handbook. Geneva: WHO; 2009.
11. National Bureau of Statistics. 2012 Population and Housing Census. Dar es Salaam: NBS; 2013.
12. Solnes Miltenburg A, Rijkers E, Maselle N, van Roosmalen J, Bunders J. Reflections on the dynamics of the coexistence of multiple knowledge cultures in a community-based maternal health project in Tanzania. Knowl Manag Dev J. 2013;9(2):162–84.
13. Vermeulen E, Solnes Miltenburg A, Barras J, Maselle N, van Elteren M, van Roosmalen J. Opportunities for male involvement during pregnancy in Magu district, rural Tanzania. BMC Pregnancy Childbirth. 2016;16:66.
14. Solnes Miltenburg A, Lambermon F, Hamelink C, Meguid T. Maternity care and Human Rights: what do women think? BMC Int Health Hum Rights. 2016;16(1):17.
15. JHPIEGO. Monitoring Birth Preparedness and complication readiness: tools and indicators for maternal and newborn health. Baltimore: JHPIEGO; 2004.
16. Magpi. Magpi online data collection tool. 2016. http://home.magpi.com. Accessed Apr-May & Dec 2014.
17. National Bureau of Statistics (NBS) and ICF Macro. Tanzania Demographic and Health Survey 2010. Dar es Salaam: NBS; 2011.
18. MoHCDGEC. The National Road Map Strategic Plan to Improve Reproductive, Maternal, Newborn, Child & Adolescent Health in Tanzania (2016–2020). One Plan II. Dar es Salaam: Ministry of Health (MoH); 2016.
19. Lobis S, Mbaruku G, Kamwendo F, McAuliffe E, Austin J, de Pinho H. Expected to deliver: alignment of regulation, training, and actual performance of emergency obstetric care providers in Malawi and Tanzania. Int J Gynaecol Obstet. 2011;115(3):322–7.
20. Ueno E, Adegoke AA, Masenga G, Fimbo J, Msuya SE. Skilled birth attendants in Tanzania: a descriptive study of cadres and emergency obstetric care signal functions performed. Matern Child Health J. 2015;19(1):155–69.
21. Hanson C, Ronsmans C, Penfold S, Maokola W, Manzi F, Jaribu J, et al. Health system support for childbirth care in Southern Tanzania: results from a health facility census. BMC Res Notes. 2013;6:435.
22. Sorensen BL, Elsass P, Nielsen BB, Massawe S, Nyakina J, Rasch V. Substandard emergency obstetric care - a confidential enquiry into maternal deaths at a regional hospital in Tanzania. Trop Med Int Health. 2010;15(8):894–900.
23. Campbell OMR, Calvert C, Testa A, Strehlow M, Benova L, Keyes E, et al. The scale, scope, coverage, and capability of childbirth care. Lancet. 2016;6736(16):1–16.
24. UNICEF, WHO. Every newborn: an action plan to end preventable newborn deaths. 2013. www.everynewborn.org.
25. Lawn J, Shibuya K, Stein C. No cry at birth: global estimates of intrapartum stillbirths and intrapartum-related neonatal deaths. Bull World Health Organ. 2005;83:409–17.
26. Banke-Thomas A, Wright K, Sonoiki O, Banke-Thomas O, Ajayi B, Ilozumba O, et al. Assessing emergency obstetric care provision in low- and middle-income countries: a systematic review of the application of global guidelines. Glob Health Action. 2016;9:31880.
27. Magu District Management Team. Annual Report Magu District Hospital 2013. Magu: DHMT; 2014.
28. Magoma M, Massinde A, Majinge C, Rumanyika R, Kihunrwa A, Gomodoka B. Maternal death reviews at Bugando hospital north-western Tanzania: a 2008–2012 retrospective analysis. BMC Pregnancy Childbirth. 2015;15:333.
29. Mkoka DA, Goicolea I, Kiwara A, Mwangu M, Hurtig A. Availability of drugs and medical supplies for emergency obstetric care: experience of health facility managers in a rural District of Tanzania. BMC Pregnancy Childbirth. 2014;14(1):108.
30. Mselle LT, Moland KM, Mvungi A, Evjen-olsen B, Kohi TW. Why give birth in health facility ? Users ' and providers ' accounts of poor quality of birth care in Tanzania. BMC Health Serv Res. 2013;13(1):174.
31. Mkoka DA, Mahiti GR, Kiwara A, Mwangu M, Goicolea I, Hurtig A-K. "Once the government employs you, it forgets you": Health workers' and managers' perspectives on factors influencing working conditions for provision of maternal health care services in a rural district of Tanzania. Hum Resour Health. 2015;13(77):1–13.
32. Penfold S, Shamba D, Hanson C, Jaribu J, Manzi F, Marchant T, et al. Staff experiences of providing maternity services in rural southern Tanzania - a focus on equipment, drug and supply issues. BMC Health Serv Res. 2013;13(1):61.
33. Nyamtema AS, Urassa DP, Massawe S, Massawe A, Lindmark G, van Roosmalen J. Partogram use in the Dar es Salaam perinatal care study. Int J Gynaecol Obstet. 2008;100(1):37–40.
34. Jaffré Y. Towards an anthropology of public health priorities: maternal mortality in four obstetric emergency services in West Africa. Soc Anthropol. 2012;20(1):3–18.
35. Spangler SA. Assessing skilled birth attendants and emergency obstetric care in rural Tanzania: the inadequacy of using global standards and indicators to measure local realities. Reprod Health Matters. 2012;20(39):133–41.
36. Graham W, Woodd S, Byass P, Filippi V, Gon G, Virgo S, et al. Diversity and divergence: the dynamic burden of poor maternal health. Lancet. 2016; 6736(16):1–12.

Measuring oral health during pregnancy: sensitivity and specificity of a maternal oral screening (MOS) tool

Ajesh George[1*], Hannah G. Dahlen[2], Anthony Blinkhorn[3], Shilpi Ajwani[4], Sameer Bhole[4], Sharon Ellis[5], Anthony Yeo[6], Emma Elcombe[7], Ayesha Sadozai[8] and Maree Johnson[9]

Abstract

Background: Midwives can play a key role in promoting the oral health of pregnant women and assessing their oral health status. A maternal oral assessment tool (MOS) was developed and pilot tested by the study investigators to assist midwives in this role and the results were promising. The aim of this study was to undertake further sensitivity and specificity assessment of the MOS tool using two-comparison approaches- the longer oral health screening tool known as the Oral Health Impact Profile (OHIP-14) and an oral assessment by trained study dentists.

Methods: Pregnant women were recruited for this study as part of a larger randomised controlled trial of a Midwifery Initiated Oral Health (MIOH) program. Pregnant women completed the MOS and OHIP-14 as part of their initial assessment undertaken by 38 trained and accredited midwives. A dental assessment was conducted for all women in the intervention group using three trained study dentists with high inter rater reliability.

Results: Two hundred and eleven pregnant women participated in the validation of the MOS tool. Results from both approaches found the MOS tool to have high sensitivity, correctly identifying 88–94 % of women at risk of poor dental health, and low specificity (14–21 %).

Conclusions: This study has shown that the MOS tool can be successfully implemented by midwives during a woman's first antenatal visit and can identify up to 94 % of women at risk of poor oral health and needing a dental referral. The tool has the potential to be transferable to other antenatal care providers and could be incorporated into hospital obstetric database systems.

Keywords: Oral health, Pregnancy, Midwives, Antenatal care, Prenatal care, Validation

Background

Population oral health experts within Australian and internationally have developed guidelines [1–4] that emphasise the importance of oral health screening for women during pregnancy. Pregnancy increases the risk of oral health problems (periodontal disease and tooth decay) due to physiological changes associated with pregnancy [5, 6]. In addition, early screening of women for oral health problems, provides an opportunity for women to learn about how to prevent decay for themselves and also for their future or existing children [1, 7]. The initial comprehensive review of women's health is conducted at the antenatal clinic by midwives for most Australian women [8]. This provides a unique opportunity to assess and intervene to improve the oral health of women and their children. The potential for midwives and other antenatal care providers to also undertake an assessment of women's health at that initial visit (primary care settings) has been supported in other studies [3, 4, 9]. The availability of a valid, simple to administer, oral health assessment tool with demonstrated sensitivity and specificity, would facilitate the identification of women with oral health

* Correspondence: a.george@westernsydney.edu.au
[1]Collaboration for Oral Health Outcomes, Research Translation and Evaluation (COHORTE) Research Group, Western Sydney University, South Western Sydney Local Health District, Ingham Institute Applied Medical Research, University of Sydney, Liverpool BC, Locked Bag 7103, Liverpool, NSW 1871, Australia
Full list of author information is available at the end of the article

problems and potentiate early dental interventions through referral during the optimal treatment time of the first trimester [10, 11].

Concerns raised about oral health during pregnancy go beyond dental caries. Systematic reviews have shown a positive association between adverse pregnancy outcomes such as preterm delivery and periodontal disease, although a cause and effect relationship has not been established (11, 12). Several trials have been conducted within Australia to intervene during pregnancy in an attempt to reduce the incidence of adverse birth outcomes such as the SMILE study [12] and the Midwifery Initiated Oral Health (MIOH) trial [13]. As part of the MIOH Trial we have included several instruments, and undertaken oral health assessments by dentists to determine the sensitivity and specificity of the Maternal Oral Screening (MOS) Tool.

The MOS tool was developed following a comprehensive literature review of screening items for oral health during pregnancy [10]. The result was a preferred two-item tool: item 1 referring to commonly reported dental problem during pregnancy and those caused by oral diseases [10, 14]; item 2 referring to how often the woman has seen a dentist in the last 12 months [10, 14]. A total score of ≥1 (having a dental problem or not seen a dentist in the previous 12 months) indicated that women were at risk of poor oral health and required a referral to a dentist. A visual inspection was optional for confirming the presence of dental problems and was only undertaken if a problem was identified by the pregnant women (See Table 1 below). An important part of the development process was the measurement of the tools sensitivity and specificity which indicates whether a patient will be screened in for an intervention (in this case dental treatment) or screened out (in this case having good oral health). A tool that allows for both situations to be considered with appropriate proportions is always an aspiration, however, in some clinical situations this may not always be possible [15]. Therefore the emphasis is often placed on whether the tool captures populations at risk of the condition, in this case women with poor oral health. Clinical evaluation of sensitivity and specificity is frequently used as the gold standard in clinical conditions where clinical assessment is a key diagnostic step [16]. We had previously pilot tested the MOS tool and found that it was promising in a sample of 56 women [10]. The pilot results suggested that the tool was acceptable to pregnant women and midwives and was sensitive (98 %) to identifying dental problems and facilitating dental referrals. However, further evaluation of the tool in a larger sample was warranted.

Table 1 Maternal Oral Screening tool for antenatal clinics

The maternal oral screening tool
Item 1. Do you have bleeding gums, swelling, sensitive teeth, loose teeth, holes in your teeth, broken teeth, toothache or any other problems in your mouth?
Yes □ (1)
No □ (0)
If yes, visual inspection of oral cavity (optional to confirm Item 1)
Item 2. Have you seen a dentist in the last 12 months?
Yes □ (0)
No □ (1)

Items 1 and 2 are scored either 0 or 1. Participants with a total score ≥ 1 are referred for a dental check-up.

Aim

This study sought to undertake sensitivity and specificity assessment of the maternal oral health screening tool using two comparison approaches- the 14 item oral health screening tool known as the Oral Health Impact Profile (OHIP-14) and a clinical oral assessment by trained study dentists.

Methods

This study was undertaken as part of an existing multicenter randomized controlled trial that is evaluating the effectiveness of a midwifery initiated oral health program in improving the uptake of dental services, oral health knowledge, quality of life and oral health status of pregnant women (Trial ID ACTRN12612001271897). At the initial assessment, pregnant women, undergo screening and referral (where appropriate) by appropriately accredited midwives [17].

Sample and setting

The pregnant women were recruited from three large antenatal clinics in Sydney. The eligibility criteria for the MIOH trial have been reported elsewhere [13] and included low risk women with a single pregnancy (more than 12 and less than 20 weeks gestation). These women were screened at their initial antenatal appointment and provided dental referrals by accredited midwives who had completed the MIOH education program [17, 18]. One group of women in the trial was referred to study dentists for a clinical examination regardless of whether they were screened to be at risk of poor oral health. These women formed the study sample for the testing of the MOS tool.

Characteristics of women attending the three antenatal clinics

Two hundred and eleven participants were recruited for this study. The majority of participants were Australian born (n = 128, 61 %) with a mean age of 29 years (SD = 5.7, range = 18–43 years). Most women were multiparous (65 %), partnered (81 %) and in their second trimester (n = 387, 92 %). The highest level of education recorded was university (18 %) followed by trade school (35 %). Most participants were not working (56 %) or working part time (22 %). More than 40 % of participants ($n = 83$) had a combined annual household income of less than $60,000 and a high proportion (50 %) lived in areas of low socio-economic advantage (lowest Socio-Economic Index for Area quintile as measured through the Australian Bureau of Statistics).

Characteristics of midwives undertaking the screening and referral of women

Thirty-eight midwives successfully completed the MIOH education program and undertook the screening and referral of the pregnant women. The midwives had a mean age of 43.4 years (SD 11.5) and an average of 15.8 years of clinical practice experience (SD 11.7). Nearly half the midwives (47.4 %) had postgraduate qualifications.

OHIP-14

The OHIP-14 is a subjective measure of oral health that has been found to be a precise, valid and reliable instrument ($\alpha = 0.88$) [19]. It has been used previously as a 'gold standard' measure for validating other oral assessment tools [20]. OHIP-14 contains 14 questions assessed on a 5-point Likert scale and the total scores range from 0 to 56 with higher scores indicating poorer oral health. This tool was developed based on a conceptual model defined by Locker [21] focusing on seven domains- functional limitation, physical pain, psychological discomfort, physical disability, psychological disability, social disability and handicap (see Additional file 1).

Clinical examination by study dentists

Three experienced dentists were recruited to the study from health services where the study was conducted. Several reliable measures were used to assess the extent of dental problems in pregnant women. These included the decay, missing and filled teeth (DMFT) index [22] and the periodontal screening and reporting (PSR) index (24). The DMFT index identified whether decay was present while the PSR index (scoring 0–4) assessed the health of the gums with a score of two and above indicating gum disease requiring treatment [23]. Pregnant women were determined to have poor oral health if they had any dental decay and a PSR score of greater than two. One of the investigators (SA) undertook to train all dentists on a standard assessment and intervention protocol. The dentists were assessed on five patients for various measures with >80 % inter-rater reliability in the key study measures (DMFT and PSR).

Procedure

The items for the MOS and OHIP-14 were included in the initial assessment undertaken by the midwife with the consenting woman presenting to the antenatal clinic. The data collection procedures for the MIOH Trial are more fully described within the protocol [13]. The dental assessment was conducted for all women in the intervention group that had access to the study dentists [13]. Ethical approval was obtained from the Human Research and Ethics Committees of Sydney Local Health District (reference no HREC/11/CRGH/28) and Western Sydney University (reference no H9709). Written consent to participate in the trial was obtained from women attending the antenatal clinic at the initial presenting visit.

Data management and analysis

Statistical analysis was completed using SPSS v22. Descriptive statistics were used to describe the demographic information of the sample population. The relationships between the screening tools were assessed using chi-squared analyses after variable dichotomisation. The level of significance (α) was set at 0.05. Sensitivity, specificity, positive predictive value (PPV) and negative predictive value (NPV) were computed using conditional probabilities based on a two-way table. Confidence intervals were determined using the central limit theorem formulation.

Results

MOS tool

In total, an average of 67 % ($n = 141$) of women reported having a current problem or concern with their teeth, gums or mouth, and 39 % reported seeing a dentist in the previous 12 months. Using the screening criteria (Table 1), 86 % of women were deemed at risk of poor oral health (Table 2).

Table 2 Women's responses to the MOS tool, OHIP-14 and Dental Assessment

	No. (%)
Maternal Oral Screening Tool ($n = 207$)	
Item 1: Do you have problems in your mouth? [Yes]	141 (66.8 %)
Item 2: Have you seen a dentist in the last 12 months? [No]	128 (60.7 %)
'At risk' of poor oral health[1]	181 (85.8 %)
OHIP-14 (Self-report) ($n = 207$)	
Score > 4	90 (43.5 %)
Dental Assessment ($n = 131$)	
Any tooth decay detected? [Yes]	81 (62 %)
PSR rating ≥ 2 [Yes]	118 (90 %)
Women with poor oral health[2]	74 (56 %)

PSR Periodontal screening and recording index
[1]Participants considered 'At risk' of poor oral health if they reported a problem with their teeth, gums or mouth OR if they had not seen a dentist in the previous 12 months, $n = 207$
[2]Participants considered to have poor oral health if they had dental decay detected and had a PSR score of ≥ 2, $n = 131$

Approach 1 –OHIP- 14

A total of 207 (98 %) participants satisfactorily completed the OHIP-14. The mean OHIP-14 score was 6.8 (SD = 8.6, median = 4.0, range 0–38). As cut-off scores for identifying patients at risk of poor oral health has not been established with the OHIP-14, the total score for each participant was dichotomised using the median split as described by Locker et al. [24] categorised as either 'At risk' (score greater than 4) or 'Not at risk' (score 0 to 4) (Table 2).

Approach 2 - dental assessment

Of the 207 participants referred, 131 women completed the dental assessments. Analysis of these data found 90 % ($n = 118$) of women had a PSR rating of two or more, 62 % ($n = 81$) had dental decay, and 56 % ($n = 74$) of women had both of these and were considered to have poor oral health.

Sensitivity and specificity

The MOS data was assessed against two gold standard measures of oral health; the 14 item OHIP questionnaire and a clinical oral health check. Both analyses found the MOS tool to have high sensitivity (88–93 %) for detecting women at risk of poor oral health. More specifically, analysis of the MOS tool against the OHIP-14 found that Item 1 of the MOS gave the highest sensitivity (82.2 %) while Item 2 gave the highest specificity (56.4 %). When items 1 and 2 were combined the sensitivity increased to 93.3 % while the specificity decreased (Table 3). A similar pattern of results was seen when the MOS tool was compared to the Clinical oral assessment with the highest sensitivity (87.8 %) being achieved by combining items 1 and 2. Overall, combining items 1 and 2 of the MOS tool resulted in relatively low specificities (Dental assessment = 14.0 % and OHIP-14 = 20.5 %).

Table 3 Sensitivity and specificity of Maternal Oral Screening Tool compared with OHIP-14 and Dental Assessment

	MOS - Item 1 % (95 % CI)	MOS - Item 2 % (95 % CI)	Combined % (95 % CI)
OHIP-14 (Self-report)[1] ($n = 207$)			
Sensitivity	82.2 (74.3–89.1)	32.2 (22.6–40.7)	93.3 (88.2–97.9)
Specificity	46.2 (37.1–55.2)	56.4 (47.4–65.4)	20.5 (13.2–27.8)
PPV	54.0 (45.7–62.4)	36.3 (25.7–46.8)	47.5 (40.1–54.8)
NPV	77.1 (67.3–87.0)	52.0 (43.3–60.7)	80.0 (65.7–94.3)
Dental assessment (PSR > 2 and Decay present) ($n = 131$)			
Sensitivity	70.3 (59.9–82.1)	41.9 (30.7–54.7)	87.8 (80.4–96.3)
Specificity	29.8 (17.9–41.7)	68.4 (56.4–80.5)	14.0 (5.0–23.1)
PPV	56.5 (46.4–66.7)	63.3 (49.8–76.8)	57.0 (47.9–66.1)
NPV	43.6 (28.0–59.2)	47.6 (36.8–58.4)	47.1 (23.3–70.8)

[1]Item 1 = Do you currently have any problems with your teeth Gums or mouth?, Item 2 = Have you had a dental check up in the last 12 months?
CI Confidence interval, *PPN* Positive predictive value, *NPV* Negative predictive value

Discussion

The focus of this study was to further validate a maternal oral health screening tool for pregnant women. Developing such a tool is important because of the high prevalence of poor oral health among pregnant women and its impact on maternal and infant outcomes (5). Further, current guidelines advocate the need for all antenatal care providers to undertake oral health education, assessment and referral during early pregnancy (1–3). Initial piloting of the MOS tool suggested that it was easy to administer by midwives and had good sensitivity in identifying dental problems in pregnant women and facilitating referrals (15). However, the pilot study had limited sample size and further testing of the sensitivity and specificity was warranted.

This study used a two staged approach using a larger sample size to validate the MOS tool. Current practice during the first antenatal visit involves midwives assessing multiple health areas at one time, thus consideration of time constraints was an important factor in assessing oral health during this visit (25). This was one of the main reasons why only three items were considered during the development phase of the tool (15), only two of which were used in this study. The study results reiterate earlier suggestions that the 2-item tool (which is part of the MIOH education program) was easy to administer by midwives and comprehend by pregnant women (16, 18, 19).

Validation of the MOS tool (2-item) showed high sensitivity across both gold standards (88–97 %) which is similar to results of the pilot study (75–98 %). This combined with moderated NPV's of 47–80 % confirm that the MOS tool is reliable and able to correctly identify the majority of women in need of a dental referral. The specificity of the tool remained low even with increased sample size (14–19 %), however when interpreting this value consideration must be given to the purpose to the tool. In this situation correct identification of women at risk of poor oral health, compared to identifying those with good oral health, is of paramount importance especially considering that it is recommended that all women should see a dentist early in their pregnancy even if they are unaware of any dental problems (1, 12). The positive predictive value of the MOS tool indicates that around 50 % of the women referred for a dental assessment, will in fact be in need of dental care. In addition it should be noted that low specificity values are not uncommon in oral health screening tools with values ranging from 2.9 to 37.5 % observed in studies addressing oral health in early childhood (27) and HIV patients (26).

The study reinforces earlier suggestions (15) that the MOS tool can be easily administered by midwives. The fact that the education that accompanies the assessment tool has been successfully implemented in other states in Australia (19) indicates a level of tool transference. In the future this tool could be used by other antenatal care providers as an assessment tool. In addition, there is no restriction on this tool being used solely by midwives, therefore other health care professionals who have contact with mothers early in the antenatal period may also be able to successfully undergo the training and administered the MOS tool. Further the tool could also be incorporated into existing obstetric systems to increase the number women captured/screened across the country.

Although the tool has low specificity, in the current Australian system, where we have strict eligibility criteria's for public dental services (28) as opposed to a free universal dental scheme for pregnant women, the impact of over referral will be mostly borne by the individual rather than the government. The potential cost benefits however is not to be disregarded; the encouragement of women to access dental services earlier during pregnancy is likely to have flow on health benefits, improving maternal health and quality of life (29), child oral health (30) and potentially birth outcomes (31) which ultimately could reduce the overall cost burden to society.

Lastly, it should be noted that although the OHIP- 14 is frequently used as a gold standard for measures in a variety of populations such as older people [19, 25] and HIV patients [20] it may not be as appropriate for this population. Only 6 of the 14 OHIP items were scored frequently >0 in the study population. These items were related to the physical pain, psychological discomfort and psychological disability domains of the OHIP-14. As the OHIP tool is derived from the conceptual understanding of Locker et al. [21] focusing on disability, the remaining domains and related items may not be as suitable for this sample of healthy women. Further studies should be conducted to develop or modify the OHIP-14 for this population of predominantly young healthy women. Similarly as suggested by Locker et al. [24] longitudinal studies should be undertaken to identify the ability of the OHIP tool to measure changes over time.

Limitations

This study was undertaken in South West Sydney and the findings may deliver differing results in other populations of pregnant women from higher socio-economic backgrounds, or indeed from other countries. Similarly this study has focused on only one aspect of psychometric assessment of a tool and other aspects such as construct validity was not undertaken within this sample. We also note that although the OHIP-14 was used as a gold standard, similar results in terms of sensitivity and specificity were also demonstrated with clinical examination by dentists.

Conclusion

The MOS (2-item) provides a sensitive screening tool that is easy to use by midwives and potentially other antenatal care providers including general practitioners. The items are easily administered and provide an opportunity to raise awareness with women about the importance of oral health to their overall health as well as the health of the unborn fetus. This simple initial screening approach conducted by a non-oral health professional, with specialized training, complements the service provided by dentists where more thorough examination of oral health risk can be undertaken. Further studies should examine the potential for the OHIP-14 or other modifications of the OHIP to more appropriately target items of relevance for young healthy pregnant women.

Abbreviations

DMFT: Decay, missing and filled teeth; MIOH: Midwifery Initiated Oral Health program; MOS: Maternal oral assessment tool; NPV: Negative predictive value; OHIP-14: Oral Health Impact Profile; PPV: Positive predictive value; PSR: Periodontal screening and reporting

Funding

This work was supported by the Australian National Health and Medical Research Council Project Grant (APP1022007).

Authors' contributions

AG and MJ prepared the first draft of the manuscript. AY, EE and AS performed the quantitative data analysis and AG, EE and MJ performed the synthesis and interpretation. AG, HD, AB, SA, SB, SE and MJ conceived and designed the study. All authors (AG, HD, AB, SA, SB, SE, AY, EE, AS and MJ) provided input into versions of the manuscript and read and approved the final manuscript.

Competing interests

The authors declare that they have no competing interests.

Author details

[1]Collaboration for Oral Health Outcomes, Research Translation and Evaluation (COHORTE) Research Group, Western Sydney University, South Western Sydney Local Health District, Ingham Institute Applied Medical Research, University of Sydney, Liverpool BC, Locked Bag 7103, Liverpool, NSW 1871, Australia. [2]School of Nursing & Midwifery, Western Sydney University, Ingham Institute Applied Medical Research, Parramatta 2150, Australia. [3]Faculty of Dentistry, University of Sydney, Sydney 2006, Australia. [4]Sydney Local Health District Oral Health Services, Sydney Dental Hospital, University of Sydney, Sydney 2010, Australia. [5]Antenatal Services, Camden and Campbelltown Hospitals, South Western Sydney Local Health District, Campbelltown 2560, Australia. [6]School of Nursing & Midwifery, Western Sydney University, Parramatta 2150, Australia. [7]Western Sydney University, University of New South Wales, Ingham Institute Applied Medical Research, Liverpool 2170,

Australia. [8]Centre for Applied Nursing Research, Western Sydney University, South Western Sydney Local Health District, Ingham Institute Applied Medical Research, Liverpool 1871, Australia. [9]Faculty of Health Sciences, Australian Catholic University, Ingham Institute Applied Medical Research, Sydney 2060, Australia.

References

1. New South Wales Health. In: Department of Health NSW, editor. Early childhood oral health guidelines for child health professionals. 3rd ed. New South Wales: Centre for Oral Health Strategy; 2014.
2. National Health Service Health Scotland. Maternal and early years for early years workers: How can I help address oral health problems in pregnancy? National Health Service Health Scotland. 2013. http://www.maternal-and-early-years.org.uk/how-can-i-help-address-oral-health-problems-in-pregnancy. Accessed October 2015.
3. Oral Health Care During Pregnancy Expert Workshop. Oral health care during pregnancy: a national consensus statement. Washington DC: National Maternal and Child Oral Health Resource Center; 2012.
4. Sanz M, Kornman K, working group 3 of the joint EFPAAPw. Periodontitis and adverse pregnancy outcomes: consensus report of the joint EFP/AAP workshop on periodontitis and systemic diseases. J Clin Periodontol. 2013;40:S164–9. doi:10.1111/jcpe.12083.
5. George A, Johnson M, Blinkhorn A, Ellis S, Bhole S, Ajwani S. Promoting oral health during pregnancy: current evidence and implications for Australian midwives. J Clin Nurs. 2010;19(23–24):3324–33. doi:10.1111/j.1365-2702.2010.03426.x.
6. Silk H, Douglass AB, Douglass JM, Silk L. Oral health during pregnancy. Am Fam Physician. 2008;77(8):1139–44.
7. Weintraub J, Prakash P, Shain S, Laccabue M, Gansky S. Mothers' caries increases odds of children's caries. J Dent Res. 2010;89(9):954–8.
8. Midwives ACo. National midwifery guidelines for consultation and referral. 2nd ed. Deakin West ACT: Australian College of Midwives Inc; 2008.
9. Australian Health Ministers Advisory council. Clinical practice guidelines: antenatal care- Module 1. In: Ageing AGDoHa, editor. Canberra. 2012.
10. George A, Ajwani S, Johnson M, Dahlen H, Blinkhorn A, Bhole S, et al. Developing and testing of an oral health screening tool for midwives to assess pregnant woman. Health Care Women Int. 2015;36(10):1160–74. doi:10.1080/07399332.2014.959170.
11. George A, Duff M, Johnson M, Dahlen H, Blinkhorn A, Ellis S, et al. Piloting of an oral health education programme and knowledge test for midwives. Contemp Nurse. 2014;46(2):180–6.
12. Newnham J, Newnham IA, Ball CM, Wright M, Pennell CE, Swain J, Doherty DA. Treatment of periodontal disease during pregnancy *a randomized controlled trial*. Obstet Gynecol. 2009;114(6):1239–48.
13. Johnson M, George A, Dahlen H, Ajwani S, Bhole S, Blinkhorn A, et al. The midwifery initiated oral health dental service protocol: an intervention to improve oral health outcomes for pregnant women. BMC Oral Health. 2015;15:2. doi:10.1186/1472-6831-15-2.
14. Health NYSDo. Oral health care during pregnancy & early childhood: Practice guidelines. Albany: Health NYSDo; 2006.
15. Donaldson LJ, Donaldson RJ. Choosing the screening test. Essential public health. 2nd (Revised) ed. Berkshire: LibraPharm Limited; 2003. p. 120–3.
16. Ramos RQ, Bastos JL, Peres MA. Diagnostic validity of self-reported oral health outcomes in population surveys: literature review. Rev Bras Epidemiol. 2013;16:716–28.
17. George A, Lang G, Johnson M, Ridge A, De Silva A, Ajwani S, et al. The evaluation of an oral health education program for midwives in Australia. Women Birth. 2016;29(3):208–213.
18. George A, Duff M, Johnson M, Dahlen H, Blinkhorn A, Ellis S, et al. Piloting of an oral health education program and knowledge test for midwives. Contemp Nurse. 2014;46(2):184–90.
19. Slade GD. Derivation and validation of a short-form oral health impact profile. Community Dent Oral Epidemiol. 1997;25(4):284–90. doi:10.1111/j.1600-0528.1997.tb00941.x.
20. Jeganathan S, Purnomo J, Houtzager L, Batterham M, Begley K. Development and validation of a three-item questionnaire for dietitians to screen for poor oral health in people living with human immunodeficiency virus and facilitate dental referral. Nutr Diet. 2010;67(3):177–81. doi:10.1111/j.1747-0080.2010.01452.x.
21. David L. Measuring oral health; a conceptual framework. Community Dent Health. 1988;5:5–13.
22. Aggeryd T. Goals for oral health in the year 2000: cooperation between WHO, FDI and the national dental associations. Int Dent J. 1983;33(1):55–9.
23. Mitchell TV. Periodontal screening and recording: Early detection of periodontal diseases. 2014. https://www.dentalcare.com/en-us/professional-education/ce-courses/ce53. Accessed Nov 2016.
24. Locker D, Matear D, Stephens M, Lawrence H, Payne B. Comparison of the GOHAI and OHIP-14 as measures of the oral health-related quality of life of the elderly. Community Dent Oral Epidemiol. 2001;29(5):373–81.
25. Locker D, Jokovic A, Clarke M. Assessing the responsiveness of measures of oral health-related quality of life. Community Dent Oral Epidemiol. 2004;32(1):10–8.

20

eRegistries: indicators for the WHO Essential Interventions for reproductive, maternal, newborn and child health

Vicki Flenady[1,2*], Aleena M. Wojcieszek[1,2], Ingvild Fjeldheim[3], Ingrid K. Friberg[3], Victoria Nankabirwa[4,5], Jagrati V. Jani[3,5], Sonja Myhre[3], Philippa Middleton[2,6], Caroline Crowther[6,7], David Ellwood[2,8], David Tudehope[1], Robert Pattinson[9], Jacqueline Ho[10], Jiji Matthews[11], Aurora Bermudez Ortega[12], Mahima Venkateswaran[3,5], Doris Chou[13], Lale Say[13], Garret Mehl[13] and J. Frederik Frøen[2,3,5]

Abstract

Background: Electronic health registries – *eRegistries* - can systematically collect relevant information at the point of care for reproductive, maternal, newborn and child health (RMNCH). However, a suite of process and outcome indicators is needed for RMNCH to monitor care and to ensure comparability between settings. Here we report on the assessment of current global indicators and the development of a suite of indicators for the WHO *Essential Interventions* for use at various levels of health care systems nationally and globally.

Methods: Currently available indicators from both household and facility surveys were collated through publicly available global databases and respective survey instruments. We then developed a suite of potential indicators and associated data points for the 45 WHO *Essential Interventions* spanning preconception to newborn care. Four types of performance indicators were identified (where applicable): process (i.e. coverage) and outcome (i.e. impact) indicators for both screening and treatment/prevention. Indicators were evaluated by an international expert panel against the *eRegistries* indicator evaluation criteria and further refined based on feedback by the *eRegistries* technical team.

Results: Of the 45 WHO Essential Interventions, only 16 were addressed in any of the household survey data available. A set of 216 potential indicators was developed. These indicators were generally evaluated favourably by the panel, but difficulties in data ascertainment, including for outcome measures of cause-specific morbidity and mortality, were frequently reported as barriers to the feasibility of indicators. Indicators were refined based on feedback, culminating in the final list of 193 total unique indicators: 93 for preconception and antenatal care; 53 for childbirth and postpartum care; and 47 for newborn and small and ill baby care.

Conclusions: Large gaps exist in the availability of information currently collected to support the implementation of the WHO *Essential Interventions*. The development of this suite of indicators can be used to support the implementation of *eRegistries* and other data platforms, to ensure that data are utilised to support evidence-based practice, facilitate measurement and accountability, and improve maternal and child health outcomes.

Keywords: Performance indicators, Process indicators, Outcome indicators, Intervention coverage, ehealth, Registries, Maternal health, Perinatal health, Newborn health

* Correspondence: vicki.flenady@mater.uq.edu.au
[1]Mater Research Institute, The University of Queensland (MRI-UQ), Brisbane, Australia
[2]International Stillbirth Alliance, Bristol, UK
Full list of author information is available at the end of the article

Background

Lack of quality data on the health status of individuals is a major contributor to poor health outcomes at a population level [1]. Progress towards the United Nations recently proposed Sustainable Development Goals (SDGs) [2] can only be monitored with efficient and effective health information systems. Despite this obvious need, most low- and middle-income countries (LMIC) have insufficient systems in place for the collection, analysis and reporting of health data, severely hampering both health system and policy-level decision-making [3].

Improvement of data collection is ongoing in many countries with the advent of electronic methods of data collection, including electronic medical records to replace paper-based systems. The *eRegistries* Initiative aims to support a safe and efficient transition to integrated electronic health information systems in LMIC [4, 5] (Frost M, Hodne Titlestad O, Lewis J, Mehl G, Frøen JF: eRegistries: Architecture and Free Open Source Software for maternal and child health Registries, submitted). *eRegistries* should collect and manage information that is adapted both to the health system's information needs, as well as the data collection and real-time analysis methodology. Many existing indicators for monitoring health have been designed and constructed to be reliably measured from household and facility surveys [6, 7]; for example, breastfeeding rates for children <6 months of age. While these surveys are critical for national and global monitoring needs [8], the historically weak data-collection capabilities of LMIC [9, 10] render the utility of such indicators limited in the context of the current global transition to more robust health information systems.

Further, while these indicators are designed to guide national policy level decisions and are collected through relatively infrequent population surveys, improvement in service delivery is not their primary aim. Similarly, many facility-based surveys only include indicators to assess readiness to deliver healthcare, leaving little attention paid to quality of care. There are gaps in the specific indicators needed to monitor and improve quality of care, which are needed to supplement the existing facility readiness and the population health indicators.

The Donabedian framework [11] describes three types of indicators typically needed for monitoring the provision of healthcare: structure, process and outcome. In this framework, 'structure' refers to the assets needed to support health care, also known as 'inputs' and 'outputs' in monitoring and evaluation frameworks [12], and include access, supplies and personnel. Process indicators refer to actions/activities performed during the delivery of health care and may be known as coverage (or, as in monitoring and evaluation frameworks, outcome) indicators. The Donabedian framework uses 'outcomes' indicators to refer to the endpoint of the individual health status, community or population; these are often termed impact indicators by monitoring and evaluation frameworks. 'Bottleneck analyses' consider six factors to assess how to change impact: three structural (access, availability, training) and three process (initial coverage, continued coverage, effective coverage) indicators [13, 14]. Effective coverage indicators attempt to include all aspects of quality within a single final indicator that summarises the proportion of patients receiving high-quality of care.

In this second paper of *eRegistries* series, we report on indicators for use in monitoring the WHO *Essential Interventions Commodities and Guidelines for RMNCH* [15], which aim to improve quality of care and health outcomes in reproductive, maternal and newborn care.

This component of the *eRegistries* Initiative had two main aims:

1. to assess the status of global indicators by describing the data that are currently available to address the WHO *Essential Interventions*, and
2. to develop a robust suite of indicators and respective data points to monitor WHO *Essential Interventions* – both screening and management components – for use in *eRegistries*.

We considered the 45 *WHO Essential Interventions* delivered up to 6 weeks post-partum, including those for: (1) preconception and periconceptual care; (2) antenatal care; (3) childbirth care; (4) postpartum care (of the mother); (5) immediate care of the newborn; (6) neonatal infection management; and (7) care for small and ill babies.

Methods

Assessment of the current status of global indicators

We first assessed the extent to which the 45 WHO *Essential Interventions* [15] were being addressed in either household or facility surveys, to better understand the landscape of current data needs and gaps that our indicator development project should address. Our search focussed on the most recently reported process and outcome indicators identified from globally recognised sources. First, we examined the common international databases which compile indicators from various sources. These included the Countdown to 2015 databases, UNICEF databases, WHO observatory, and UNAIDS. These sources typically reported household surveys, primarily the large scale multi-country initiatives of the Demographic and Health Surveys (DHS) and Multiple Indicator Cluster Survey (MICS). The DHS and MICS websites were then assessed for additional information which was not yet available in the large compilations already mentioned. The average value for the most recent estimate of each indicator was calculated in Microsoft Excel (Redmond, WA).

As household surveys are not designed for, nor capable of, assessing process indicators relevant to care delivered at facilities, we also assessed the availability of indicators of key interventions directly from facility-based sources. Eight survey instruments were identified which collected data through either direct observations of patients or via medical records review; we did not consider routine health information systems as each country has their own unique set of indicators that may or may not be available in the public domain. Two published reviews [16, 17] which identified available survey tools or instruments were sourced. Surveys mentioned in these two sources that did not focus on health, or were not used in multiple LMIC, were excluded. In addition, to ensure accuracy, two facility survey programs were directly contacted for supplemental information. These facility surveys have several purposes, one of which is to assess the readiness of a facility to implement quality emergency obstetric care. The survey instruments ultimately included were: Service Provision Assessment (SPA) (2012 version), Averting Maternal Death and Disability (AMDD), the Maternal and Child Health Integrated Program Quality of Care survey (MCHIP-QoC), the Postpartum Hemorrhage Prevention and Treatment questionnaire on Active Management of the third stage of Labor (POPPHI), the World Bank's Service Delivery Indicators tool (SDI) (2012 Kenya version), WHOs Service Availability and Readiness Assessment (SARA) (version 2.1), as well as the WHO's surveys on Perinatal Health and on Maternal and newborn health from 2007 and 2010, respectively. All documents reviewed were the most recent versions available in November 2014, unless otherwise stated. One instrument included information on management of post-partum haemorrhage and was only included in our results as a denominator for relevant interventions. Data were extracted from website materials or survey instruments. Where information was unavailable, survey support staff were interviewed to identify the number of national facility surveys performed for the specified interventions. For each intervention, three domains related to process indicators were assessed: training and knowledge, availability of supplies (inventory), and whether the intervention was actually performed. The number of survey instruments collecting any information relevant to each of the 45 *Essential Interventions* in each of these three domains was measured through careful reading of each survey module.

Defining indicators and data points

For each of the 45 *Essential Interventions*, we conducted a comprehensive search of existing WHO indicators, followed by indicators from other professional bodies (Table 1). Existing indicators were adapted or developed as required by the *eRegistries* technical team with reference to the practice guidelines and training manuals cited within each WHO *Essential Intervention*, and other resources where appropriate.

Four types of indicators were defined for each WHO intervention:

- *process indicator/s for screening/risk identification* (the proportion of patients for whom screening tests/risk identification measures were performed);
- *outcome indicator/s for screening/risk identification* (the proportion of patients screening positive/ identified as 'at-risk');
- *process indicator/s for treatment/management* (the proportion of patients treated); and
- *outcome indicator/s for treatment/management* (the proportion of patients with adverse outcomes in the population).

For some interventions, screening/risk assessment indicators were not applicable. We considered screening/risk indicators not applicable where the given treatment/management was recommended to all women or babies of a given clearly defined population (e.g. Antenatal care essential package for all pregnant

Table 1 Major sources for identifying existing indicators

WHO and UNAIDS indicators	Other indicators
• The World Health Statistics 2011 Indicator Code Book [28] • WHO indicator registry (http://www.who.int/gho/indicator_registry/en/index.html) • WHO Global Health Observatory (http://apps.who.int/gho/data/#) • Indicator registries relevant to monitoring and evaluation for specific Essential Interventions (e.g. UNAIDS Indicator Registry: http://www.indicatorregistry.org/) • The World Health Organization's near-miss approach for maternal health [29] • Monitoring emergency obstetric care: a handbook [30] • Inter-agency Field Manual on Reproductive Health in Humanitarian Settings [31] • Countdown to 2015 - Building a Future for Women and Children report [32] • Indicators obtained from relevant reports on monitoring and evaluation of the specific intervention (e.g., the 'WHO World Malaria Report') found from general search of the WHO website (http://www.who.int/en/)	• The official list of MDG Indicators (mdgs.un.org) • NICE menu of indicators: (www.nice.org.uk/standards-and-indicators) • New Zealand Guidelines Group website: (www.health.govt.nz/about-ministry/ministry-health-websites/new-zealand-guidelines-group) • National Center for Health Statistics Heath indicators warehouse (www.healthindicators.gov/Indicators/) • AHRQ National guidelines clearinghouse (guideline.gov/index.aspx) • Royal College of Obstetricians and Gynaecologists Guidelines (www.rcog.org.uk/guidelines/)

Website links correct as at July 2015, we acknowledge links may be updated in future women; Provision of thermal care for all newborns to prevent hypothermia; Early initiation and exclusive breastfeeding).

By data points we refer to the primary data being captured at the point of care, which is the source of information for numerator or denominator. Data points that could be readily collected using an electronic form addressing each of the process and outcome indicators were included. Data items specifically measuring each indicator (numerator and denominator) were developed balancing specificity and feasibility by country resource level. To maximise the feasibility of data collection, for defined conditions such as preeclampsia, simple data points referring to the diagnosis (yes/no) of the condition were accepted, rather than delineated by the individual components of the clinical and laboratory diagnosis.

Evaluation and refinement of indicators

Evaluation and refinement of the indicators occurred via two stages: 1) Expert panel evaluation and; 2) Response to feedback and refinement within the *eRegistries* technical team.

Expert panel evaluation

An international group of 47 experts in maternal and child health was assembled via the network of the International Stillbirth Alliance. Thirty-four panel members were invited to participate in consultation round 1; 35 in consultation round 2; and 44 in consultation round 3. Invited evaluators included researchers, senior clinicians and academics, obstetricians, neonatologists, maternal-fetal medicine specialists, epidemiologists, consumer advocates and others.

The *eRegistries* indicator evaluation tool assessing 10 domains was developed. The domains were derived by the *eRegistries* technical team after reviewing several existing indicator evaluation frameworks, including the New Economics Foundation AIMS criteria for indicators [18, 19], the Agency for Healthcare Research and Quality standards by which to judge quality indicator performance [20], Indicators to Monitor Maternal Health Goals [21], and the SMART criteria [22]. The evaluation tool (Additional file 1) was simplified based on pilot testing with a subsample of the expert panel, culminating in the final evaluation tool assessing the below five domains.

eRegistries indicator evaluation criteria:

- *Action focused:* "It is clear what needs to be done to improve outcomes associated with this indicator (e.g., immunised with tetanus toxoid to reduce neonatal tetanus)"
- *Important:* "The indicator and the data generated will make a relevant and significant contribution to determining how to effectively respond to the problem"
- *Operational:* "The indicator is quantifiable; definitions are precise and reference standards are developed and tested or it is feasible to do so"
- *Feasible:* "It is feasible to collect data required for indicator in the relevant setting"
- *Simple and valued:* "The people involved in the service can understand and value indicator"

Panel members were asked to indicate via categorical response their agreement with each of five statements addressing the above domains *(Yes/Probably/Unsure/Possibly/No/Do not wish to respond).* A comment box was provided for each indicator to enable detailed feedback. Panel members were invited to suggest other indicators or adjustments to the existing indicators. Data were analysed descriptively in Microsoft Excel by tallying the number of responses for each response category.

Indicators were evaluated in three consultation rounds: (1) Preconception/periconceptual care and antenatal care; (2) Childbirth care and postpartum care (of the mother) and; (3) Immediate newborn care, neonatal infection management, and care for small and ill babies. Additional file 2 presents a list of interventions addressed, including the number of indicators within each intervention, and where the indicators were sourced. Panel members were assigned 3 to 4 interventions in each round each and asked to evaluate all indicators within the given intervention. Interventions were assigned to evaluators randomly, unless the panel member indicated a preference based on their area of expertise.

For each intervention the panel members were given a detailed breakdown of the indicators which included definitions, numerators and denominators, data points, and references. An evidence summary for the interventions was provided based on the evidence cited in the Essential Interventions (predominantly Cochrane systematic reviews). Panel members were given an evaluation sheet along with a separate document containing background information and evaluation instructions, including further detail on the *eRegistries* indicator evaluation tool development. Evaluation materials were sent to and returned by panel members by email.

We adopted a quasi-anonymous approach for indicator evaluation; that is, while individual panel members may have known the names of other members in the group, individual responses were not identifiable to the group and panel members were not aware which interventions had been assigned for evaluation to whom.

Response to feedback and refinement within the eRegistries technical team

Following descriptive analyses, indicators that consistently failed to meet (or 'probably' meet) the defined criteria were amended based on the evaluators' comments, or else removed if deemed unnecessary for effective monitoring and evaluation of the given intervention. A series of meetings of the *eRegistries* technical team was held to review the updated indicators to ensure consistency in nomenclature across indicators and their data points, numerators and denominators.

Graphical display of potential utilisation of the eRegistries indicators

To inform the plausible utilisation of these indicators, a power graph was created reflecting different use cases. The power to detect a significant change in a given indicator was graphed in association with the indicator prevalence and a given sample size. Three scenarios of different sample sizes were assumed: 200 births annually, 10,000 births annually and 500,000 births annually, to reflect a typical rural clinic, a typical district and a typical LMIC. The graphed indicator prevalence ranged from 75 % to 0.01 %. The most likely value for each of the indicators was calculated (Additional file 3) and placed alongside the graph.

Results

Assessment of the current status of global indicators

Of the 45 WHO *Essential Interventions*, only 16 were addressed in any of the household survey data available. Of these 16 interventions, only 7 had more than one indicator for screening and management available. In addition to the indicators themselves, data were often available on contact between a woman and the health system during either antenatal care (one or four antenatal care visits) or during care at birth (either facility delivery or skilled birth attendance) (Table 2, population data). For example, data were available for caesarean section, ANC visits, skilled birth attendance, and facility delivery from 70, 73, 75, and 75 countries, respectively, with at least 75 % of these data from 2010–2015.

The facility-based instruments did collect data on process indicators for many of the *Essential Interventions*, but were more focused on readiness to deliver antenatal care and emergency obstetric care; outcome indicators were rarely included. The availability of supplies was universally available from the survey instruments for only four interventions, while the supplies available for seven interventions were not tracked in any of the instruments. Similar results were observed for training relative to the *Essential Interventions* and for whether the intervention was actually performed. In addition, eight of the WHO *Essential Interventions* were not able to be tracked at facilities by any of the identified facility survey instruments (Table 2, facility data).

Compilation and expert assessment

A total of 216 indicators were assembled across the following areas: 107 for preconception and antenatal care; 53 for childbirth and postpartum care; and 56 for care for newborns and small and ill babies. Of these, 122 were sourced or modified from existing indicators identified in instruments from available data sources and 94 were developed by the *eRegistries* technical team. Indicators were subsequently independently reviewed by evaluators. Response rates across the evaluation rounds were 23, 21, and 25 (68 %, 60 %, and 57 % respectively), with 31 evaluators in total participating (see Fig. 1 for distribution of countries represented). Some evaluators agreed to score a second set of indicators within the same round.

Indicators for preconception/periconceptual care and antenatal care generally fulfilled the criteria 'Action focused', Important', and 'Simple and valued'. Indicators were less often deemed 'Operational' and 'Feasible', particularly for cause-specific mortality where capacity in some regions to accurately attribute death to specific conditions was considered lacking. The lack of availability of resources and skilled health personnel in LMIC settings was also seen as a barrier to the utility of many indicators. Figure 2 presents evaluation data for the treatment outcome indicator 'Malaria-specific stillbirth rate (per 100,000 births)', which represents the typical pattern of results received across evaluation rounds.

Indicators for childbirth care and postpartum care (of the mother) interventions were deemed to meet (or probably meet) all criteria by the majority of evaluators. Indicators consistently scored lowest on the criteria 'Feasible' and (less often) 'Operational', with variable evaluations on the criteria 'Action focused', 'Important', and 'Simple and valued'. Panel members raised concerns around the feasibility of data collection in LMIC where many births occur at home and where follow-up is difficult. Difficulty accurately attributing cause of death for specific conditions/complications was again raised for all settings, but particularly in LMIC. The feasibility and appropriateness of the maternal near-miss indicators introduced in this round was questioned. A number of panel members thought that health workers may lack understanding and/or appreciation of the concept of near-miss, and some anticipated the indicators may lead to data manipulation in order to conceal what may be perceived as suboptimal care. Some of the indicators associated with the HIV interventions appeared too complex and needed clarification and simplification.

Indicators around newborn care received more mixed evaluations across the criteria, again, with feasibility a clear impediment. Evaluations varied on the criteria 'Action focused', 'Important', and 'Simple and valued'.

Table 2 Current status of use of global indicators for the 45 included WHO Essential Interventions

Intervention		Population data (Percent of the population)				Facility data (Number of survey instruments)		
		Screening process indicator	Screening outcome indicator	COVERAGE/Management process indicator	Management outcome indicator	Availability of supplies	Staff ever trained	Ever performed at this facility
Preconception/ Periconception and Pregnancy	Folic acid supplementation or fortification	NA	NA	–	–	5 of 7[i]	4 of 7	3 of 7
	Family planning[a]	–	22 %	31 %	4 %	5 of 7	4 of 7	3 of 7
	Prevention and management of STIs and HIV	–	–	–	–	1 of 7	2 of 7	2 of 7
	Safe abortion services	–	–	26 %	–	4 of 7	2 of 7	4 of 7
	Post-abortion care	–	–	–	–	2 of 7	2 of 7	2 of7
	Antenatal care visit (1+) (contact)	NA	NA	84 %	–	NA	NA	NA
	Antenatal care visit (4+) (contact)	NA	NA	57 %	–	NA	NA	NA
	Essential package[b]	NA	NA	–	–	4 of 7	4 of 7	3 of 7
	Iron and folic acid supplementation[c]	NA	NA	26 %	–	4 of 7	2 of 7	3 of 7
	Tetanus toxoid vaccination[d]	NA	NA	81 %	–	4 of 7	0 of 7	3 of 7
	Prevention of malaria with prophylactic antimalarials	NA	NA	27 %	–	4 of 7	4 of 7	4 of 7
	Prevention of malaria with ITN	NA	NA	37 %	–			
	Smoking cessation during pregnancy	–	–	–	–	0 of 7	0 of 7	0 of 7
	Detection and management of syphilis[e]	44 %	2 %	37 %	–	5 of 7	5 of 7	5 of 7
	Detection and management of HIV (including PMTCT)[f]	–	3 %	67 %	*17 %*	6 of 7	4 of 7	6 of 7
	Calcium supplementation for deficient women in pregnancy	–	–	–	–	1 of 7	0 of 7	0 of 7
	Aspirin for pre-eclampsia prevention			–	–	1 of 7	0 of 7	0 of 7
	Antihypertensive drugs for hypertension in pregnancy			–	–	3 of 7	0 of 7	1 of 7
	Anticonvulsants (i.e., $MgSO_4$)	–	–	–	–	7 of 7	2 of 7	3 of 7
	External cephalic version	–	–	–	–	0 of 7	0 of 7	0 of 7
	Induction of labor after pPRoM	–	–	–	–	0 of 7	0 of 7	1 of 7
	Antibiotics for pPRoM	–	–	–	–	6 of 7	0 of 7	3 of 7
	Antenatal corticosteroids	–	–	–	–	4 of 7	0 of 7	1 of 7

Table 2 Current status of use of global indicators for the 45 included WHO Essential Interventions *(Continued)*

Childbirth and postpartum care	Skilled attendant at birth (contact)	NA	NA	66 %	–	NA	NA	NA
	Facility delivery (contact)	NA	NA	63 %	–	NA	NA	NA
	Social support during childbirth	NA	NA	–	–	0 of 7	0 of 7	0 of 7
	Prophylactic antibiotics for cesarean section	–	–	–	–	5 of 7	1 of 7	3 of 7
	Cesarean section	–	–	10 %	–	3 of 7	2 of 7	4 of 7
	Uterotonics for prevention of hemorrhage	NA	NA	–	–	8 of 8	5 of 8	6 of 8
	Active management of the 3rd stage of labor	NA	NA	–	–	8 of 8	5 of 8	4 of 8
	Induction at ≥ 41 weeks of gestation	–	–	–	–	0 of 7	0 of 7	1 of 7
	Uterotonics for treatment of hemorrhage	–	–	–	–	8 of 8	2 of 8	5 of 8
	Manual removal of the placenta	–	–	–	–	4 of 7	2 of 7	3 of 7
	Initiation or continuation of HIV therapy for HIV positive women[f] (see above)[a]	–	3 %	67 %	17 %	6 of 7	4 of 7	6 of 7
	Family planning and advice for contraceptives[a] (See above)[a]	–	22 %	31 %	4.00 %	5 of 7	4 of 7	3 of 7
	Screen for and initiate or continue antiretroviral therapy for HIV[f] (see above) [a]	–	3 %	67 %	17 %	6 of 7	4 of 7	6 of 7
	Treat maternal anemia[g]	–	40 %	–	–	0 of 7	0 of 7	0 of 7
	Detect and manage postpartum sepsis	–	–	–	–	0 of 7	1 of 7	1 of 7
Newborns and small and ill babies	Immediate thermal care	–	–	–	–	4 of 7	3 of 7	2 of 7
	Promotion and support for early Initiation of breastfeeding	NA	NA	50 %	–	1 of 7	4 of 7	3 of 7
	Promotion and provision of hygienic cord and skin care	NA	NA	–	–	1 of 7	2 of 7	2 of 7
	Neonatal resuscitation	–	–	–	–	6 of 7	3 of 7	6 of 7
	Newborn Immunization[h]	NA	NA	91 %/37 %	–	2 of 7	0 of 7	1 of 7
	Presumptive antibiotic therapy for newborns at risk of bacterial infection	–	–	–	–	2 of 7	1 of 7	2 of 7
	Case management of neonatal sepsis, meningitis, and pneumonia	–	–	–	–	2 of 7	1 of 7	2 of 7
	Initiation of ART in babies born to HIV infected mother[f] (see above)[a]	–	3 %	67 %	17 %	6 of 7	4 of 7	6 of 7

Table 2 Current status of use of global indicators for the 45 included WHO Essential Interventions *(Continued)*

	Kangaroo mother care for preterm and for <2000 g babies	–	–	–	–	1 of 7	1 of 7	1 of 7
	Extra support for feeding the small and preterm baby	–	–	–	–	0 of 7	0 of 7	1 of 7
	Prophylactic and therapeutic use of surfactant	–	–	–	–	0 of 7	0 of 7	1 of 7
	Continuous positive airway pressure (CPAP) for RDS	–	–	–	–	0 of 7	0 of 7	1 of 7
	Management of newborns with Jaundice	–	–	–	–	1 of 7	0 of 7	1 of 7

[a]Screening outcome indicator is unmet need for family planning; coverage indicator is contraceptive prevalence rate; management outcome is total fertility rate
[b]Should include measurement of blood pressure, anaemia, and identification of pre-eclampsia
[c]indicator is percent of women taking 90+ days of iron supplementation, available from household surveys
[d]Source: data.unicef.org; defined as percent of neonates protected at birth from tetanus infection
[e]Source: WHO Global observatory; 56 countries with Process indicator, 62 with outcome, 31 with coverage able to be estimated
[f]Screening outcome is modelled results of HIV prevalence, available from aidsinfoonline.org/devinfo/libraries/aspx/Home.aspx; coverage indicator is percent of population in need with HIV managed, available from data.unicef.org; Management indicator is Paediatric transmission rate, available from data.unicef.org
[g]Anaemia prevalence in any woman of reproductive age, available from household surveys
[h]Source: data.unicef.org; BCG and Hepatitis B birth dose vaccinations
[i]The number of survey instruments which cover this topic out of all the survey instruments which could have covered this topic. Thus 7 survey instruments were identified for all topics except for haemorrhage for which 8 survey instruments were identified
[α]Duplicate indicators

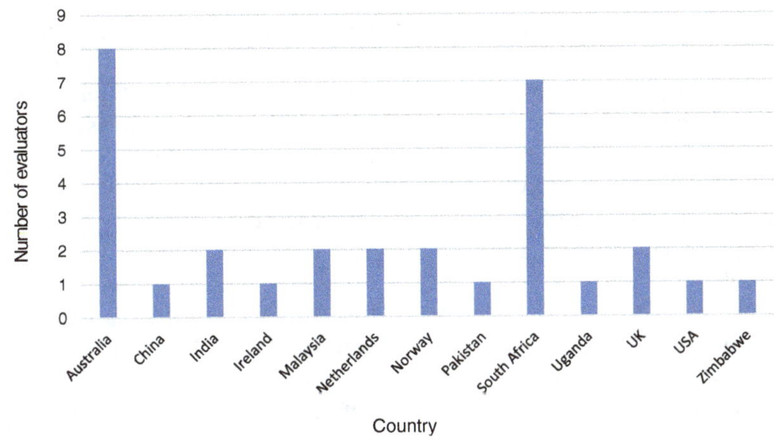

Fig. 1 Countries represented by expert panel across scoring rounds ($N = 31$)

Response to feedback and refinement within the eRegistries technical team

Amendments were made to a number of indicator titles, data points and definitions based on feedback from the expert panel (see Additional file 4 for examples). Amendments to indicators and definitions involved better operationalisation of key terms (e.g. breastfeeding counselling, 'successful' ECV, continuous support during labour). Indicators were reworded and redefined to improve direct measurability (e.g. Antenatal detection of breech presentation was revised to 'Proportion of pregnant women who have presentation of baby checked by skilled birth attendant at or after 37 weeks of gestation'). Indicators and data points were also altered in some cases to ensure applicability in different settings; for example, the indicator measuring the proportion of women with postpartum haemorrhage who received therapeutic oxytocin was deemed too restrictive for settings where other uterotonics such as misoprostol are used.

Following refinements, there were a total of 193 unique indicators: 93 addressing preconception and antenatal care; 53 addressing childbirth and postpartum care; and 47 addressing care for newborns and small and ill babies Additional file 5 presents the final list of

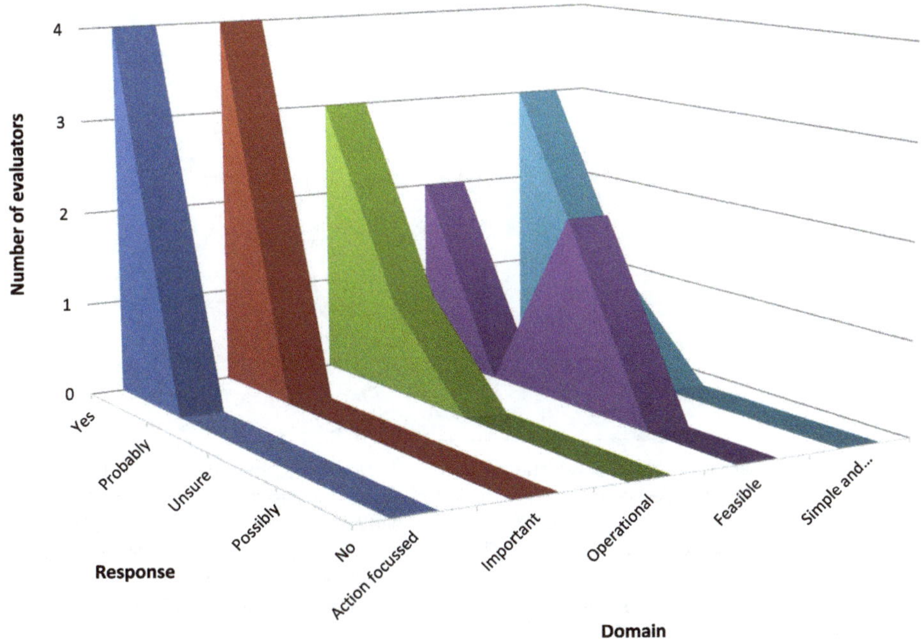

Fig. 2 Evaluation for prophylactic antimalarial for preventing malaria in pregnancy treatment outcome indicator #3: *Malaria-specific stillbirth rate (per 100,000 births) (n = 4)*

indicators including definitions, data points and sources (full indicator reports are available from the authors on request).

A series of meetings of the *eRegistries* technical team was held to review the updated indicators to ensure consistency in nomenclature across indicators and their data points, numerators and denominators. We established a set of definitions to guide the use of denominators and data points to ensure consistency across the indicator suite (Additional file 6).

Display of utilisation of the indicators

Figure 3 demonstrates the association between statistical power, sample size and the prevalence of an indicator. As shown, there is likely to be insufficient power when measured at a clinic or district levels to determine differences in rare outcomes such as mortality, while adequate power would exist at national levels. In small clinics, there is likely to be sufficient power to measure differences in common management indicators, such as skilled birth attendance and iron supplementation.

Discussion

We used the Donabedian framework [11] to determine the indicators required to successfully monitor the WHO *Essential Interventions*. This framework encompasses the intuitive relationship between three related concepts: first, the *structures* of health care are defined as the physical and organisational aspects of care settings (e.g., facilities, equipment, personnel); second, the *processes* of patient care in order to

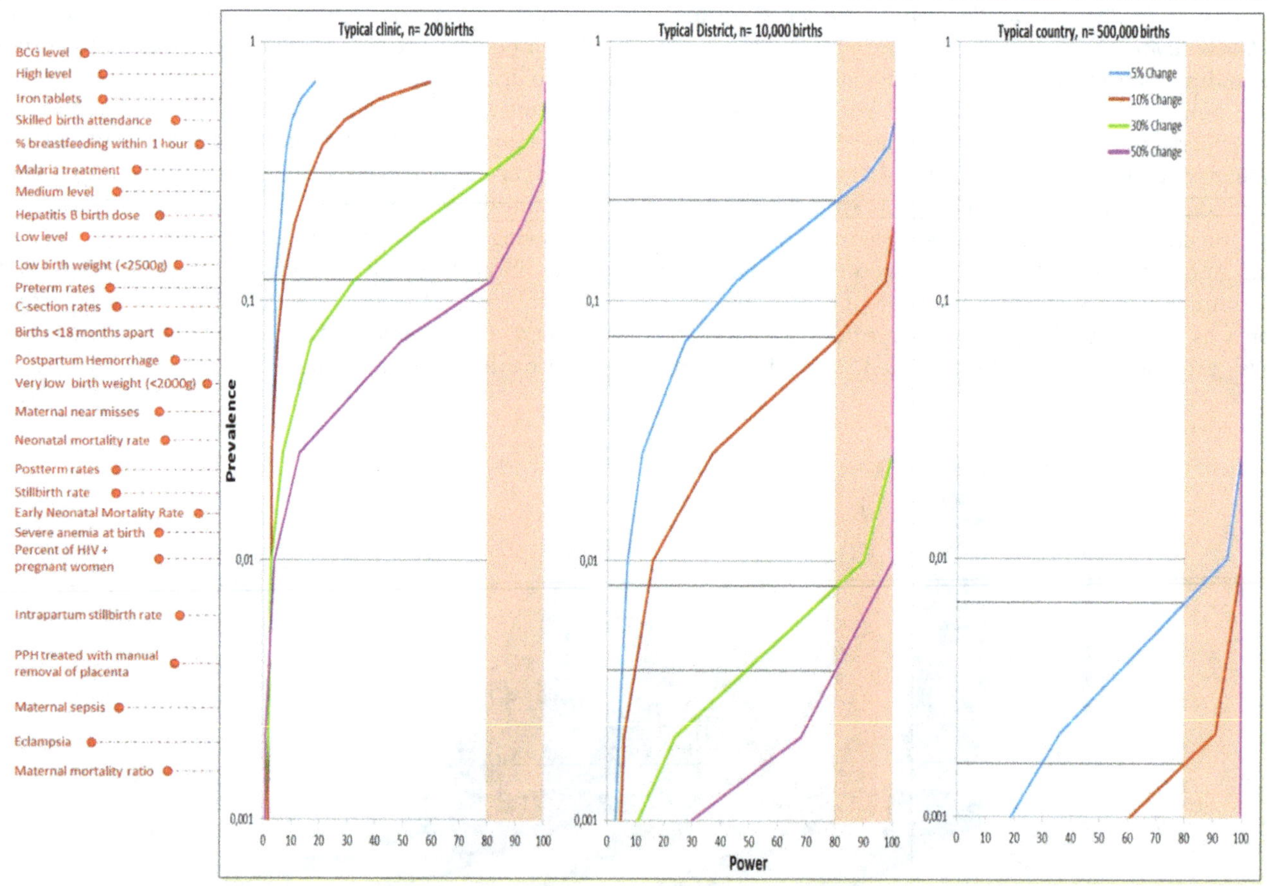

Fig. 3 Correlation between indicator prevalence, statistical power and population size. Not all available indicators should be used equally when evaluating different levels of a health system. The selection of evaluation indicators should vary based on whether there is adequate power to measure a significant change and whether the outcome is modifiable by that level of the health system, a different set of indicators is appropriate for quality improvement at clinics than for national planning purposes. The figure indicates that a typical clinic (e.g. a facility with 200 births per year) only has adequate power to identify large differences in relatively frequent events, such as process indicators for interventions needed universally (i.e. SBA, immediate breastfeeding). Districts (10,000 births annually) have the ability to monitor relatively rare process indicators (management of maternal haemorrhage) as well as relatively common impacts (i.e. stillbirths) while populations the size of a typical country (e.g. 500,000 births annually) are needed to monitor rare outcomes (i.e. cause specific maternal mortality ratios or early neonatal mortality rates). All levels of the health system should be aware of the full range of indicators, but should only be evaluated on those which are appropriate at that specific level

improve patient health; and, third, the well-known concepts of *outcomes* of medical care. Four groups of indicators were needed to clearly identify areas for quality improvement: process indicator/s for screening/risk identification (i.e. the proportion of screening tests/risk identification measures that were performed); outcome indicator/s for screening/risk identification (i.e. the proportion of women screening positive/identified as at risk); process indicator/s for treatment/management (i.e. the proportion of women treated); and outcome indicator/s for treatment/management (i.e. the proportion of adverse outcomes in the population). This work also drew upon health service 'bottleneck analyses' [13, 14], which consider structural and process factors that influence service delivery.

Our review of existing household and facility surveys which aredesigned to support national and global decision making, revealed a large gap in the availability of information to support the implementation of the WHO Essential Interventions, showing a critical need for improvements in data collection to monitor these interventions consistently across countries. Many of the needed indicators cannot be assessed retrospectively at the population level due to recall issues and lack of medical knowledge. On the other hand, many of the facility surveys focus narrowly on the structures of health care delivery. This leaves a large gap specifically in the arena of process indicators. In addition, the survey results and instruments evaluated demonstrate that several key interventions are not being monitored at all, even within the domains of structure or outcome. For example, there is no population level information to monitor antibiotics for pPRoM, while family planning activities and prevention and treatment of HIV are monitored relatively comprehensively. Although smoking cessation is recommended, none of the facility survey instruments included questions to assess this intervention and only one survey included questions on structural components to support the availability and utilization of calcium supplementation. These large gaps indicate that there is insufficient information available to guide countries and programs as they attempt to ensure the availability of the WHO *Essential Interventions* in their facilities and for their populations. There is a minimum of information to support the decision making at any of facility, national or global levels. It is this gap which the current indicator selection attempts to address.

We assembled a set of clearly defined process and outcome indicators, with a comprehensive suite of synergistic and consistent data points for effective measurement, for the 45 WHO *Essential Interventions* spanning preconception to newborn care, which can be collected from routine sources or facility surveys. Further, the *eRegistries* indicator evaluation tool makes a unique contribution to the metrics field, as it enables a priori assessment of the 'likely' or 'potential' utility of novel indicators. In our literature review, we found a paucity of information on indicator evaluation approaches to that did not rely on post-hoc review of the data generated by the indicator.

Feasibility in LMIC (informed by the direct experiences of many expert panel members) was a clear concern throughout the indicator evaluation process. Indeed, household surveys would, for example, not be able to assess all indicators proposed. Not all denominators would be measureable, making the results uninterpretable, and unattended home births would skew the numbers dramatically. However, the purpose of the proposed indicators is to facilitate uniform data collection in the presence of health workers documenting their actual work in a setting that accommodates an *eRegistry* or similarly-structured system for prospective data collection. Therefore, that a service (e.g. induction of labour for prolonged pregnancy) is not offered in a particular setting does not necessarily pose a problem for feasibility of data collection inherent in the indicator itself.

This study has several limitations. Although the expert panel consisted of members from low, middle and high-income settings, it did not include health systems specialists or programme managers, who may offer additional expertise. A legitimate feasibility problem may be posed by the use of cause-specific morbidity and mortality indicators, due to difficulty ascertaining cause of death, especially in some low-resource settings. This underscores the critical need for a quality, international, standardised cause of death classification system for maternal and perinatal mortality. Consistent application of the WHO's International Classification of Diseases for Maternal Mortality and Perinatal Mortality (ICD-MM and ICD-PM) [23] may therefore enhance the utility of some of the indicators.

The indicators presented here are important for understanding the interplay between the patient and the health system, and how health system improvement can be achieved. The indicators presented do not represent an exhaustive list of the necessary indicators for all population-based or facility-based assessments, and should not be used in isolation. While these indicators are designed for use in settings with a functional health system collecting information on care-provision provision across the continuum of care, they are developed to minimise erroneous estimates in settings where a significant proportion of individuals do not attend a health system, and thus may not be included in denominators of the population. For example, where pregnancies in need of

ANC are used in the denominator for ANC indicators, we define an eligible pregnancy as "a *woman having one documented ANC visit (unless the ANC visit is only for termination of pregnancy), OR any data documenting a pregnancy outcome or infant at any point of care*" (Additional file 6). This means that in an *eRegistry* setting tracking individuals, only individuals who are not in contact with any professional care provider from the health system through pregnancy, childbirth, post-partum care, newborn and infant care including vaccinations, will be missed as a population denominator.

In addition, these indicators are not a comprehensive set of indicators required to monitor a health system. These indicators are those that can be *collected through an eRegistry* and are necessary to address the 45 WHO *Essential Interventions*. Additional indicators for other components of a health system are clearly needed, as the WHO list does not include all interventions delivered by a health system (e.g. the management of diabetes in pregnancy). Other data sources, and potentially other indicators, should be utilized to understand the full continuum of availability, coverage and quality of community based activities, not only as stand-alone activities but also linked with facility-based activities.

The development of the *eRegistries* indicators is part of a global push to increase quality of care through an increased focus on measurement. The WHO recently published their vision for quality of care for maternal and newborn health [24], drawing partially upon the frameworks discussed in this paper, and have begun developing metrics to address quality of care. Two global action agendas, ('Strategies toward Ending Preventable Maternal Mortality' (EPMM) and the 'Every Newborn Action plan' (ENAP)) are also in the process of finalizing consensus metrics to increase the global ability to measure quality of care. These strategies contributed to the development of UN Secretary General's Global Strategy for Women's Children's and Adolescents' Health (2016–2030) which addresses relevant issues across the health in order to attain the related SDGs.

The *eRegistries* indicators contribute to the Indicator and Monitoring Framework [25] developed to support monitoring progress in implementation of the Global Strategy for Women's Children's and Adolescents' Health (2016–2030) [26]. 'Quality indicators' are needed for monitoring healthcare, whether for internal quality improvement or for external accountability [27]. The *eRegistries* technical team developed this set of indicators to provide guidance on core indicators that should be part of routine information systems to ensure that a comparable, consistent and comprehensive set of indicators is available to countries as they attempt to link their new electronic data collection systems with the older household survey-based data sources. Importantly, any implementation of an *eRegistry* must adhere to national guidelines, and include careful development of customised indicators and associated data points. This set of indicators should serve as a warehouse or library of indicators for use whenever possible to ensure comparability with WHO standards for care. These indicators should not be used en masse to monitor all levels of a health system equally. Different indicators will have different uses as well as different characteristics, dependent on the size of the population which is being monitored and the type of decisions needed at various levels of the health system. As evidenced from the graphic display of the association between power, sample size and indicator prevalence, the selected indicators can vary dramatically in usefulness for the different levels of the health system. Indicators relevant for individual clinics will typically relate to those activities being undertaken at the clinic for all women. Small sample sizes related to rare complications and outcomes will make some indicators less useful for understanding practices within specific individual clinics, but collection of these data is nonetheless highly relevant for monitoring of public health at the national-level.

Conclusions

With many countries in transition from paper to electronic data collection, more effort needs to be made to collect useable data at the point of data creation, and to minimise issues with recall, transcription and bias. The development of this suite of indicators can be used to support the implementation of *eRegistries* and other data platforms, to ensure that data are utilised to support evidence-based practice, facilitate measurement and accountability, and improve maternal and child health outcomes.

Additional files

Additional file 1: Example score sheet with indicator criteria.

Additional file 2: Evaluation rounds, interventions addressed with number of indicators and indicator sources.

Additional file 3: Likely indicator values for power comparison displayed in Fig. 3.

Additional file 4: Response to feedback – examples of indicator amendments.

Additional file 5: List of final indicators.

Additional file 6: Glossary of denominator units and definitions.

Abbreviations

ANC: Antenatal care; DHS: Demographic and health surveys; ECV: External cephalic version; ICD PM: International classification of diseases perinatal mortality; ISA: International stillbirth alliance; LMIC: Low- and middle-income countries; MICS: Multiple indicator cluster survey; PROM: Prelabour rupture of membranes; RMNCH: Reproductive, maternal, newborn and child health; SDG: Sustainable development goals; ToP: Termination of pregnancy; UHC: Universal health care; UNAIDS: Joint United Nations, Programme on

HIV/AIDS; UNICEF: The United Nations Children's Fund; WHO: World Health Organisation; WHS: World health statistics

Acknowledgments
We thank the *eRegistries indicators expert panel* for participating in indicators scoring and feedback: Zulfiqar Bhutta; Eckhart Buchmann; Sheila Clow; Ruth Davidge; Declan Devane; David Ellwood; Jan Jaap Erwich; Adrienne Gordon; Gill Gyte; Jane Hirst; Alexander Heazell; Jacqueline Ho; Dell Horey; Rachel Koshy; Carin Maree; Jiji Matthews; Elizabeth McClure; Philippa Middleton; Coceka Mnyani; Shadi Mphahlele; Stephen Munjanja; Linda Murray; Victoria Nankabirwa; Harriet Nabudere; Thanh Ha Nguyen; Robert Pattinson; Ranjan Kumar Pejaver; Haroon Saloojee; Thach Tran; David Tudehope; Mariet van Diem; and Xiaoying Zheng.
We thank Liam Flenady for technical support.

Funding
The Norwegian Agency for Development Cooperation (Norad) funded the harmonized Reproductive Health Registries project (GLO-4279 QZA 12/0355 harmonized Reproductive Health Registries) that led to the *eRegistries* Initiative (QZA-14/0022 Every Mother and Child Counts). This was led in partnership by the Norwegian Institute of Public Health and the WHO Department for Reproductive Health and the Mater Research Institute, University of Queensland (Australia), the University of Oxford (UK), and the Health Information Systems Program (Vietnam).
The contribution by JFF and JVJ was supported in part by the Centre for Intervention Science in Maternal and Child Health (CISMAC; project number 223269), which is funded by the Research Council of Norway through its Centers of Excellence scheme and the University of Bergen, Norway.

Authors' contributions
VF, AW, VN, IF, DC and JFF collaboratively developed the project plan. IKF, IF, JVJ and JFF undertook the review of current use of indicators. DC, LS and GM provided advice on the design and conduct of the project from the global and WHO perspective. PM, RP, CC, JM, DE, DT, JH and ABO provided technical and clinical advice on indicators with the technical team that refined the final indicators (VF, AW, IF, JVJ and JFF). VF, AW, PM, CC, and JFF developed the *eRegistries* indicator evaluation tool. AW managed the compilation and development of indicators and scoring by the expert panel. IKF assisted in literature reviews. MV developed the power calculations relating to indicator use. All authors assisted with preparation of the manuscript and read and approved the final version for publication.

Competing interests
The authors declare that they have no conflicts of interest. The views expressed in this article do not necessarily represent the decisions, policy, or views of the authors' affiliations.

Consent for publication
Not applicable.

Author details
[1]Mater Research Institute, The University of Queensland (MRI-UQ), Brisbane, Australia. [2]International Stillbirth Alliance, Bristol, UK. [3]Department of International Public Health, Norwegian Institute of Public Health, Oslo, Norway. [4]Department of Epidemiology and Biostatics, School of Public Health, College of Health Sciences, Makerere University, Kampala, Uganda. [5]Centre for Intervention Science in Maternal and Child Health (CISMAC), Centre for International health, University of Bergen, Bergen, Norway. [6]South Australian Health and Medical Research Institute (SAHMRI), Adelaide, Australia. [7]Liggins Institute, University of Auckland, Auckland, New Zealand. [8]Griffith University & Gold Coast University Hospital, Gold Coast, Australia. [9]Medical Research Council, University of Pretoria, Pretoria, South Africa. [10]Penang Medical College and Penang Hospital, Penang, Malaysia. [11]Christian Medical College, Vellore, Tamil Nadu, India. [12]The Australian Nurse Family Partnership Program National Program Centre, Abt Australia, Brisbane, Australia. [13]Department of Reproductive Health and Research, World Health Organization, Geneva, Switzerland.

References
1. Haazen DS, Slote A, Shorbaji A, D'Adamo M. eHealth Technical Paper: Measurement and accountability for results in health: A common agenda for the post-2015 era; 2015. http://www.healthdatacollaborative.org/resources/.
2. United Nations. Transforming our world: The 2030 agenda for sustainable development. Geneva: United Nations, Department of Economic and Social Affairs; 2015.
3. World Bank, WHO, USAID. Health measurement and accountability post 2015: Five-point Call to Action: Measurement and accountability for results in health: A common agenda for the post-2015 era; 2015. http://www.healthdatacollaborative.org/resources/.
4. Frøen JF, Myhre SL, Frost MJ, Chou D, Mehl G, Say L, et al. eRegistries: Electronic registries for maternal and child health. BMC Pregnancy Childbirth. 2016;16(1):1–15.
5. Myhre SL, Kaye J, Bygrave LA, Aanestad M, Ghanem B, Mechael P, et al. eRegistries: governance for electronic maternal and child health registries. BMC Preg Childbirth. 2016;16(1):1–11.
6. Bryce J, Arnold F, Blanc A, Hancioglu A, Newby H, Requejo J, et al. Measuring coverage in MNCH: new findings, new strategies, and recommendations for action. PLoS Med. 2013;10(5):e1001423.
7. Hancioglu A, Arnold F. Measuring coverage in MNCH: Tracking progress in health for women and children using DHS and MICS household surveys. PLoS Med. 2013;10(5):e1001391.
8. Requejo JH, Newby H, Bryce J. Measuring coverage in MNCH: Challenges and opportunities in the selection of coverage indicators for global monitoring. PLoS Med. 2013;10(5):e1001416.
9. Ndabarora E, Chipps JA, Uys L. Systematic review of health data quality management and best practices at community and district levels in LMIC. Inf Dev. 2014;30(2):103–20.
10. World Health Organisation. Monitoring maternal, newborn and child health: understanding key progress indicators. Geneva: Health Metrics Network and World Health Organisation; 2011.
11. Donabedian A. The quality of care: How can it be assessed? JAMA. 1988;260(12):1743–8.
12. World Health Organization. Monitoring, evaluation and review of national health strategies: a country-led platform for information and accountability. Geneva: World Health Organization; 2011.
13. Tanahashi T. Health service coverage and its evaluation. Bull World Health Organ. 1978;56(2):295–303.
14. UNICEF. Reaching Universal Health Coverage through District Health System Strengthening: Using a modified Tanahashi model sub-nationally to attain equitable and effective coverage. New York: United Nations Children's Fund Knowledge Management and Implementation Research Unit, Health Section, Program Division; 2013.
15. PMNCH. A global review of key interventions related to reproductive, maternal, newborn and child health (RMNCH). Geneva: The partnership for maternal, newborn and child health; 2011.
16. Measure Evaluation USAID. Profiles of health facility assessment methods. Arlington: Health Facility Assessment Technical Working Group (HFA TWG); 2005.
17. Nickerson JW, Adams O, Attaran A, Hatcher-Roberts J, Tugwell P. Monitoring the ability to deliver care in low- and middle-income countries: a systematic review of health facility assessment tools. Health Policy Plan. 2015;30(5):675–86.
18. The New Economics Foundation. Prove it! Measuring the effect of neighbourhood renewal on local people. Birmingham: Groundwork and The New Economics Foundation; 2000.
19. UNAIDS. Monitoring and Evaluation Fundamentals: An Introduction to Indicators. Geneva: UNAIDS; 2010.
20. Agency for Healthcare Research and Quality. Refinement of the HCUP Quality Indicators. Rockville: Agency for Healthcare Research and Quality; 2001.
21. World Health Organisation. Indicators to monitor maternal health goals: report of a technical working group Geneva, 8–12 November 1993. Geneva: World Health Organisation; 1994.

22. Performance Indicators in Community Health Project Working Group. Performance Indicators in Community Health: Development of a Process. Adelaide: Department of Human Services and Community Health Services South Australia; 2002.
23. Allanson ER, Tunçalp Ö, Gardosi J, Pattinson RC, Vogel JP, Erwich JJHM, Flenady VJ, Frøen JF, Neilson J, Quach A, Francis A, Chou D, Mathai M, Say L, Gülmezoglu AM. Giving a voice to millions: developing the WHO application of ICD-10 to deaths during the perinatal period: ICD-PM. BJOG. 2016. doi:10.1111/1471-0528.14243.
24. Tunçalp Ö, Were WM, MacLennan C, Oladapo OT, Gülmezoglu AM, Bahl R, et al. Quality of care for pregnant women and newborns—the WHO vision. BJOG. 2015;122(8):1045–9.
25. World Health Organization. Indicator and monitoring framework for the global strategy for women's, children's and adolescents' health (2016–2030). Geneva: World Health Organization; 2016.
26. Every Woman Every Child. The global strategy for women's, children's, and adolescents' health (2016–2030). New York: Every Woman Every Child; 2015.
27. Freeman T. Using performance indicators to improve health care quality in the public sector: a review of the literature. Health Serv Manage Res. 2002;15(2):126–37.
28. World Health Organisation. Indicator Code Book: World Health Statistics - World Health Statistics indicators. Geneva: World Health Organisation; 2011.
29. World Health Organization. Evaluating the quality of care for severe pregnancy complications: The WHO near-miss approach for maternal health. Geneva: World Health Organization; 2011.
30. World Health Organization, United Nations Population Fund, UNICEF, Mailman School of Public Health. Averting Maternal Death and Disability. Monitoring emergency obstetric care: a handbook. Geneva: World Health Organization; 2009.
31. Inter-agency Working Group on Reproductive Health in Crises: Inter-agency Field Manual on Reproductive Health in Humanitarian Settings - 2010 Revision for Field Review. Geneva: Inter-agency Working Group on Reproductive Health in Crises; 2010.
32. World Health Organization and UNICEF. Countdown to 2015 - Maternal, Newborn and Child Survival: Building a Future for Women and Children. Geneva: World Health Organization and UNICEF; 2012.

21

Antenatal depressive symptoms and maternal health care utilisation: a population-based study of pregnant women in Ethiopia

Tesera Bitew[1,2*], Charlotte Hanlon[1,3], Eskinder Kebede[4], Girmay Medhin[5] and Abebaw Fekadu[1,6,7]

Abstract

Background: Depressive symptoms during pregnancy can have multiple adverse effects on perinatal outcomes, including maternal morbidity and mortality. The potential impact of antenatal depressive symptoms on maternal health care use, however, has been little explored in low and middle-income countries (LMICs). This paper investigates whether maternal health care utilisation varies as a function of antenatal depressive symptoms.

Methods: In a population-based cross-sectional survey, 1311 women in the second or third trimesters of pregnancy were recruited in Sodo district, Gurage Zone, southern Ethiopia. Depressive symptoms were measured using a locally validated version of the Patient Health Questionnaire (PHQ-9). The association between antenatal depressive symptoms and number of antenatal care (ANC) visits was examined using Poisson regression and the association of depression symptoms with emergency health care visits using negative binomial regression. Binary logistic regression was used to investigate the association of depressive symptoms with initiation, frequency and adequacy of antenatal care.

Results: At PHQ-9 cut off of five or more, 29.5 % of participants had depressive symptoms. The majority (60.5 %) of women had attended for one or more ANC visits. Women with depressive symptoms had an increased risk of having more non-scheduled ANC visits (adjusted Risk Ratio (aRR) = 1.41, 95 % CI: 1.20, 1.65), as well as an increased number of emergency health care visits to both traditional providers (aRR = 1.64, 95 % CI: 1.17, 2.31) and biomedical providers (aRR = 1.31, 95 % CI: 1.04, 1.69) for pregnancy-related emergencies. However, antenatal depressive symptoms were not significantly associated with initiation of ANC.

Conclusions: Increased non-scheduled ANC and emergency health care visits may be indicators of undetected depression in antenatal women, and have the potential to overwhelm the capacity and resources of health care systems, particularly in LMICs. Establishment of a system for detection, referral and treatment of antenatal depression, integrated within existing antenatal care, may reduce antenatal morbidity and treatment costs and promote efficiency of the health care system.

Keywords: Maternal health care use, Antenatal care utilization, Antenatal care, Antenatal depression, Maternal depression, Sub-Saharan Africa, Ethiopia

* Correspondence: tesera_bitew@dmu.edu.et
[1]Department of Psychiatry, College of Health Sciences School of Medicine, Addis Ababa University, Addis Ababa, Ethiopia
[2]Department of Psychology, College of Social Science and Humanities, Debre Markos University, Debre Markos, Ethiopia
Full list of author information is available at the end of the article

Background

Maternal mortality remains a major public health challenge despite the encouraging changes achieved through the Millennium Development Goals [1, 2]. Nearly 99 % of global maternal deaths occur in low- and middle-income countries [1]. High maternal mortality is attributed to low antenatal health service utilization [3–7], high rates of home delivery [8–12] and low use of family planning services [1, 13]. Ethiopia contributes to between 3 and 5 % of global maternal mortality [5, 14]. Within Ethiopia, approximately three-quarters of these deaths are considered to be the result of undetected and untreated antenatal causes of obstetric complications, such as hemorrhage [15], infection [15], unsafe abortion, hypertension [15] and risk factors for obstructed labor [16–18]. To reduce the risk of pregnancy and obstetric complications, the World Health Organization recommends that women should attend at least four antenatal visits during pregnancy and deliver at a health facility [1].

In the African region, between 2000 and 2009, only 47 % of births were attended by skilled personnel and only 44 % of pregnant women had at least four antenatal care visits [19]. The situation is of major concern in Ethiopia [3, 4, 8, 11, 20–22], where only 11.7 % of births are attended by skilled health personnel, only 34 % of pregnant women attend for the recommended number of antenatal care visits [5] and there has been inadequate reduction in maternal mortality [23]. The total number of disability adjusted life years (DALYs) attributed to maternal mortality (10.6 %) in a rural area of Ethiopia exceeded that of malaria (10.4 %), tuberculosis (7 %), depression (6.5 %) or HIV (3.5 %) [24].

Maternal mortality and morbidity are established global public health challenges, but evidence is also emerging of the public health importance of maternal depression [25–30]. Antenatal depression is estimated to affect about 20 % of pregnant women in LMICs [31–35], compared to about 10 % in high-income countries [36, 37]. The adverse effects of maternal depression on productivity of mothers, child growth, health and behavioral outcomes, as well as perinatal outcomes, have been well documented [38–40].

Antenatal depressive symptoms have the potential to impact negatively upon health service utilization and thereby contribute to increased perinatal complications and maternal mortality. However, studies investigating the impact of antenatal depressive symptoms on health service utilization have been small in number and conducted almost exclusively in high-income countries. In these studies, antenatal depression has been found to be associated with increased unscheduled gynecological and obstetrician visits [25, 41], although no association was seen with initiation of antenatal care visits [42]. In studies examining the adequacy of antenatal care utilization, defined as attendance for 50 % or more of the expected ANC reviews [41, 43], no association was found between antenatal depression and adequate use of ANC. In the only study from Africa that the authors are aware of, a non-significant association was found between antenatal depression and antenatal care attendance [44].

There is, therefore, a clear gap in understanding the impact of depressive symptoms on antenatal care use, particularly in LMICs where perinatal outcomes are poor. Improved detection and treatment of antenatal depression is not prioritized in most LMIC health systems [45] but may improve ANC use, and therefore obstetric outcomes. Indeed, better evidence is needed to support greater priority to mental health care. In this paper, we report findings from a study that aimed to investigate whether antenatal depressive symptoms are associated with initiation, frequency and adequacy of ANC visits, and adherence with recommended schedules of ANC visits, in a rural Ethiopian setting. We hypothesised that ANC utilisation would vary as a function of antenatal depressive symptoms.

Methods

The study was a cross-sectional, population-based survey.

Study setting

The study was conducted in the Sodo District, Gurage Zone, Southern Nations, Nationalities and People's Region (SNNPR) of Ethiopia, located about 100 km from the capital, Addis Ababa. The district is administratively divided into 58 kebeles or sub-districts (54 rural and four urban), the smallest administrative unit in Ethiopia. Sodo has a varied topography (40 % plains, 7 % mountainous, 30 % undulating and 23 % valleys) and agriculture is the main mode of subsistence in the area (Tafesse, 2002, personal communication). The population of the district was estimated to be 161,952 persons (79,356 men; 82,596 women) in 2007 [46]. The majority of the inhabitants belong to the Sodo Gurage ethnic group (85 %) [47, 48]. The remaining population are mostly Oromo and Amhara in ethnicity [48]. The official language of the region and the district is Amharic.

Sample size estimation and recruitment of participants

A total of 1311 women were recruited into the study between September and November 2014. Eligibility criteria for women were as follows: (1) in the second or third trimester of pregnancy; (2) continuous residence in the area for at least the preceding 6 months; (3) not having hearing or cognitive impairment to the extent of impairing capacity to communicate adequately, and (4) giving informed consent to take part in the study.

EpiInfo version 7 software (EpiInfo; CDC, 2000) was used to estimate the sample size assuming a statistical power of 80 % with a two tailed 5 % margin of error for three dependent variables (ANC use, delivery care use and pregnancy complications). ANC utilization as the dependent variable yielded the greatest sample size: 276 women with depressive symptoms, the exposure or independent variable, assuming 34 % antenatal care utilization [5] among the unexposed and a 6 % difference between exposed and unexposed groups. To obtain 276 pregnant women with antenatal depressive symptoms, assuming a prevalence of 19.9 % [32], 1387 pregnant women needed to be screened for depression.

Locating participants

In the Ethiopian health system, community-based health workers (Health Extension Workers; HEWs) are responsible for health prevention and promotion activities. HEWs collect community-based data for the health information system, especially information about maternal health. During their 3-monthly house-to-house visits of the population living in their sub-district, they are expected to identify and monitor pregnant mothers and to keep accurate and up-to-date maternal records in the health posts (primary care facilities at the sub-district level). In addition, the health development army (a community-based network of health education volunteers, each of whom covers five families) are required to report pregnant women in their respective units to the HEWs. For this study, HEWs, health development army leaders, community leaders and pregnant women themselves acted as key informants to identify all pregnant women living in their sub-district. The data collectors then carried out home visits to the identified pregnant women, gave them information about the study, obtained informed consent and then conducted the interview. Women were visited three times before they were considered unavailable to participate in the study.

Data collection and quality control

There were 40 data collectors and four supervisors, all of whom had previous experience of data collection for other projects in the same district. The data collectors were trained for 2 days by the main study co-ordinator (TB) on administration of the instruments, the objectives of the study and ethical issues. Lectures, demonstrations and role plays were the methods used to train the data collectors. The main coordinator of the study also held weekly meetings with the data collectors and supervisors. The conduct of the study was closely monitored and supervised. Completed questionnaires were checked carefully on a daily basis for consistency, adherence to instructions and missing data, first by the supervisors, then by main coordinator and finally by the data entry clerks. Questionnaires deemed to have problems were returned back to the data collectors for investigation, and if necessary for correction or reassessment. Finally, data were computerized using a double data entry with EpiData version 3.1 (EpiData; CDC, 2000).

Measurement

Outcomes

Utilisation of ANC services was assessed in relation to four dimensions of antenatal care: initiation of antenatal care (i.e., time of the first ANC visit), frequency of ANC attendance, adequacy of ANC attendance and adherence to ANC schedules.

Initiation of ANC and frequency of ANC attendance were assessed by an item in a self-report questionnaire asking about the gestational age at which the women attended for each of their ANC visits. Any ANC initiated before or at the 16th week of gestation was labeled as "timely initiation" and visits after this time were labeled "late" based on WHO recommendations. Adherence to ANC attendance schedules was estimated in relation to WHO guidance, which proposes that the first ANC attendance should take place before the 16th week of gestation; second ANC attendance between weeks 24 and 28; third ANC between weeks 30 and 32; and fourth ANC visit between weeks 36 and 40. Any visits out of these proposed intervals were considered to be non-scheduled. Women who initiated ANC visits between 24 and 28 weeks of gestation and continued the remaining visits as recommended were considered to be non-adherent for the first ANC schedules but adherent for the remaining ANC schedules. Finally, the numbers of scheduled and non-scheduled ANC visits were counted for each respondent. Respondents were asked about the number of emergency contacts for pregnancy complications with a range of specified types of traditional healers or biomedical health service providers available in the area [49].

The frequency of antenatal care visits was expressed as the ratio of the number of actual ANC visits to the total number of ANC visits recommended by WHO at the given gestational age. WHO proposes one, two, three and four ANC contacts for women at the 16th, 28th, 32nd and 40th week of gestation, respectively. Finally a ratio of 125 % or more of the recommended number of ANC visits was categorized as "increased use of ANC" and otherwise as "expected use of ANC". Adequacy of ANC use was also categorized based on Kotlchuk's index [50]. Women with 50 % or more ANC attendance and timely initiation (during or before the 16th week of gestation), as defined by WHO, were described as receiving "adequate ANC" while those with either late initiation or less than a 50 % expected attendance of ANC were defined as receiving "inadequate ANC".

Exposure

Antenatal depressive symptoms were assessed with a locally validated Amharic version of the Patient Health Questionnaire (PHQ-9) [51]. A score of five or more was considered to be indicative of high antenatal depressive symptoms (the optimal score for increased probability of major depressive disorder in the criterion validation study). In Ethiopia, the PHQ-9 was found to have good internal consistency (Cronbach's alpha = 0.81) and excellent intra-class correlation of 0.92 in a study of 926 outpatients in a major referral hospital in Addis Ababa [52]. Measures of depression specific to the perinatal period were considered; however, a validation study in rural Ethiopia concluded that Edinburgh Postnatal Depression Scale had low criterion validity and poor internal consistency [53]. Although previous Ethiopian studies had used the locally-validated Self-Reporting Questionnaire (SRQ-20) for measurement of common mental disorders [34], the PHQ-9 was preferred due to its focus on depressive symptoms [53].

Potential confounders

Intimate partner violence (IPV) was assessed using a five item scale, the Women's Abuse Screening Test (WAST) [54, 55]. The scale was chosen for its brevity and the acceptability of the wording. Social support was measured using the Oslo Social Support Scale (OSSS-3) [56], a three item scale which asks about concern from others, ease of getting help and the number of supporting persons that participants can count on. Stressful life events were measured with the list of threatening experiences (LTE), a 12-item self-report questionnaire. The LTE has good test-retest reliability and internal consistency [57]. Both the OSSS-3 and LTE have been used in a community based study in the same setting [47].

Respondents were asked about the number of previous stillbirths, miscarriages, neonatal and infant mortality. The items were adapted from the Ethiopian Demographic Health Survey of 2011 [5]. Women were also asked whether they had chronic medical conditions, including HIV, tuberculosis, renal or cardiac diseases, hypertension, anemia or gastritis. Items asking the number of emergency health care provider visits to biomedical and traditional health care providers were used to assess women's emergency health care use for pregnancy-related complications.

An item from the Ethiopian Demographic Health Survey was used to ask whether the woman wanted the pregnancy (labeled as "wanted") or would have preferred it to happen at a future date (labeled as "mistimed") or if she had never wanted to be pregnant at all (labeled as "unwanted"). Accessibility of health care was measured by using seven items asking respondents about the level of difficulty and distance to reach the nearest health facility and travel time to their respective nearest health facility, as well as affordability and availability of health care facilities [58]. Finally, self-reported pregnancy complications included a list of key danger signs during pregnancy, including bleeding, swollen hands/face, blurred vision, convulsions, high fever, loss of consciousness, severe abdominal pain, premature rupture of membranes, and discharge with unusual odor, pain during urination, severe headache and severe weakness. Closed ended questions were used to assess socio-demographic and socio-economic variables, including residence, marital status, estimated monthly income and educational level of participants.

Data analysis

Data were analysed using the Statistical Packages for Social Sciences, version 20 (SPSS 20; IBM Corp 2012) and Stata version 13 (Stata Corp, 2013). A total of eight missing data [PHQ (1 missing), IPV (3 missing), accessibility to health care facility (3 missing) and LTE (1 missing)] were found. We included an average of observed scores of a respective variable to fill the missed item in the variables. Residence was categorized into urban/rural; marital status into married and single (never married, divorced and widowed) categories; Educational level into "non-literate", "primary schooling (Grade 1–8)" and "Secondary Schooling" (Grade 9 and above) categories. Monthly income was categorized into tertiles as "high", "medium", and "low". The profile of predictors and outcomes was described using simple descriptive summary values.

Poisson regression was used to examine the association between antenatal depressive symptoms and components of antenatal care use (number of non-scheduled and total number of ANC visits) after testing the assumption of equality of the variance and the mean. Negative binomial regression was used to examine the association between antenatal depressive symptoms and number of traditional and biomedical emergency health care provider visits. Socio-demographic and socioeconomic variables, interpersonal and life adversities, obstetric and medical conditions were included in all analyses as potential confounders. Gestational age was controlled as an offset variable in all poisson and negative binomial regression models. Binary logistic regression was used to test the relation between antenatal depressive symptoms and frequency, adequacy and initiation of antenatal health care use.

Results

Amongst 1321 women identified as potentially eligible, 44 were excluded because they were in the first trimester of pregnancy; three refused participation and seven couldn't be accessed despite three trials to find from their location.

Characteristics of participants

Among study participants 98.6 % were married, 67.0 % were non-literate, and 92.1 % were rural residents. The mean age was 26.8 years (Table 1). With respect to ANC attendance, 60.5 % had initiated ANC (37.0 % by 16 weeks gestation). About one third of women fulfilled criteria for adequate antenatal care. Nearly 30.0 % of women had PHQ-9 score of five or more, indicating probable depression. Forty four percent of the participants reported an unintended pregnancy (36.2 % unwanted and 7.8 % mistimed) and 27.0 % had a history of adverse perinatal outcomes during their previous pregnancy.

Antenatal depressive symptoms and adherence to ANC visits

Depressive symptoms during pregnancy were associated significantly with increased risk of having more non-scheduled ANC visits (aRR = 1.41, 95 % CI: 1.20, 1.65) and an increased number of total ANC visits (aRR = 1.23, 95 % CI: 1.12, 1.36) (Table 2).

Greater accessibility of the primary health care facility was associated with increased risk of having more non-scheduled ANC visits (aRR = 1.06 95 % CI: 1.02, 1.09) as well as with an increased number of total ANC visits (aRR = 1.04, 1.02, 1.06). Similarly, women with experience of ANC use in the past pregnancy had increased risk of more non-scheduled ANC visits (aRR = 1.28,

Table 1 Characteristic of respondents ($N = 1311$)

Characteristics	Values	Number	Percent
Marital Status	[c]Single	18	1.4
	Married	1293	98.6
Pregnancy Intention	Unwanted	475	36.2
	Mistimed	102	7.8
	Wanted	734	56.0
Monthly Income category	High	429	32.7
	Medium	423	32.3
	Low	459	35.0
Residence	Rural	1208	92.1
	Urban	103	7.9
Mother's Education	Grade 9–12 and above	53	4.0
	Grade 1–8	380	29.0
	Non-literate	878	67.0
Patient Health Questionnaire Status	PHQ ≥ 5	387	29.5
	PHQ < 5	924	70.5
Use of ANC during Past Pregnancy	Yes	793	60.5
	No	518	39.5
Number of Chronic Illnesses	One or more	440	33.6
	None	871	66.4
Past experience of adverse perinatal outcomes	1 or more	356	27.2
	None	955	72.8
Number of ANC Visits	Never initiated ANC	461	35.2
	Once or more	850	64.8
Self-reported pregnancy complications	None	655	50.1
	One or more	656	49.9
Adequacy of Antenatal Care	[a]Inadequate	861	65.7
	[b]Adequate	450	34.3
Time of Initiation of ANC	Timely (Up to 16th week of gestation)	455	37.7
	Late (After 16th week of gestation)	856	62.3

Mean age = 26.8 years
[a]Inadequate = less than 50 % of expected ANC attendance or late initiation
[b]Adequate = more than 50 % of expected ANC attendance and timely initiation
[c]Unmarried, divorced, widowed

Table 2 The association of antenatal depression with total and non-scheduled number of ANC visits

Characteristics		Total number of ANC Visits		Number of Non-scheduled ANC visits	
		CRR (95 % CI)	ARR (95 % CI)	CRR (95 % CI)	ARR (95 % CI)
Antenatal Depression:	PHQ-9 ≥ 5	1.12 (1.02, 1.23)[a]	1.23 (1.12, 1.36)[b]	1.21 (1.04, 1.40)[a]	1.41 (1.20, 1.65)[b]
	PHQ-9 < 5	1	1	1	1
Accessibility of Health facility		1.06 (1.03, 1.09)[a]	1.04 (1.02, 1.06)[b]	1.09 (1.04, 1.23)[b]	1.06 (1.02, 1.09)[b]
Marital Status:	Single	1.03 (0.72, 1.47)	0.99 (0.69, 1.42)	1.13 (0.60, 2.15)	1.04 (0.59, 1.82)
	Married	1	1	1	1
Residence:	Rural	0.65 (0.51, 0.83)[a]	0.85 (0.72, 1.01)	0.50 (0.40, 0.61)[b]	0.65 (0.51, 0.85)[b]
	Urban	1	1	1	1
Income:	High	1.15 (0.97, 1.37)	1.13 (1.00, 1.26)[a]	1.37 (1.11, 1.70)[a]	1.29 (1.07, 1.56)[a]
	Medium	1.06 (0.89, 1.26)	1.03 (0.92, 1.15)	1.13 (0.89, 1.43)	1.05 (0.88, 1.26)
	Low	1	1	1	1
Education:	Grade 9–12 and above	1.79 (1.28, 2.50)[b]	1.16 (0.92 (1.48)	2.06 (1.52, 2.81)[b]	0.99 (0.69, 1.43)
	Grade 1–8	1.27 (0.90, 1.49)	1.08 (0.96, 1.20)	1.13 (0.89, 1.43)	1.10 (0.92, 1.32)
	Non-literate	1	1	1	1
Intimate Partner Violence		1.01 (0.98, 1.03)	1.01 (0.99, 1.03)	1.00 (0.97, 1.03)	1.00 (0.97, 1.02)
Social Support		1.02 (0.99, 1.06)	1.02 (1.00, 1.04)	1.03 (0.99, 1.08)	1.03 (0.99, 1.07)
Number of Life threatening Events		1.01 (0.96, 1.06)	1.01 (0.98, 1.04)	1.05 (0.98, 1.17)	1.05 (1.00, 1.10)
Parity		0.93 (0.90, 0.96)[b]	0.94 (0.92, 0.97)[b]	0.89 (0.85, 0.94)[b]	0.91 (0.86, 0.95)[b]
Pregnancy Intention:	Unwanted	0.75 (0.65, 0.88)[b]	0.84 (0.75, 0.93)[b]	0.75 (0.61, 0.91)[a]	0.89 (0.75, 1.06)
	Mistimed	0.89 (0.68, 1.17)	0.91 (0.77, 1.09)	0.78 (0.56, 1.10)	0.86 (0.64, 1.15)
	Wanted	1	1	1	1
Adverse Perinatal outcomes: ≥1[c]		0.90 (0.77, 1.06)	0.94 (0.84, 1.04)	0.79 (0.64, 0.97)[a]	0.85 (0.71, 1.02)
ANC visit in past pregnancy: ≥1[c]		1.08 (0.94, 1.25)	1.19 (1.08, 1.31)[b]	1.10 (0.91, 1.33)	1.28 (1.09, 1.51)[a]
Chronic Medical conditions: ≥1[c]		1.08 (0.94, 1.25)	1.07 (0.97, 1.17)	1.14 (0.95, 1.37)	1.10 (0.95, 1.28)

[a]Statistically significant at < 0.05
[b]Statistically significant at < 0.001
[c]Reference group was "none"

95 % CI: 1.09, 1.51) as well as total number of ANC visits (aRR = 1.19, 95 % CI: 1.08, 1.31) compared to those without experience of ANC use. Each increment in parity was associated with reduced risk of non-scheduled ANC visits (aRR = 0.91, 95 % CI: 0.86, 0.95) and a lower total number of ANC visits (aRR = 0.94, 95 % CI: 0.92, 0.97). Rural residence and low income were associated with reduced levels of non-scheduled ANC visits.

Antenatal depressive symptoms and initiation, frequency and adequacy of ANC use

Antenatal depressive symptoms were associated with increased odds of ANC attendance beyond that recommended in ANC schedules (aOR = 1.86, 95 % CI: 1.29, 2.68). Increased access to the health facility (aOR = 1.16, 95 % CI: 1.07, 1.25) and experience of ANC in a previous pregnancy (aOR = 1.65, 95 % CI, 1.14, 2.41) were associated with increased ANC visits. Increasing parity (aOR = 0.84, 95 % CI: 0.75, 0.94) was associated with lower than expected ANC attendance. Increased parity (aOR = 0.90, 95 % CI: 0.83, 0.96) and unwanted pregnancy (aOR = 0.63, 95 % CI: 0.48, 0.83) were associated with lower levels of adequate ANC care (Table 3).

Antenatal depressive symptoms were not associated with timely initiation of ANC visits (aOR = 1.24, 95 % CI: 0.95, 1.63) (Table 3). Increased accessibility of the health facility (aOR = 1.07, 95 % CI: 1.02, 1.13) and having one or more chronic conditions (aOR = 1.28, 95 % CI: 1.00, 1.62) were associated significantly with increased timely initiation of ANC. Increased parity (aOR = 0.99, 95 % CI: 0.83, 0.96) and unwanted pregnancy (aOR = 0.65, 95 % CI: 0.49, 0.86) were associated significantly with delayed initiation of ANC.

Antenatal depressive symptoms and emergency health care use

Antenatal depressive symptoms were associated with increased risk of a greater number of traditional emergency health care provider visits (aRR = 1.64, 95 % CI: 1.17, 2.31), biomedical health care provider visits (aRR =

Table 3 The association of antenatal depression with initiation of ANC, frequency of ANC follow ups and adequacy of ANC

Characterstics		Initiation of ANC		ANC Visits higher than expected in a given Gestational Age		Adequacy of ANC Use	
		COR (95 % CI)	AOR (95 % CI)	COR (95 % CI)	AOR (95 % CI)	COR (95 % CI)	AOR (95 % CI)
PHQ 9 Score: PHQ-9 ≥ 5		1.10 (0.93, 1.24)	1.24 (0.95, 1.63)	1.45 (1.05, 2.05)[a]	1.86 (1.29, 2.68)[a]	1.09 (0.0.85, 1.39)	1.24 (0.94, 1.62)
		1	1	1	1	1	1
Access to Healthcare		1.10 (1.04, 1.15)[b]	1.07 (1.02, 1.13)[a]	1.18 (1.10, 1.27)[b]	1.16 (1.07, 1.25)[b]	1.10 (1.04, 1.15)[b]	1.07 (1.02, 1.13)[a]
Marital Status:	Married	1.20 (0.46, 3.12)	1.26 (0.47, 3.39)	1.31 (0.38, 4.58)	1.08 (0.29, 3.98)	0.96 (0.36, 2.56)	1.03 (0.37,2.86)
	Single	1	1	1	1	1	1
Residence: Rural		0.47 (0.31, 0.70)[b]	0.80 (0.48, 1.32)	0.39 (0.24, 0.62)[b]	0.62 (0.34, 1.14)	0.48 (0.32, 0.72)[b]	0.82 (0.49, 1.36)
Income:	High	1.14 (0.87, 1.51)	1.08 (0.80, 1.47)	1.19 (0.81, 1.75)	1.18 (0.77, 1.820)	1.16 (0.88, 1.54)	1.09 (0.80, 1.48)
	Medium	1.11 (0.84, 1.46)	1.05 (0.78, 1.40)	1.05 (0.71, 1.57)	0.97 (0.64, 1.47)	1.11 (0.84, 1.47)	1.04 (0.78, 1.40)
	Low	1	1	1	1	1	1
Education:	Non-literate	0.32 (0.18, 0.57)[b]	0.64 (0.32, 1.26)	0.39 (0.20, 0.76)[a]	1.06 (0.45, 2.50)	0.32 (0.18, 0.56)[b]	0.59 (0.29, 1.20)
	Elementary Schooling	0.46 (0.26, 0.82)[a]	0.61 (0.30, 1.23)	0.60 (0.30, 1.19)	1.10 (0.49, 2.47)	0.44 (0.25, 0.79)[a]	0.61 (0.31, 1.20)
	Secondary Schooling	1	1	1	1	1	1
Intimate Partner Violence		1.01 (0.97, 1.05)	1.02 (0.97, 1.06)	1.03 (0.99, 1.07)	1.02 (0.96, 1.08)	1.00 (0.97, 1.04)	1.01 (1.00, 1.06)
Social Support		1.04 (0.98, 1.10)	1.03 (0.97, 1.10)	1.00 (0.93, 1.09)	1.00 (0.92, 1.09)	1.04 (0.98, 1.04)	1.04 (0.97, 1.11)
Number of Life Threatening Events		1.04 (0.96, 1.13)	1.04 (0.95, 1.14)	1.04 (0.94, 1.16)	1.02 (.91, 1.16)	1.04 (0.96, 1.07)	1.04 (0.95, 1.14)
Parity		0.87 (0.82, 0.92)[b]	0.89 (0.83, 0.96)[a]	0.84 (0.77, 0.91)[b]	0.84 (0.75, 0.94)[a]	0.87 (0.82, 0.92)[b]	0.90 (0.83, 0.96)[a]
Pregnancy Intention:	Unwanted	0.54 (0.42, 0.69)[b]	0.65 (0.49, 0.86)[a]	0.62 (0.43, 0.88)[a]	0.78 (0.52, 1.15)	0.52 (0.40,0.67)[b]	0.63 (0.48, 0.83)[a]
	Mistimed	1.03 (0.67, 1.59)	1.11 (0.71, 1.71)	0.80 (0.43, 1.49)	0.84 (0.44, 1.60)	1.04 (0.68, 1.59)	1.11 (0.72, 1.72)
	Wanted	1	1	1	1	1	1
Previous Use of ANC: ≥1[c]		1.01 (0.80, 1.28)	1.14 (0.88, 1.47)	1.24 (0.89, 1.74)	1.65 (1.14, 2.41)[a]	1.04 (0.82, 1.31)	1.18 (0.91, 1.52)
Past Adverse obstetric history: ≥1[c]		0.98 (0.76, 1.26)	1.08 (0.82, 1.43)	0.72 (0.49, 1.06)	0.74 (0.49, 1.12)	0.96 (0.74, 1.24)	1.06 (0.80, 1.41)
Chronic Medical conditions: ≥1[c]		[a]1.30 (1.03, 1.64)	1.28 (1.00, 1.62)[a]	1.06 (0.77, 1.47)	1.03 (0.73, 1.45)	1.30 (1.03, 1.63)[a]	1.27 (1.00, 1.62)

[a]Statistically significant at < 0.05
[b]Statistically significant at < 0.001
[c]Reference was "none"

1.32, 95 % CI: 1.04, 1.69) and increased number of total emergency health care visits (aRR = 1.44, 95 % CI: 1.16, 1.80) (Table 4).

Having a chronic medical condition and higher income were associated with increased emergency health care visits of any type (traditional, biomedical and total number of health care visits). Increased number of traditional emergency health care provider visits was associated with rural residence (aRR = 3.87, 95 % CI: 1.54, 9.74), being in a high income category (aRR = 4.40, 95 % CI: 2.89, 6.69) and medium income categories (aRR = 1.07, 95 % CI: 1.26, 3.08), increased intimate partner violence (aRR = 1.15, 95 % CI: 1.09, 1.21), increased number of threatening life events (aRR = 1.27, 95 % CI: 1.16, 1.39) and having one or more chronic medical conditions (aRR = 2.86, 95 % CI: 0.03, 4.03). A history of adverse perinatal outcomes was associated with a lower risk of traditional health care visits (aRR = 0.53, 95 % CI: 0.36, 0.80) but not associated with emergency help-seeking from biomedical health care providers (aRR = 1.05, 95 % CI: 0.81, 1.37) (Table 4).

An increased number of biomedical health care provider visits was also associated with increased access to health care facility (aRR = 1.34 95 % CI: 1.00, 1.79), high income (aRR = 1.46, 95 % CI: 1.15, 1.84) and having one or more chronic medical conditions (aRR = 1.11, 95 % CI: 1.06, 1.17) as shown in Table 4.

Discussion

In this community-based survey from rural Ethiopia, nearly one-third of antenatal women had high levels of depressive symptoms. Antenatal depressive symptoms were associated independently with increased number of non-scheduled ANC visits, and increased presentations for emergency health care. There was no association between antenatal depressive symptoms and initiation and adequacy of ANC.

Table 4 The association of antenatal depression and Number of traditional, modern and total number of emergency health care provider visits during pregnancy

Characteristics		Number of Traditional health care provider visits		Number of Modern health care provider visits		Number of either of both health care provider visits	
		cRR (95 % CI)	aRR (95 % CI)	cOR (95 % CI)	aRR (95 % CI)	cOR (95 % CI)	aRR (95 % CI)
PHQ 9 Score:	PHQ ≥ 5	2.15 (1.70, 2.71)[b]	1.64 (1.17, 2.31)[a]	1.29 (1.03, 1.62)[a]	1.32 (1.04, 1.69)[a]	1.63 (1.33, 1.99)[b]	1.44 (1.16, 1.80)[a]
	PHQ < 5	1	1	1	1	1	1
Access to Healthcare		0.94 (0.89, 0.98)[a]	1.07 (1.00, 1.14)	1.10 (1.06, 1.17)[b]	1.11 (1.06, 1.17)[b]	1.04 (1.00, 1.08)	1.08 (1.03, 1.13)[a]
Marital Status:	Single	0.19 (0.03, 1.37)	0.13 (0.01, 1.26)	1.17 (0.50, 2.74)	1.33 (0.56, 3.17)	0.75 (0.32, 1.72)	0.84 (0.35, 1.97)
	Married	1	1	1	1	1	1
Residence:	Rural	1.47 (0.86, 2.51)	3.87 (1.54, 9.74)[a]	060 (0.40, 0.92)[a]	0.79 (0.46, 1.34)	0.96 (0.71, 1.29)	1.17 (0.70, 1.95)
	Rural	1	1.00	1	1.00	1	1.00
Income:	High	4.44 (3.33, 5.93[a]	4.40 (2.89, 6.69)[b]	1.52 (1.15, 1.99)[a]	1.34 (1.00, 1.79)[a]	2.20 (1.72, 2.82)	1.93 (1.48, 2.51)[b]
	Medium	1.35 (0.95, 1.91)	1.97 (1.26, 3.08)[a]	1.00 (0.76, 1.32)	0.98 (0.74, 1.30)	1.11 (0.87, 1.43)	1.18 (0.91, 1.5)
	Poor	1	1	1	1	1	1
Education:	Secondary Schooling	0.98 (0.52, 1.84)	0.81 (0.25, 2.66)	1.50 (0.83 2.71)	0.96 (0.45, 2.06)	1.27 (0.73, 2.20)	0.92 (0.45, 1.88)
	Elementary Schooling	0.92 (0.72, 1.78)	1.07 (0.68, 1.7)	0.85 (0.66, 1.10)	0.86 (0.63, 1.16)	0.96 (0.77, 1.20)	0.96 (0.73, 1.28)
	Non-literate	1	1	1	1	1	1
Intimate Partner Violence		1.13 (1.10, 1.16)[b]	1.15 (1.09, 1.21)[b]	1.00 (0.96, 1.04)	0.99 (0.95, 1.03)	1.07 (1.04, 1.11)[b]	1.05 (1.02, 1.09)[a]
Social Support		0.96 (0.91, 1.01)	1.00 (0.92, 1.09)	1.04 (0.99, 1.10)	1.05 (0.99, 1.12)	1.01 (0.96, 1.06)	1.03 (0.97, 1.09)
Number of Life Threatening Events		1.30 (1.25, 1.350)[b]	1.27 (1.16, 1.39)[b]	1.10 (1.02, 1.17)[a]	1.07 (1.00, 1.16)	1.16 (1.09, 1.23)[b]	1.10 (1.03, 1.18)[a]
Parity		1.17 (1.11, 1.23)[b]	1.04 (0.94, 1.14)	1.04 (0.99, 1.10)	1.03 (0.95, 1.11)	1.07 (1.03, 1.13) [b]	1.04 (0.98, 1.11)
Pregnancy Intention:	Unwanted	1.94 (1.53, 2.451)[b]	1.26 (0.86, 1.85)	0.95 (0.75, 1.21)	0.94 (0.72, 1.23)	1.17 (0.95, 1.44)	0.97 (0.76, 1.24)
	Mistimed	1.18 (0.76, 1.84)	0.72 (0.39, 1.34)	0.97 (0.64, 1.47)	0.98 (0.63, 1.51)	0.99 (0.68, 1.44)	0.89 (0.60, 1.32)
	Wanted	1	1	1	1	1	1
Past Adverse obstetric history: Yes[c]		0.71 (0.55, 0.92)[a]	0.53 (0.36, 0.80)[a]	1.10 (0.86, 1.40)	1.05 (0.81, 1.37)	0.97 (0.78, 1.21)	0.89 (0.70, 1.14)
Chronic Medical conditions: Yes[c]		3.51 (2.73, 4.51)[b]	2.86 (2.03, 4.03)[b]	1.58 (1.26, 1.98)[a]	1.46 (1.15, 1.84)[b]	2.14 (1.75, 2.63)[b]	1.84 (1.49, 2.28)[b]

[a]Statistically significant at < 0.05
[b]Statistically significant at < 0.001
[c]Reference was "none"

Prevalence of antenatal depressive symptoms

The prevalence of depressive symptom s among antenatal women varies across LMIC studies. Our finding of a relatively high prevalence of depressive symptoms (29.5 %) during pregnancy accorded with studies from South Africa [59], Ghana [31], Viet Nam [33] and south Brazil [60] where the prevalence of antenatal depression was 39, 26, 29.9 and 32.8 %, respectively. However, the prevalence of antenatal depressive symptoms in this study was higher than that seen in previous community studies from Ethiopia. In a study from south-western Ethiopia [32], which used the Edinburgh Postnatal Depression Scale (not validated for a rural Ethiopian population) the prevalence of antenatal depression was found to be 19.9 %. However, in a study in Butajira (a district on the southern border of Sodo) the prevalence of depressive and anxiety symptoms measured with the validated Self Reporting Questionnaire (SRQ-20) was found to be 12.0 % [34]. Normal symptoms of pregnancy which overlap with depressive symptoms in PHQ-9 may explain the relatively high prevalence of antenatal depressive symptoms in our study. Nonetheless, we have also noted the importance of somatic symptoms in the presentation of perinatal depression in this population [30]. Despite these variations, depressive symptoms in the perinatal period are important public health issues in LMICs, with the potential to affect not only health and functioning but also service use.

Antenatal depression and ANC attendance

Our finding of increased non-scheduled ANC visits and total number of ANC visits in women with antenatal depressive symptoms were broadly consistent with the few reports from high income countries [25, 41, 61]. Increased non-scheduled ANC visits in our study is also in keeping with meta-analyses and systematic reviews of depression in general, where depression was associated with around a three times increase in non-adherence to medical recommendations [62, 63]. The increased non-scheduled ANC visits among women with depressive symptoms may be explained by somatic symptoms of depression motivating them to seek help. Our finding of an increased number of total ANC visits among women with depressive symptoms was mainly through non-scheduled ANC visits. The increased number of ANC visits among women with higher socio-economic status is in keeping with a study from Ghana [64].

Antenatal depressive symptoms vs initiation and adequacy of ANC use

In the current study, antenatal depressive symptoms were not associated significantly with initiation of ANC visits in either univariate or multivariable models. This differs from the finding of delayed initiation of ANC in depressed women in the USA [42]. Timely initiation of ANC for some women might have preceded the onset of depressive symptoms since we recruited women in the second and third trimesters and consequently screened depressive symptoms after 16th week of gestation (a cut off time point of timely or delayed initiation of ANC) for most women. This might be the reason for the non-significant finding of the association between antenatal depressive symptoms and initiation of ANC in our study.

Antenatal depressive symptoms were associated with a higher overall number ANC visits than expected but non-significantly associated with adequacy of antenatal care visits after adjusting for potential confounders. The study replicated the non-significant association of antenatal depression and adequacy of antenatal health care visits in hospital based studies from the USA [41, 43].

Antenatal depressive symptoms and emergency health care use

The finding of a significant association between antenatal depressive symptoms and number of emergency visits to traditional and biomedical health care provider visits is in keeping with hospital-based studies in Australia [65], Sweden [25] and the USA [41]. In those countries, antenatal depressive symptoms were associated with increased obstetrician visits and increased use of planned Caesarean section [25, 41].

Various explanations have been provided to understand increased emergency health care provider visits. First, reduced self-care [63], social support [66] and reduced cognition and motivation [67, 68] among people with depressive symptoms increase their vulnerability to other medical conditions and complications that consequently increase the chance of needing emergency intervention [63]. Second, women with depressive symptoms may delay timely help-seeking due to reduced social support [66], lower satisfaction with health care services [65], poorer motivation and memory of schedules [67, 68] and reduced self-care [63] which means that the condition is more likely to progress and lead to presentation as an emergency. Third, women with depression may worry more about perinatal symptoms [69–71] so that they seek emergency care. This has been reported previously in postnatal women in HICs, in which emergency healthcare utilization may be increased substantially, including visits to psychiatrists, paediatricians, general practitioners and traditional providers [65, 72].

Although selection bias was minimized in this population based study, recall bias is an important issue because of low literacy and poor record keeping in this predominantly rural population. Nevertheless, by conducting the study in the antenatal period, the risk of recall bias is reduced especially for measurement of the outcome variables. The risk of social desirability bias was minimized by training the data collectors so that they would clearly explain about the study and its objective to the participants before conducting interview, encouraging them to be frank in their responses. Though we used robust method to identify all cases during the study period, we cannot be certain whether all pregnant women in the district have been identified. Furthermore, we assessed women's adherence to WHO's recommendations on ANC attendance but not the adherence of health professionals to WHO's recommendations to ANC.

Conclusions

This study offers an insight to health planners about the potential effects of antenatal depressive symptoms on antenatal service utilization. Our finding of a strong association between antenatal depressive symptoms and use of ANC services, mostly through non-scheduled visits, is important, given the relatively high prevalence of depressive symptoms in this population. First, the limited service available for antenatal women could be overwhelmed. Secondly, the increase in non-scheduled visits could potentially be associated with undetected and untreated pregnancy complications as a result of inadequate antenatal care. Thirdly, depressive symptoms are associated with an increase in medically unexplained somatic complaints [63, 73], which may result in increased non-scheduled visits. Thus, establishing a system for improved detection, referral and treatments of antenatal depression may promote efficiency in the health system and may potentially reduce morbidity, mortality and cost.

Abbreviations

ANC: Antenatal care; ANDS: Antenatal depressive symptoms; aOR: adjusted Odds Ratio; aRR: adjusted Risk Ratio; ARR: Adjusted Risk Ratio; CI: Confidence Interval; CRR: Crude Risk Ratio; GA: Gestational age; LMIC: Low and middle income countries; LMP: Last Menstrual period

Acknowledgment
We thank Dr. Simone Honikman for commenting on an earlier draft of the manuscript and Professor Martin Prince, Professor Larry Wissow and Dr Rosie Mayston for their comments during the inception and design of the study. We would also like to acknowledge the Sodo District Health Bureau for their technical and administrative support. We would like to thank PRIME for the financial support. Finally, we would like to thank all of the participants of this study for their time and patience in responding to our interviews.

Funding
The study was funded by the Department for International Development (UKAID) (PO 5248). This particular study was supported through the small grant's initiative of the Programme for Improving Mental health care (PRIME) provided to TB. However, the funding body did not play any role in the design of study, data collection, interpretation of data or in writing or submission of the manuscript.

Authors' contributions
TB, CH, EK and AF were involved in designing the study. TB, CH and AF participated in data collection. TB, CH, GM and AF participated in analysis. TB prepared first draft. TB, CH, EK, GM and AF revised drafts of the paper. TB, CH, GM, AF read and approved the final manuscript.

Authors' information
TB: PhD fellow, Addis Ababa University, College of Health Sciences, Department of Psychiatry; Lecturer in Debre Markos University, College of Social Science and Humanities, Department of Psychology.
CH: Associate Professor of Psychiatry (MD, PhD, MRCPsych), Addis Ababa University, Addis Ababa, Ethiopia.
EK: Assistant professor of obstetrics and gynecology (MD), Addis Ababa University, Addis Ababa, Ethiopia.
GM: Associate Professor of Epidemiology and Biostatistics, (PhD), Aklilu Lemma Institute of Pathobiology, Addis Ababa University, Addis Ababa, Ethiopia.
AF: Associate Professor of Psychiatry (MD, PhD, MRCPsych), Addis Ababa University, Addis Ababa, Ethiopia. He is also MRC African Research Leader.

Competing interests
The authors declare that they have no competing interests.

Author details
[1]Department of Psychiatry, College of Health Sciences School of Medicine, Addis Ababa University, Addis Ababa, Ethiopia. [2]Department of Psychology, College of Social Science and Humanities, Debre Markos University, Debre Markos, Ethiopia. [3]Global Mental Health, Centre for Global Mental Health, Health Services and Population Research Department, Institute of Psychiatry, King's College London, London, UK. [4]Department of Obstetrics and Gynecology, College of Health Sciences, Addis Ababa University, Addis Ababa, Ethiopia. [5]Aklilu Lemma Institute of Pathobiology, Addis Ababa University, Addis Ababa, Ethiopia. [6]Center for Innovative Drug Development and Therapeutic Trials for Africa (CDT-Africa), Addis Ababa University, Addis Ababa, Ethiopia. [7]Department of Psychological Medicine, Centre for Affective Disorders, Institute of Psychiatry, Psychology and Neuroscience, King's College London, London, UK.

References

1. WHO. Trends in Maternal Mortality: 1990 to 2010. Geneva: WHO, UNICEF, UNFPA and The World Bank estimates; 2012.
2. Hogan M, Foreman K, Naghavi M, Ahn S, Wang M, Makela S, et al. Maternal Mortality for 181 Countries, 1980–2008: A systematic analysis of progress towards Millenium Development Goal 5 (MDG-5). Lancet. 2010;375(9726):1609–23.
3. Aktar S. Health Care Seeking Behavior for safe motherhood: Findings from Rural Bangladesh. Bangladesh e-J Soc. 2012;9(2):57–70.
4. Babalola S, Fatusi F. Determinants of use of maternal health services in Nigeria–looking beyond individual and household factors. BMC Pregnancy Childbirth. 2009;9:43.
5. CSA. Ethiopia Demographic and Health Survey. Addis Ababa: ICF International; 2011.
6. Regassa N. Antenatal and postnatal care service utilization in southern Ethiopia: a population-based study. Afr Health Sci. 2011;11(3):390–7.
7. Simkhada B, Teijlingen E, Porter M, Simkhada P. Factors affecting the utilization of antenatal care in developing countries: systematic review of the literature. J Adv Nurs. 2007;6(13):244–60.
8. Abebe F. Factors associated with home delivery in Bahirdar, Ethiopia: A case control study. BMC Res Notes. 2012;5:653.
9. Worku A, Fantahun M. Factors affecting utilization of skilled maternal care in Northwest Ethiopia: a multilevel analysis. BMC Int Health Hum Rights. 2013;13:20.
10. Worku A, Yalew A, Afework M. Maternal Complications and Women's Behavior in Seeking Care from Skilled Providers in North Gondar, Ethiopia. PLoS One. 2013;8(3):e60171.
11. Abera M, G/mariam A, Belachew T. Predictors of safe deliery serice utilizion in Arsi Zone, South-East Ethiopia. Ethiop J Health Sci. 2011; 21(Special Issue):95–106.
12. Tefera A, Alemu FM, Woldeyohannes SM. Institutional delivery service utilization and associated factors among mothers who gave birth in the last 12 months in Sekela District, North West of Ethiopia: A community-based cross sectional study. BMC Pregnancy Childbirth. 2012;12:74.
13. Fisher J, de Mello MC, Izutsu T, Tran T. The Ha Noi Expert Statement: Recognition of Maternal Mental Health in Resource Constrained is essential for achieveing the milinium development goals. Int J Ment Heal Syst. 2011;5:2.
14. CSA. Ethiopia: Improved Capacity of Training Institutions for Health Workers. Addis Ababa: Ethiopian society of population studies; 2005.
15. Mersha A, Jira C, Demessie S. Community based study on maternal mortality in Jimma town, south western Ethiopia. Indian J Public Health. 1996;40(2):30–4.
16. Garomssa H, Dwivedi A. Maternal mortality in Ambo Hospital: a five year retrospective review. Ethiop J Reprod Health. 2008;2(1):1–13.
17. Gaym A. Maternal mortality studies in Ethiopia—magnitude, causes and trends. Ethiop Med J. 2009;47(2):95–108.
18. Say L, Chou D, Gemmill A, Tuncalp O, Moller A, Daniels J, et al. Global causes of maternal death: a WHO systematic analysis. Lancet Glob Health. 2014;2(6):323–33.
19. WHO. Health Situation Analysis in the African Region: Atlas of Health Statistics. In: Africa WRof, editor. 2011.
20. Ahmed F, Moussa K, Petterson K, Asamoah B. Assessing knowledge, attitude, and practice of emergency contraception: a cross-sectional study among Ethiopian undergraduate female students. BMC Public Health. 2012;12:110.
21. Bradley E, Byam P, Alpern R, Thompson J, Zerihun A, Abeb Y, et al. A Systems Approach to Improving Rural Care in Ethiopia. PLoS ONE. 2012; 7(4):e35042.
22. Farnes C, Beckstrand RL, Callister LC. Help-Seeking Behaviors in Childbearing women in Ghana, West Africa. Int Nurs Rev. 2011;58:491–7.
23. Berhan Y, Berhan A. Review of Maternal Mortality in Ethiopia: A story of the past 30 years. Ethiop J Health Sci. 2014;(Speicla Issue):3–14.
24. Abdulahi H, Mariam DH, Kebede D. Burden of Disease Analysis in Rural Ethiopia. Ethiop Med J. 2001;39:271–81.
25. Andersson L, Sundstrom-Poromaa I, Wulff M, Astrom M, Bixo M. Implications of antenatal depression and anxiety for obstetric outcome. Obstet Gynecol. 2004;104(3):467–76.

26. Dayan J, Creveuil C, Herlicoviez M, Herbel C, Baranger E, Savoye C, et al. Role of anxiety and depression in the onset of spontaneous preterm labor. Am J Epidemiol. 2002;155(4):293–301.
27. Grigoriadis S, VonderPorten EH, Mamisashvili L, Tomlinson G, Dennis CL, et al. The Impact of Maternal Depression during pregnancy on Perinatal Outcomes: A systematic Review and Meta-analysis. J Clin Psychiatry. 2013; 74(4):e321–41.
28. Grote N, Bridge J, Gavin A, Melville J, Iyengar S, Katon W. A Meta-analysis of Depression During Pregnancy and the Risk of Preterm Birth, Low Birth Weight, and Intrauterine Growth Restriction. Arch Gen Psychiatry. 2010; 67(10):1012 21.
29. Hanlon C, Medihin G, Alem A, Tesfaye F, Lakew Z, Worku B. Impact of antenatal common mental disorders upon perinatal outcomes in Ethiopia: The P-MaMiE Population-based cohort study. Trop Med Int Health. 2008; 14(2):156–66.
30. Senturk V, Hanlon C, Medihin G, Dewey M, Araya M, Alem A, Prince M, Stewart R. Impact of Perinatal somatic and common mental disorder symptoms on functioning on Ethiopian Women: The P-MaMiE population based cohort study. J Affect Disord. 2012;136:340–3349.
31. Bindt C, Appiah-Poku J, Te Bonle M, Schoppen S, Feldt T, Barkmann C, et al. Antepartum depression and anxiety associated with disability in African women: cross-sectional results from the CDS study in Ghana and Cote d'Ivoire. PLoS One. 2012;7(10):e48396.
32. Dibaba Y, Fantahun M, Hindin M. The association of unwanted pregnancy and social support with depressive symptoms in pregnancy: evidence from rural Southwestern Ethiopia. BMC Pregnancy Childbirth. 2013;13:135.
33. Fisher J, Tran T, La B, Kriitma K, Rossenthal D, Tran T. Common Perinatal Mental disorders in Northern Viet Nam: Community Prevalence and Health Care Use. Bull World Health Organ. 2010;88:737–45.
34. Medihin G, Hanlon C, Dewey M, Alem A, Tesfaye F, Lakew Z, et al. The effect of Maternal common mental disorders on infant undernutrition in Butajira, Ethiopa: P-MaMiE study. BMC Psychiatry. 2010;10:32.
35. Situala S, Shakya R, Shyangwa P. Depression during Pregnancy in a Tertiary Care Center of Eastern Nepal. J Nepal Med Assoc. 2008;47(171):128–31.
36. Lancaster C, Gold K, Flynn H, Yoo H, et al. Risk factors for depressive symptoms during pregnancy: a systematic review. Am J Obstet Gynecol. 2010;202(1):5–14.
37. WHO. Millenium Development Goal 5: Improving maternal health. Geneva: Department of Mental Health and Substance Abuse; 2008.
38. Bonari L, Pinto N, Einarson A, Steinereir M, Koren G. Perinatal Risks of Untreated Depression During Pregnancy. Can J Psychiatry. 2004;49(11):726–35.
39. Rahman A, Bunn J, Lovel H, Creed F. Association between antenatal depression and low birthweight in a developing country. Acta Psychiatr Scand. 2007;115:481–6.
40. Stein A, Pearson R, Goodman S, Rapa E, Rahman A, McCallum M, et al. Effects of perinatal mental disorders on the fetus and child. Lancet. 2014; 384:1800–19.
41. Magriples U, Kershaw T, Rising S, Massey Z, Ickovics J. Prenatal health care beyond the obstetrics service: Utilization and predictors of unscheduled care. Am J Obstet Gynecol. 2008;198(1):75.e1–e7.
42. Chandler D. Late Entry into Prenatal care in a Rural Setting. J Midwifery Womens Health. 2002;47:28–34.
43. Kim H, Mandell M, Crandall C, Kuskowski M, Dieperink B, Buchberger R. Antenatal psychiatric illness and adequacy of prenatal care in an ethnically diverse inner-city obstetric population. Arch Womens Ment Health. 2006;9(2):103–7.
44. Weobong B, Asbroek A, Soremekun S, Manu A, Owusu-Agyei S, Prince M, et al. Association of Antenatal Depression with Adverse Consequences for the Mother and Newborn in Rural Ghana: Findings from the DON Population-Based Cohort Study. PLoS ONE. 2014;9(12):e116333.
45. Baron E, Hanlon C, Mall S, Honikman S, Breuer E, Kathree T, et al. Mental health in primary care in five low and middle income countries: a situtational analysis. BMC Health Serv Res. 2016;16:53. doi:10.1186/s12913-016-1291-z.
46. CSA. Statistical Abstracts (2011/2012): Annual Statistical Reports. 2011.
47. Fekadu A, Medhin G, Selamu M, Hailemariam M, Alem A, Giorgis TW, et al. Population level mental distress in rural Ethiopia. BMC Psychiatry. 2014;14:194.
48. CSA. The 2007 Poulation and Housing Census of Ethiopia: Resullts for SNNPR. In: Statistical Report on population Size and Characterstics. 2010. Part I.
49. Selamu M, Asher L, Hanlon C, Medihin G, Hailemariam M, Patel V, et al. Beyond the Biomedical: Community resources for mental health care in rural Ethiopia. PLoS ONE. 2015;10(5):e0126666.
50. Kotelchuck M. The Adequacy of Prenatal Care Utilization Index: Its US Distribution and Association with Low Birthweight. Public Health Brief. 1994;9(9).
51. Kroenke K, Spitzer R, Wiliams J. Validity of a Brief Depression Severity Measure. J Gen Intern Med. 2001;16:606–13.
52. Gelaye B, Williams M, Lemma S, Deyessa N, Bahretibeb Y, Shibre T, et al. Validity of the patient health questionnaire-9 for depression screening and diagnosis in East Africa. Psychiatry Res. 2013;210(2):653–61.
53. Hanlon C, Medihin G, Alem A, Araya M, Abdulahi A, Tesfaye M. Measuring Common Mental Disorders in Women in Ethiopia: Reliability and construct Validity of Comprehensive Psychopathological rating Scale. Soc Psychiatry Psychiaric Epidemiol. 2008;43:653–9.
54. Rabin R, Jennings J, Campbell J, Bair-Merritt M. Intimate Partner Violence Screening Tools. Am J Prev Med. 2009;36(5):439–45.
55. Zink T, Levin L, Putnam F, Beckstrom A. Accuracy of Five Domestic Violence Screening Questions With Nongraphic Language. Clin Pediatr. 2007;46(2):127 31.
56. Boen H. Characteristics of senior centre users–and the impact of a group programme on social support and late-life depression. Norsk Epidemiologi. 2012;22(2):261–9.
57. Brugha TS, Cragg D. The List of Threatening Experiences: the reliability and validity of a brief life events questionnaire. Acta Psychiatr Scand. 1990;82(1):77–81.
58. Fotso J, Mukiira C. Perceived quality of and access to care among poor urban women in Kenya and their utilization of delivery care: harnessing the potential of private clinics? Health Policy Plan. 2011;1–11.
59. Hartley M, Tomlinson M, Greco E, Comulada S, Stewart J, Roux J, Mbewu N, Rotheram-Borus N. Depressed mood in pregnancy: Prevalence and correlates in two Cape Town peri-urban settlements. Reprod Health J. 2011;8:9.
60. Anselmi L, Barros F, Minten G, Gigante D, Horta B, Victora C. Prevalence and early deteminants of common mental disorders in the 1982 birth cohort, Pelotas, South Brazil. Rev Saude Publica. 2008;42(12):26–33.
61. Alder J, Fink N, Urech C, Hosli I, Bitzer J. Identification of antenatal depression in obstetric care. Arch Gynecol Obstet. 2011;284(6):1403–9. Epub 2011/03/23. eng.
62. Katon W. Epidemiology and treatment of depression in patients with chronic medical illness. Dialogues Clin Neurosci. 2011;13(1):7–23.
63. DiMatteo R, Lepper H, Croghan T. Depression Is a Risk Factor for Noncompliance With Medical Treatment Meta-analysis of the Effects of Anxiety and Depression on Patient Adherence. Arch Intern Med. 2000;160:2101–7.
64. Arthur E. Wealth and antenatal care use: implications for maternal health care utilisation in Ghana. Heal Econ Rev. 2012;2:14.
65. Webster J, Pritchard M, Linnane J, Roberts J, Hinson J, Starrenburg S. Postnatal depression: use of health services and satisfaction with health-care providers. J Qual Clin Pract. 2001;21(4):144–8.
66. Zuckerman B, Amaro H, Bauchner H, Cabral H. Depressive symptoms during pregnancy: relationship to poor health behaviors. Am J Obstet Gynecol. 1989;160(5):1107–11.
67. Airaksinen E, Larsson M, Forsell L. Cognitive functions in depressive disorders: evidence from a population-based study. Psychol Med. 2004;34:83–91.
68. Nauatin M, Mitchel P, Goodwin G. Cognitive Deficits in Depression: A review article. BJP. 2001;178:200–6.
69. Hanlon C, Whitley R, Wondimagegn D, Alem A, Prince M. Between life and death: exploring the socio-cultural aspect of antenatal mental distress in rural Ethiopia. Arch Womens Ment Health. 2010;13(5):385–93.
70. Stewart R, Umar E, Gleadow-Ware S, Creed F, Bristow K. Perinatal distress and depression in Malawi: an exploratory qualitative study of stressors, supports and symptoms. Arch Womens Ment Health. 2015;18:177–85.
71. Mwape L, McGuiness T, Dixey R, Johnson S. Socio-cultural factors surounding Mental distress during the perinatal period in Zambia: a qualitative investigation. Int J Ment Health Syst. 2012;6(12):1–10.
72. Dennis C. Influence of depressive symptomatology on maternal health service utilization and general health. Arch Womens Ment Health. 2004;7:183–91.
73. Mogga S, Prince M, Alem A, Kebede D, Stewart R, Glozier N, et al. Outcome Of major Depression In Ethiopia Population-Based Study. Br J Psychiatry. 2006;189:241–6.

Growing inequities in maternal health in South Africa: a comparison of serial national household surveys

Njeri Wabiri[1*], Matthew Chersich[2], Olive Shisana[3,4], Duane Blaauw[5], Helen Rees[2] and Ntabozuko Dwane[1]

Abstract

Background: Rates of maternal mortality and morbidity vary markedly, both between and within countries. Documenting these variations, in a very unequal society like South Africa, provides useful information to direct initiatives to improve services. The study describes inequalities over time in access to maternal health services in South Africa, and identifies differences in maternal health outcomes between population groups and across geographical areas.

Methods: Data were analysed from serial population-level household surveys that applied multistage-stratified sampling. Access to maternal health services and health outcomes in 2008 ($n = 1121$) were compared with those in 2012 ($n = 1648$). Differences between socio-economic quartiles were quantified using the relative (RII) and slope (SII) index of inequality, based on survey weights.

Results: High levels of inequalities were noted in most measures of service access in both 2008 and 2012. Inequalities between socio-economic quartiles worsened over time in antenatal clinic attendance, with overall coverage falling from 97.0 to 90.2 %. Nationally, skilled birth attendance remained about 95 %, with persistent high inequalities (SII = 0.11, RII = 1.12 in 2012). In 2012, having a doctor present at childbirth was higher than in 2008 (34.4 % versus 27.8 %), but inequalities worsened. Countrywide, levels of planned pregnancy declined from 44.6 % in 2008 to 34.7 % in 2012. The RII and SII rose over this period and in 2012, only 22.4 % of the poorest quartile had a planned pregnancy. HIV testing increased substantially by 2012, though remains low in groups with a high HIV prevalence, such as women in rural formal areas, and from Gauteng and Mpumalanga provinces. Marked deficiencies in service access were noted in the Eastern Cape ad North West provinces.

Conclusions: Though some population-level improvements occurred in access to services, inequalities generally worsened. Low levels of planned pregnancy, antenatal clinic access and having a doctor present at childbirth among poor women are of most concern. Policy makers should carefully balance efforts to increase service access nationally, against the need for programs targeting underserved populations.

Keywords: Maternal health, South Africa, Equity gap, Access, National household survey, Relative inequalities

Background

South Africa is one of the most inequitable countries in the world, by almost any measure. The wealthiest 10 percent of the population, for example, accounts for more than half the country's income [1]. Indices of health, and especially of maternal health, clearly reflect the inequalities in access and health outcomes that mark the country. Maternal mortality varies considerably between provinces, for instance, with the institutional-level maternal mortality rates (MMR; maternal deaths per 100,000 live births) ranging from 69 in the Western Cape to 185 in the North West Province [2]. The prevalence of HIV also differs substantially between geographical areas. The 2012 national antenatal survey found that the HIV prevalence at district level ranges from 1.5 to 40.7 %, around a national average of 29.2 %[3].

Maternal mortality has fluctuated over the past decades. Institutional MMR progressively escalated from the late

* Correspondence: nwabiri@hsrc.ac.za
[1]Epidemiology and Strategic Information Unit, Human Sciences Research Council, Pretoria, South Africa
Full list of author information is available at the end of the article

1990s onwards, up to levels of 176 nationally in the 2008–2010 triennium, but dropped thereafter to 147 by 2012 [4, 5]. The wide scale-up of antiretroviral treatment (ART) across the country, and especially among pregnant women, is credited with these reductions [5, 6]. While HIV-related mortality has decreased, maternal deaths due to haemorrhage have actually risen, especially among women who had a caesarean section [5]. The increase in these and other deaths from direct obstetric causes, are ascribed to deficiencies in the quality of maternal health services, most notably in patient transport, the availability of intensive care units and the provision of emergency obstetric care [5].

Health service data are available to guide improvements in the quality of services. The district monitoring systems have been strengthened [2] and the factors contributing to maternal deaths are frequently assessed [4, 6, 7]. What we lack, however, is an assessment of access to maternal health services at a population level, disaggregated by population group, and assessed over time. Analysing data from national household surveys can fill these gaps. A survey in 2008 [8] highlighted marked differences in maternal health status across socio-economic and other population groups, especially between rural and urban areas. Using data from a follow-up survey in 2012, the study presented here updates the 2008 findings and examines how inequalities have changed since then. The analysis focuses primarily on absolute and relative differentials between socio-economic groups, but also on the influence of factors such as rural–urban location, race and HIV status. More broadly, by determining the distribution and outcomes of maternal health services over time, the study identifies the underserved groups and geographical areas. This information can be used to help direct health system resources and initiatives to raise the quality of services.

Methods

Survey sampling, field and laboratory procedures

This paper is a sub-analysis of the third (2008) and fourth (2012) South African National HIV Prevalence, Incidence, Behaviour and Communication Surveys [9, 10]. The two surveys employed multistage stratified sampling, taking into account province; locality (urban formal, urban informal, rural formal including commercial farms, and rural informal or tribal areas); and race groups. Full details of the survey methods, response rates and ethical procedures are detailed elsewhere [9, 11]. In brief, the sampling frames were based on enumerator areas (EAs) used in the South Africa national census. The primary sampling units consisted of 1000 EAs, which were selected from a database of 86,000 EAs. Fifteen households within each selected EA constituted the secondary sampling units (15,000 households). The same EAs were used in both surveys, but different households were selected. The final sampling unit was made up of eligible individuals within households. Anyone who slept in the household on the night preceding the survey (including visitors) was considered a household member. In 2008, only four persons were eligible to participate from each household; one in each age group (0–1, 2–11, 12–14, and above 15 years) [8]. In the 2012 survey, all persons in the selected households were eligible. Consenting participants responded to individual questionnaires. Dried blood spot specimens were collected from consenting participants, tested for HIV antibodies and linked anonymously with the questionnaires administered to study participants [12].

Study variables and measures

The analysis includes data collected from two groups of women aged 15–55 years: those who had been pregnant in the preceding 2 years and those interviewed as the parent or guardian of a child below two years. The study variables are described in the publication of the 2008 survey findings [8], and are only overviewed here. Socio-economic quartiles (SEQ) were derived from an asset score based on measures of household-living standards, and were generated using multiple correspondence analysis [13, 14]. Quartiles were preferred over quintiles as the socio-economic differentials are very narrow in many areas of the country, given that many women perform the same income-generation activities and thus have similar incomes and asset levels [8, 15]. Quintiles would thus have been unable to differentiate between women in Q1 and Q2, who have essentially the same living standards.

Access to maternal health services was measured by: utilisation of antenatal clinics; HIV testing coverage; and the presence of a skilled birth attendant (SBA) or doctor at birth [8]. Maternal health status was not assessed in detail within the survey, thus proxy indicators were used. Women who said they had a fair or poor health status were categorised as having a lower self-assessed health status, and compared with those reporting good or excellent health. Planned pregnancy, multiparity (five or more children), and prevalence of HIV infection were used as indicators of maternal health status, given their links with pregnancy outcomes for women and children [16].

Though the study focused on the distribution of access and outcomes by SEQ, variation was also assessed across other categories of social differentiation. The applicable categories of the PROGRESS-Plus acronym were used, namely: **P**lace of Residence (province;

locality as urban formal and informal, and rural formal and informal), **R**ace, **O**ccupation, **E**ducation, **S**ocio-economic Status (SEQ and employment of the mother), and Age and HIV status representing the **Plus** category [17]. We also examined whether there were systematic differences in access to services between those with and without HIV infection.

Statistical models and measures of inequality by socioeconomic status

Data were analysed using Stata version 13.0 (College Station, Texas, United States [18]), taking into account the complex multilevel sampling design (by age, race group and province) and participant non-response. Summary indices for descriptive analysis are weighted percentages, while unweighted counts are provided. Clustering was not accounted for given that the large number of primary sampling units (1000) in the study is comparable to respondent number, diminishing such effects [8].

Socio-economic inequalities in maternal health were calculated using three inequality measures: the Slope Index of Inequality (SII) for quantifying absolute inequalities, and the Relative Index of Inequality (RII) and Concentration Index (CI) for assessing the magnitude of relative inequalities [19–21]. ArcGIS Desktop Version 10.0 was used to show the geographical variation in access to antenatal services and a skilled birth attendant, planned pregnancy and health status.

Slope index of inequality and the relative index of inequality

The SII and RII indices are regression based and take the whole wealth distribution into account, rather than only comparing the two most extreme groups (e.g., the wealthiest and poorest quartiles), such as done with a rate difference and rate ratio [20]. The RII and SII are "recommended when making comparisons over time or across populations" [22, 23]. While most trend studies focus on relative, as opposed to absolute inequalities [24], the use of both provides a more complete assessment of patterns of inequalities and changes over time [25, 26].

To derive the SII and RII, each woman in the study population was assigned a notional socio-economic rank score, scaled to take values between 0 (bottom of hierarchy (Q1)) and 1 (top of hierarchy (Q4)) [8]. The rank score equals the midpoint of the range in the cumulative distribution of the population of participants in a given SEQ [24]. For example, if the Q1 women comprise 34.5 % of the population, the women in this category are assigned a rank score of 0.17 (0.345/2), and if the Q2 women comprises 32.5 % of the population, the corresponding rank score is 0.51 (0.345 + [0.325/2]) and so forth. The generated individual data is self-weighted and the only weight applied in the analysis is the survey weight to correct for survey sample design.

We then used generalised linear models (GLM) to fit binomial models (Eq. 1) to generate inequality measures, as has been suggested by several authors [24, 27–30].

$$g(Y) = \beta_0 + \beta_1 rscore + \beta_2 survey + \varepsilon \qquad (1)$$

where Y = 1 if outcome is present and Y = 0 if absent, *g(Y) = Y* is the identity link function (i.e. binomial regression) generating SII together with the 95 % confidence and, *g(Y) = log(Y)* is log link function (i.e. log-binomial regression) generating the RII and the 95 % confidence interval, *rscore* is the notional socio-economic rank score for each woman, β_1 and β_2 are the regression coefficients. *Survey* equals 1 for the 2008 survey and 2 for the 2012 survey, and ε is the error term with a binomial distribution.

The SII, the β_1 under binomial regression, represent the estimated difference in predicted value of the outcome between those at the top (wealthiest) and those at the bottom (poorest) of the social hierarchy. SII is the absolute effect on health outcome of moving from the poorest to the wealthiest group [20, 31]. A positive SII represent inequality in favour of the wealthy, while a negative SII is inequality in favour of poor.

The RII, the exponential of the slope, $\exp(\beta_1)$ under log-binomial regression, represents the proportionate difference in outcome across the distribution of socio-economic position; or the likelihood of having an outcome, relative to one's SES level. The RII increases from zero, with higher values indicating higher inequality. An RII above one indicates that the outcome is more prevalent among wealthy women, compared to their poor counterparts. To deal with lack of model convergence, we fitted Poisson regression with robust variance [32]. Poisson regression is suitable when outcomes are not rare, as in this study where most had prevalence greater than 10 %[28]. A decline in both SII and RII is the best evidence of progress in closing the inequality gap [24].

For each outcome, the linear trends of the RII and SII over the five year period 2008–2012 were tested by estimating the p-value for an interaction term between rank score and years since baseline, i.e. 2008 survey coded 1, 2012 coded 2, to account for the different time intervals between surveys (Eq. 2). Positive and significant coefficients, β_3 greater than one, for the interaction term indicate widening RII (SII) inequalities over time.

$$g(Y) = \beta_0 + \beta_1 rscore + \beta_2 survey + \beta_3 rscore * survey + \varepsilon \qquad (2)$$

Concentration index

The concentration index is defined with reference to the concentration curve, which plots the cumulative proportion of health outcome against the cumulative proportion of the population, ranked by SEQ beginning with the poorest [8, 33]. If health access is equally distributed across SEQ, concentration curves coincide with the diagonal line of equality. The Concentration Index is given by twice the area between the concentration curve and line of equality and ranges from −1 to 1. Zero represents perfect equality, while positive values indicate richer individuals have greater coverage (or good health outcomes) than poorer individuals [33].

Results

In 2008, data were gathered on 23,308 people, and 56.0 % of those interviewed were women aged 15–55 years (8292/14,798). Of these women, 13.5 % (1121/8292) had been pregnant in the preceding 2 years, and 15.8 % (1310/8292) had a child in the past 2 years. The proportion of survey participants aged 15–55 years in 2012 was similar to that in 2008 (53.5 %; 13,187/24,659). Of these, 12.5 % (1648/13,187) had been pregnant or had a child in the past 2 years.

Variation in socio-economic characteristics of women by population group

In both surveys, about 95 % of pregnancies occurred in African or Coloured women (Table 1). White and Indian women, however, constituted 33.6 % of the wealthiest quartile in 2012, higher than levels in 2008 (23.9 %). In each survey, about 60 % of women in QI and QII were single, while this figure was only 40 % among the wealthiest women. Wealth quartile remains strongly associated with educational attainment and employment. Overall, educational attainment appears to be rising (44.2 % of women had completed secondary school in 2012, versus 40.0 % in 2008). However, still only about 10 % of the population had any post-school education in 2012. The proportion unemployed and seeking work was higher in 2012 than in 2008 in QI (51.6 versus 44.0 %) and QII (49.2 versus 33.9 %), while it decreased in the two wealthier quartiles.

Socio-economic status varies considerably between provinces, and across urban and rural divides. In each survey, pregnant women in the wealthiest two quartiles were heavily concentrated in the urban formal areas of Gauteng and Western Cape. By contrast, almost three quarters of the poorest quartile lived in rural informal locations in 2012, up from 61.0 % in 2008. In the 2012 survey, the poorest quartile mostly lives in KwaZulu Natal (20.9 %), Eastern Cape (30.9 %) and Limpopo (19.5 %). Few wealthy women inhabit the latter two provinces (they together constituted only about 5 % of the wealthiest quartile in 2012).

Inequalities in access to maternal health services

About 10 % of the overall population had not accessed ANC in 2012. Compared with 2008, *receipt of any ANC* declined in 2012 among all women and across almost all sub-groups, but especially in QI and QII women (Additional file 1: Table S1 and Fig. 1). Among those who attended ANC, the overall proportion that had *four or more ANC visits* was similar in 2008 and 2012, but inequalities within many population groups worsened. The gap between the poorest and wealthiest quartile rose from 5.7 % in 2008 to 16.0 % in 2012. In 2012, the proportion attending four or more visits rose with age and with each increase in education level (for example, from 72.9 % in those with under three years of schooling to 94.7 % in those with tertiary education), and was much higher in employed than unemployed women.

In 2012, considerably more women attended *ANC before 20 weeks* than in 2008, with double digit increases seen in most population groups, even in the poorest quartile. Though no changes were detected in inequalities over time, the SII (0.31) and RII (1.59) remained very high in 2012. Differences in 2012 were above 20 % between the sub-categories of almost all of the PROGRESS-Plus groups. Moreover, significant differences between more and less vulnerable groups were detected in early attendance for nine population subgroups in 2012, but for only three in 2008 (Additional file 1: Table S1). In the 2012 survey, ANC attendance before 20 weeks was particularly low among women under 20 years, those living in rural and urban informal areas, and in Black African women. Importantly, 75.2 % of HIV-infected women attended before 20 weeks, compared to 63.5 % of uninfected women.

The substantial levels of absolute and relative inequality in *SBA coverage* were maintained in the second survey. Relatively low SBA coverage persists in QI, Black African women, rural areas and low education groups. Based on all measures of socio-economic inequality, *doctor attending childbirth* remains the most unequal of measures (CI = 0.27 in 2012, for example). Overall, the proportion of deliveries attended by a doctor had, however, increased considerably in 2012 in almost population groups, but was accompanied by a worsening of absolute inequalities (QI-QIV range and SII). The SII measure shows a 58.7 percentage point increase between the lowest and highest income quartiles. Gaps between race groups also rose (90 % of White and Indian women had a doctor present in 2012, 20–30 % higher than in 2008, while in Black African women, these levels only increased from 23.5 % in 2008 to 28.4 % in 2012).

Marked increments were noted in *HIV testing* in 2012, with these services largely pro-poor. More than 90 % of all population sub-groups had an HIV test in the past

Table 1 Distribution of socio-economic status among women pregnant in past 2 years between 2008 and 2012; Distribution of socio-economic status among population sub-groups in women pregnant in past 2 years: analysis of the 2008 and 2012 national SABSSM survey

	Socio-economic Status								Overall total (Unweighted *N*, %)	
	QI poorest (%)		QII (%)		QIII (%)		QIV wealthiest (%)			
	2008	2012	2008	2012	2008	2012	2008	2012	2008	2012
Age categories									1111	1619**
15 to 19	12.1	14.2	13.1	9.5	9.6	9.9	4.6	4.6	11.1	10.2
20 to 29	50.4	50.8	48.6	57.8	52.4	55.3	51.4	50.6	50.5	54.0
30 to 39	32.8	26.2	36.2	28.9	35.5	31.4	37.0	39.8	35.0	30.4
40 to 55	4.7	8.8	2.1	3.8	2.4	3.5	6.9	4.9	3.4	5.3
Place of residence									1115***	1619***
Urban formal	7.8	11.3	27.6	27.1	82.0	76.8	95.7	89.7	43.2	45.7
Urban informal	20.3	11.0	16.3	12.0	7.6	9.1	1.5	1.0	13.7	9.3
Rural formal	10.9	4.8	9.7	3.1	6.3	2.9	0.3	6	8.3	3.9
Rural informal	61.0	72.8	46.4	57.8	4.2	11.3	2.5	3.3	34.8	41.1
Province									1115***	1619***
Eastern Cape	21.2	30.9	8.2	7.1	8.5	4.6	15.0	2.3	12.8	12.6
Free State	3.5	3.2	6.6	5.8	4.7	6.4	3.2	6.9	4.8	5.4
Gauteng	10.5	8.5	8.2	18.3	41.2	40.6	40.4	50.5	21.3	26.4
KwaZulu Natal	23.2	20.9	28.7	26.2	16	12.3	9.9	10.0	21.7	18.4
Limpopo	22.4	19.5	15.0	15.4	2.8	3.7	2.9	2.5	12.7	11.4
Mpumalanga	8.0	6.5	10.4	12.9	3.4	7.0	8.5	3.7	7.5	8.1
North West	7.8	6.8	13.7	8.1	8.2	6.0	1.3	4.7	9.2	6.6
Northern Cape	1.2	1.2	1.7	1.2	2.3	5.1	2.1	3.9	1.8	2.7
Western Cape	2.1	2.6	7.4	4.9	12.9	14.3	16.7	15.5	8.2	8.4
Race									1110***	1615***
African	98.4	96.9	95	95.7	77.5	82.9	60.4	49.7	88	85.7
White	0.0	0.1	0.3	0.0	8.1	2.0	17.6	23.4	4.0	4.0
Coloured	1.6	3.0	4.5	4.2	13.0	13.2	15.7	16.7	7.1	8.2
Indian	0.0	0.0	0.1	0.1	1.4	1.8	6.3	10.2	1.0	2.0
Highest education									1111***	1471***
No schooling-Gr3	7.1	3.6	5.3	2.5	1.7	1.2	0.2	1.2	4.4	2.3
Gr4-Gr7	17.8	19.0	10.1	7.9	5.4	4.2	2.8	1.8	10.4	9.2
Gr8-Gr11	58.3	60.9	51.4	44.0	34.4	40.0	13.8	20.5	45.3	44.4
Gr12	15.2	16.4	28.6	39.9	44.0	41.6	36.2	44.1	29.7	34.2
Tertiary	1.7	0.1	4.6	5.7	14.6	13.0	47.0	32.4	10.3	10.0
Employment									1096***	1589***
Housewife	26.2	17.0	21.1	11.2	13.8	12.5	11	17.5	19.6	14.2
Unemployed, not seeking work	9.6	10.9	10.0	7.6	3.4	7.0	2.0	2.3	7.3	7.6
Unemployed, seeking work	44.0	51.6	33.9	49.2	36.2	35.6	28.1	12.7	37.2	40.7
Informal sector, self-employed	4.6	0.6	6.0	3.4	6.3	7.2	9.6	7.0	6.0	4.2
Scholar or student	5.6	11.9	13.3	10.1	5.6	10.1	2.4	4.9	7.7	9.8
Part employed	6.5	3.6	4.1	5.5	4.0	7.7	4.0	14.2	4.8	6.8
Full employed	2.4	2.5	10.7	11.1	28.9	18.3	43.0	38.4	16.2	14.7
Pensioner, sick or disabled	1.2	1.9	1.0	1.9	1.8	1.7	0.1	3.0	1.2	2.0

Table 1 Distribution of socio-economic status among women pregnant in past 2 years between 2008 and 2012; Distribution of socio-economic status among population sub-groups in women pregnant in past 2 years: analysis of the 2008 and 2012 national SABSSM survey *(Continued)*

Marital status									1113**	1601***
Single	59.3	57.8	64.8	62	55.7	50.2	41.1	36.1	58.4	53.7
Married/cohabiting	36.5	38.7	32.7	35.6	43.2	48.2	55.0	63.5	38.9	44.1
Divorced/widow	4.1	3.5	2.5	2.4	1.2	1.6	3.9	0.5	2.7	2.2

Distribution of socio-economic status among population sub-groups in women pregnant in past 2 years: analysis of the 2008 and 2012 national SABSSM survey. Table shows column percentages. *P* value assesses the distribution of population group across quartiles; $^{**}P < 0.01$; $^{***}P < 0.001$

two years, considerably higher than in 2008. Of concern, however, testing levels were relatively low among some groups that had the highest HIV prevalence. For example, the following groups had an HIV prevalence above 20 % and more than 5 % had never tested: women 40–55 years, housewives, married or cohabiting women, unemployed women not seeking work, those who did not complete primary school, and women living in rural formal areas, or Gauteng and Mpumalanga Provinces. Still in 2012, some 3.9 % of HIV-infected women said they had never tested.

Distribution of planned pregnancy and fertility

The overall proportion of *pregnancies that were planned* declined from 44.6 % in 2008 to 34.7 % in 2012, with the largest drop amongst the poorest quartile (Additional file 2: Table S2 and Fig. 1). Further, in 2012, more considerable step-wise decreases were noted in the proportion of planned pregnancy with each SEQ, and the rises in SII and RII indicate growing inequalities in this outcome (RII = 1.4 in 2008 and 3.0 in 2012; and SII = 0.13 in 2008 and 0.39 in 2012; Table 2).

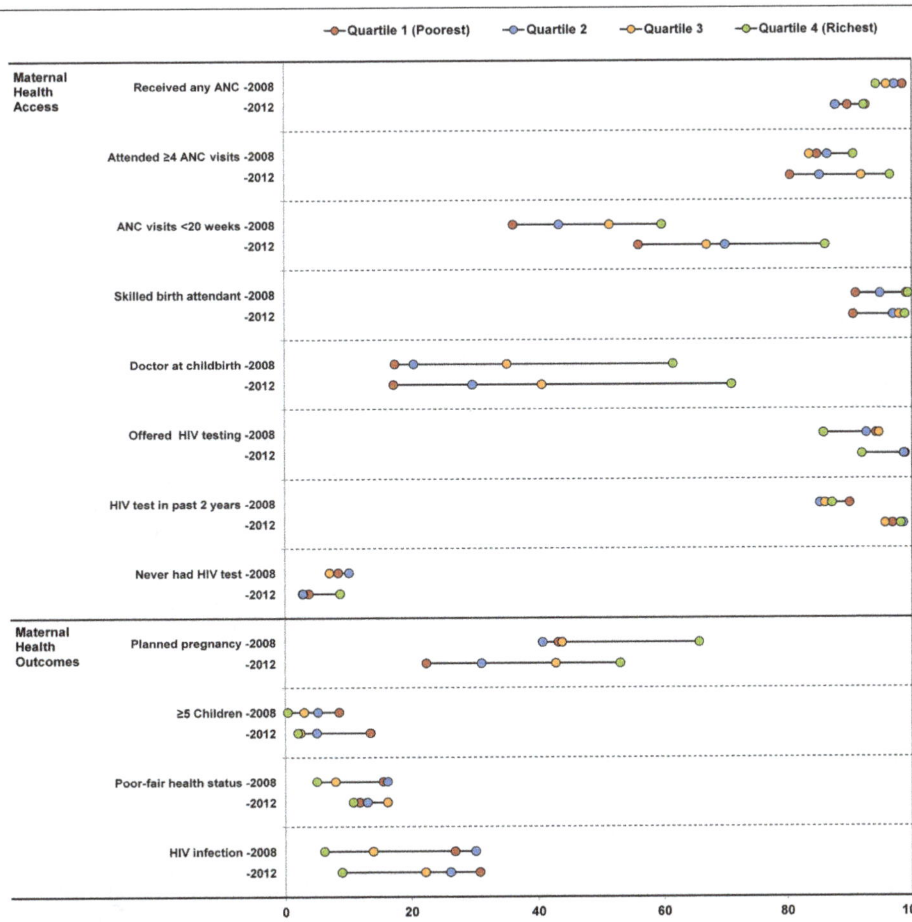

Fig. 1 Time differentials in coverage of maternal health services and health status in South Africa; Time differentials in coverage of maternal health services and in maternal health status across socio- economic quartiles in South Africa

Table 2 Trends in SII and RII in access to maternal health services and in health status; Trends in absolute and relative socio-economic inequalities in access to maternal health services and in maternal health status in South Africa

Variable	Range (Q4–Q1)		Slope of index inequality (95 % CI)			Relative index of inequality (95 % CI)			Concentration Index	
	2008	2012	2008	2012	Change in equity (*P*-value)	2008	2012	Change in equity (*P*-value)	2008	2012
Received any ANC	-4.3	2.6	−0.047** (−0.094 - -0.001)	0.051 (−0.027 - 0.130)	0.030	0.951** (0.904 - 1.000)	1.056 (0.971 - 1.149)	0.037	−0.005	0.015
Attended ≥4 ANC visits	5.7	16.0	0.024 (−0.084 - 0.132)	0.209*** (0.129 - 0.288)	0.005	1.027 (0.909 - 1.160)	1.271*** (1.139 - 1.417)	0.008	0.011	0.033
ANC visit <20 weeks gestation	23.5	30.1	0.274*** (0.106 - 0.442)	0.312*** (0.165 - 0.460)	0.741	1.831*** (1.268 - 2.644)	1.593*** (1.278 - 1.984)	0.525	0.116	0.077
Skilled birth attendant	8.5	8.4	0.121*** (0.066 - 0.176)	0.113** (0.020 - 0.207)	0.888	1.135*** (1.071 - 1.202)	1.124** (1.021 - 1.238)	0.869	0.017	0.018
Doctor attended childbirth	44	53.7	0.401*** (0.270 - 0.531)	0.587*** (0.449 - 0.724)	0.063	5.285*** (2.971 - 9.398)	5.802*** (3.856 - 8.728)	0.797	0.300	0.268
Offered HIV testing in pregnancy	−8.4	−7.0	−0.042 (−0.106 - 0.021)	−0.042 (−0.093 - 0.009)	0.999	0.951 (0.880 - 1.028)	0.940 (0.862 - 1.024)	0.833	−0.007	−0.004
HIV test in past 2 years	−2.8	1.3	−0.050 (−0.152 - 0.051)	−0.004 (−0.049 - 0.041)	0.419	0.943 (0.838 - 1.061)	0.996 (0.951 - 1.042)	0.405	0.000	−0.006
Never had HIV Test	−1.4	5.0	−0.028 (−0.120 - 0.065)	0.030 (−0.031 - 0.091)	0.297	0.739 (0.264 - 2.068)	2.631 (0.395 - 17.518)	0.236	−0.001	0.450
Planned pregnancy	22.5	30.6	0.134 (−0.032 - 0.301)	0.391*** (0.258 - 0.524)	0.009	1.391 (0.929 - 2.084)	2.999*** (2.096 - 4.292)	0.004	0.078	0.161
Five or more children	-8.2	−11.5	−0.099*** (−0.139 - -0.060)	−0.117*** (−0.162 - -0.073)	0.548	0.129*** (0.033 - 0.497)	0.045*** (0.014 - 0.144)	0.255	−0.326	−0.324
Poor-fair health status	−10.5	−1.0	−0.150*** (−0.234 - -0.066)	0.022 (−0.068 - 0.112)	0.004	0.331*** (0.167 - 0.654)	1.165 (0.631 - 2.151)	0.004	−0.043	−0.040
HIV infection	−20.6	−21.7	−0.281*** (−0.427 - -0.136)	−0.251*** (−0.372 - -0.129)	0.38	0.340*** (0.178 - 0.649)	0.372*** (0.224 - 0.620)	0.821	−0.193	−0.213

Trends in absolute and relative socio-economic inequalities in access to maternal health services and in maternal health status in South Africa: the repeated cross-sectional national SABSSM surveys 2008 and 2012
** $P < 0.01$; *** $P < 0.001$

In both surveys, only about a third of HIV-infected women reported having had a planned pregnancy. In 2012, levels of unplanned pregnancy were highest in informal areas (both rural and urban ones), which have the highest HIV prevalence of all places of residence. Among women younger than 20 years in the second survey, only 8.7 % of pregnancies were planned. Scholars and students accounted for 9.8 % of all pregnancies in 2012, while only 7.7 % in 2008.

The markedly unequal distribution of *multiparous women* across socio-economic groups persists: in 2012, 13.5 % of QI women had a parity of five or more, while this figure was 6.4 % in QIV women (Fig. 1). Also, only 3.5 % of women in formal urban areas had five or more children, compared with about 9.0 % in rural areas.

Inequalities in maternal health status and in prevalence of HIV infection

Overall, in both surveys, around 13 % of women described themselves as being in *poor or fair health*. However, unlike in 2008, the proportion of women reporting this outcome in 2012 was very similar between SEQs, thus reflecting a narrowing of relative and absolute inequalities over time (Table 2). The proportion of HIV-infected women with a poor-fair health status was lower in 2012 (20.2 %) than in 2008 (25.1 %; Additional file 2: Table S2). In 2012, however, the proportions with poor or fair health increase stepwise with age category or decrease in education group.

The distribution of HIV infection among population groups in 2012 remained markedly unequal, though inequalities between SEQs were stable. HIV status is strongly associated with demographic and socio-economic characteristics – in both surveys, there are double digit absolute percentage differentials within each of the PROGRESS-Plus groups.

Inequalities in access and outcomes between different provinces

Large differences were noted at provincial level for almost all the indicators studied, and access to services even declined in some provinces (Fig. 2). For example, compared with 2008, coverage of SBA decreased in 2012 in the Eastern Cape and North West Provinces. Gauteng had widened socioeconomic inequalities in the indicator ANC attendance before 20 weeks, while the relative inequalities in this variable narrowed in Western Cape, Eastern Cape and KwaZulu Natal (Fig. 2). Disparities also widened in 2012 compared to 2008 for self-reported health status in the North West and Gauteng provinces, but were narrower in the Western Cape. Inequalities for planned pregnancy were also wider in the Free State and North West provinces in 2012 compared to 2008. Lastly, in the two provinces with the highest HIV prevalence, KwaZulu Natal and Mpumalanga, only 21.8 % and 25.2 % of pregnancies were planned respectively.

Overall, the Eastern Cape Province still has the poorest access to services for many measures, aside from HIV testing, which had approximated national levels by 2012. Compared with the national average, in the Eastern Cape, 9.0 % fewer women had four or more ANC visits; 18.0 % less attended ANC before 20 weeks of pregnancy; and SBA coverage was 8.2 % lower. Moreover, in contrast with other provinces, coverage of some services in the Eastern Cape actually declined between 2008 and 2012. Planned pregnancy in the province decreased from 38.1 % in 2008 to 18.8 % in 2012 and HIV prevalence rose from 18.6 to 25.1 %.

Discussion

The extraordinarily high levels of inequalities noted in 2008 persist and were even exacerbated in many of the services studied. Several underlying disparities in the social determinants of health also worsened. Moreover, substantial declines took place in the overall coverage of ANC services and in planned pregnancy in the country. Encouragingly, however, some notable advances have occurred in access to maternal health services in the country as a whole. HIV testing coverage rose nationally, as did early ANC attendance and the likelihood of having a doctor present at birth. Also, inequalities detected in health status and in HIV testing in 2008 were no longer present by 2012. Improvements in health status may be due to the high coverage of ART, and consequent gains in health among HIV-infected women, who are predominately in QI and QII.

Inequalities experienced by several PROGRESS-Plus groups warrant specific mention. Overall, compared with other race groups, Black African women had poorer access to services and health outcomes on several indicators, most notably early ANC attendance, skilled birth attendance, planned pregnancy and HIV prevalence. These findings are particularly concerning given the strong links between these indicators and the risk for mother-to-child transmission of HIV (MTCT). As in 2008, education level was linked with almost all measures of access to services and health outcomes. Though the proportion of women completing secondary school in lower economic groups appears to be rising, these are matched by worsening inequities in employment. Also noteworthy, rural areas experienced several deficiencies in service delivery, particularly in access to a SBA. Poorer socio-economic groups are increasingly concentrated within the Eastern Cape, and several services there actually deteriorated over the study period. Service delivery deficiencies were also noted in North West Province, albeit to a lessor extent than the Eastern Cape. Both these provinces are plagued with corruption [34, 35].

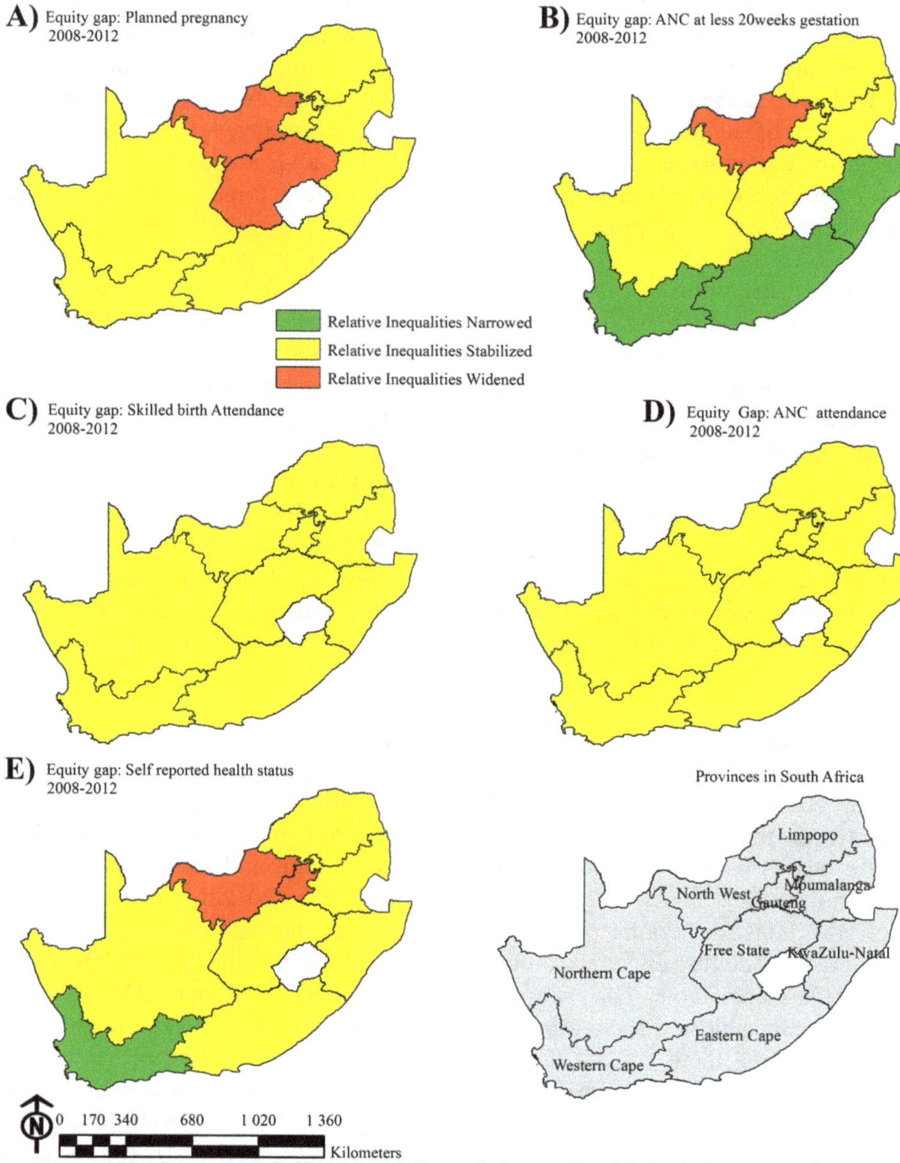

Fig. 2 RII differentials in Planned pregnancy, SBA, ANC, health status, ANC at less 20 weeks gestation; Provincial differentials in RII in Planned pregnancy, SBA, ANC, health status and ANC at less than 20 weeks gestation over 5 years period in South Africa. Yellow represent provinces with stable high RII, Green indicates provinces where RII narrowed, an improvement, and red indicate provinces where RII widened indicating a high equity gap in access between wealthy and poor women

Differentials in coverage of services must also be interpreted in the light of markedly asymmetric needs between population groups, as measured by HIV status, for example. HIV prevalence in the poorest quartile is 20 percentage points higher than in the wealthiest women, signalling the chronic deficiencies in access to high-quality health, education and social services in the country. HIV remains the preeminent risk factor for maternal morbidity and mortality in the country [36, 37] and infected women require more, not equal, levels of services. It is, however, precisely those with the highest levels of need that remain underserved. Still 5 percent of women have never accessed HIV testing, which should be universally provided for all pregnant women in the country [38]. Non-testing is even higher in some groups with a high HIV prevalence, many of whom might mistakenly perceive themselves to be at low risk, as they are older, married housewives, or feel protected by living within a rural traditional society. Information campaigns could focus on addressing these misperceptions. Gaps in HIV testing among older women also perhaps reflect the difficulties of an often considerably younger peer counsellor in discussing HIV testing and sexual matters with older women.

Timely and frequent attendance at ANC and for facility birth are especially important for preventing MTCT and conditions such as hypertension, anaemia, and fetal alcohol spectrum disorders, which require early detection and repeated interventions during pregnancy. As ART is now widely available [39], the most critical factor which determines whether a woman transmits HIV to her infant is the duration of ART during pregnancy [40, 41]. Demand- and supply-side interventions could reverse the concerning disparities noted and overall gaps in these services.

The persistent, even escalating, socially-determined inequities in service access support the call for state support during pregnancy in South Africa [42]. Moreover, the widening of unemployment differentials indicates that income-related inequities among pregnant women are actually worsening. The existing child support grant in South Africa, widely credited with improving child health in the country [43], should be initiated during pregnancy to alleviate the indirect costs of accessing services, such as transport and childcare while away from the family [42]. Grants given during pregnancy have raised service utilisation in many Latin American and South East Asian countries, and have led to marked improvements in maternal and child health outcomes [44].

Attention paid to family planning has risen in recent years, both globally and within South Africa [45]. Increases in unintended pregnancy, especially among young women and scholars, as well as a widening of inequalities in this outcome, indicate that a focus on family planning is long overdue. Improvements in family planning services would lower maternal, neonatal and infant mortality, and assist in reaching the MTCT elimination targets (nearly 70 % of pregnancies among HIV-infected women were unplanned in both surveys) [46]. It will be important to monitor whether family planning services have improved following the Contraceptive Policy introduced in South Africa in 2013.

Limitations

Aside from biological measures of HIV status, many outcomes were self-reported, and subject to social desirability and recall biases. Self-assessed health status may be especially vulnerable to misclassification. Although this measure is associated with morbidity and predicts mortality, its validity may vary across population groups [47–49]. As a further limitation, we did not adjust the socio-economic inequality measures for potential confounding variables, such as race, education and geographical areas. Indeed, the analysis largely focused on impacts of socio-economic inequalities, and only presents salient findings related to the other PROGRESS-Plus groups.

The proportion ineligible or declining participation in the surveys was substantial. Plausibly, those declining enrolment may, for example, have had different health-seeking behaviours than those who participated. Moreover, wealthier and white race groups were more likely to decline survey participation [10], groups that might incur specific forms of measurement bias. For example, wealthy women who visited a private-sector obstetrician during pregnancy may have reported not having received antenatal care during pregnancy. Finally, in future studies, measuring distance to a facility could provide a better assessment of geographical access than simple rural and urban dichotomies. This information and data from tools such as Global Positioning Systems could be used for pinpointing poorly performing areas.

Conclusions

The most striking finding is the widening of both absolute and relative inequalities in several measures of access to care. Even in measures where inequalities did not rise, substantial disparities persist. Encouragingly, differences in overall health status between quartiles narrowed.

This analysis provides actionable information by identifying which interventions and groups require most attention. Considerable gains could be made by targeting underserved groups, as well as the factors underlying the differences in access, such as poor quality services and unsatisfactory patient experiences. Clearly, the continued deficiencies, even deterioration in service delivery in the Eastern Cape and North West Provinces warrant attention. Furthermore, to reach the country's targets for elimination of HIV infection in children, government should focus on improving access to HIV testing in groups which have relatively low HIV testing coverage, but high HIV prevalence, such as older women. Strengthening of family planning services, especially for teenagers, scholars and other low uptake groups would also reduce HIV infections in children, among other sizable benefits.

Though the health system bears responsibility for narrowing gaps in access, factors outside the health sector, such as unemployment, also account for demand for care and population health more broadly [2, 50]. Demand side interventions could incentivise early and frequent ANC visits. This might be achieved by beginning the child support grant in pregnancy and requiring an ANC card as part of grant enrolment procedures. Finally, policy makers will need to choose between prioritising further overall improvements in health services (noted on several indicators in this study), or redressing the uneven improvements that have taken place.

Additional files

Additional file 1: Table S1. Results on inequalities in access to maternal health services across different populations groups in South Africa.

Additional file 2: Table S2. Results on inequalities in maternal health outcomes across different populations groups in South Africa.

Acknowledgements
We thank Dr Fiona Scorgie (PhD) and Dr Brian Williams (PhD), both academic writers and native English speakers, for assisting with the copy editing the manuscript.

Funding
Financial support for survey data used in the study was from the President's Emergency Plan for AIDS Relief (PEPFAR) through the United States Centers for Disease Control and Prevention (HHS/CDC) under the terms of Cooperative Agreement number 1 U2G PS 000570 and 3U2GGH000570. The funders had no role in study design, data collection and analysis, decision to publish, or preparation of the manuscript. The study contents are solely the responsibility of the authors and do not necessarily represent the official views of the Centers for Disease Control and Prevention (CDC).

Authors' contributions
All authors contributed to the overall study design and specific methodologies. NW MC DB conceived the study design, performed the statistical analysis, drafted the manuscript and edited the manuscript for crucial content. ND HR OS provided critical review of the manuscript. NW coordinated the finalising the manuscript. All authors read and approved the final manuscript.

Competing interests
The author(s) declare that they have no competing interests.

Author details
[1]Epidemiology and Strategic Information Unit, Human Sciences Research Council, Pretoria, South Africa. [2]Wits Reproductive Health and HIV Institute, Faculty of Health Sciences, University of the Witwatersrand, Johannesburg, South Africa. [3]Evidence Based Solutions, Cape Town, South Africa. [4]Department of Psychiatry and Mental Health, University of Cape Town, Cape Town, South Africa. [5]Centre for Health Policy, School of Public Health, Faculty of Health Sciences, University of the Witwatersrand, Johannesburg, South Africa.

References
1. The World Bank. Income share. 2011.
2. Massyn N, Day C, Peer N, Padarath A, Barron P. District Health Barometer 2013/14. Durban; 2014.
3. National Department of Health. The 2012 National Antenatal Sentinel HIV & Herpes Simplex Type-2 Prevalence Survey in South Africa. 2013.
4. Moodley J, Pattinson R, Fawcus S, Schoon M, Moran N. The confidential enquiry into maternal deaths in South Africa: a case study. Bjog. 2014;121: 53–60.
5. Department of Health. Saving Mothers: Tenth interim report on Confidential Enquiries into Maternal deaths 2011–2012. Pretoria; 2013.
6. Buchmann E, Mnyani C, Frank K, Chersich M, McIntyre J. Declining maternal mortality in the face of persistently high HIV prevalence in a middle-income country. Bjog. 2015;12:220–7.
7. Black V, Brooke SCM. Effect of human immunodeficiency virus treatment on maternal mortality at a tertiary center in South Africa: a 5-year audit. Obs Gynecol. 2009;114:292–9.
8. Wabiri N, Chersich M, Zuma K, Blaauw D, Goudge J, Dwane N. Equity in maternal health in South Africa: analysis of health service access and health status in a national household survey. PLoS One [Internet]. 2013 [cited 2013 Nov 7];8:e73864. Available from: http://www.pubmedcentral.nih.gov/articlerender.fcgi?artid=3765324&tool=pmcentrez&rendertype=abstract
9. Shisana O, Rehle T, Simbayi L, Zuma K, Jooste S, Zungu N, et al. South African national HIV prevalence, incidence, behaviour and communication survey, 2012. Cape Town: HSRC Press; 2014.
10. Shisana O, Rehle T, Simbayi L, Zuma K, Jooste S, Pillay-van-Wyk V, et al. South African National HIV Prevalence, Incidence, Behaviour and Communication Survey, 2008.A Turning Tide Among Teenagers ? [Internet]. Cape Town, South Africa: HSRC press; 2009. Available from: www.hsrcpress.ac.za
11. Shisana O, Rehle T, Simbayi L, Zuma K, Jooste S, Pillay-van-Wyk V, et al. South African national HIV prevalence, HIV incidence, behaviour and communication survey. Cape Town: HSRC press; 2005.
12. Rehle T, Hallet T, Shisana O, van Wyk V, Zuma K, Carrara H, et al. Decline in New HIV Infections in South Africa: Estimating HIV Incidence from Three National HIV Surveys in 2002, 2005 and 2008. PLoS One [Internet]. 2010;5. Available from: e11094. doi:10.1371/journal.pone.0011094.
13. Bartholomew D, Steele F, Moustaki I, Galbraith J. The analysis and interpretation of multivariate data for social scientists. London: Chapman & Hall/CRC; 2002.
14. Howe LD, Hargreaves JR, Huttly SR. Issues in the construction of wealth indices for the measurement of socio-economic position in low-income countries. Emerg. Themes Epidemiol. [Internet]. 2008 [cited 2012 Mar 28];5:3. Available from: http://www.pubmedcentral.nih.gov/articlerender.fcgi?artid=2248177&tool=pmcentrez&rendertype=abstract
15. Onwujekwe O, Uzochukwu B, Eze S, Obikeze E, Okoli C, Ochonma O. Improving equity in malaria treatment: relationship of socio-economic status with health seeking as well as with perceptions of ease of using the services of different providers for the treatment of malaria in Nigeria. Malar. J. [Internet]. 2008 [cited 2012 Jul 25];7:5. Available from: http://www.pubmedcentral.nih.gov/articlerender.fcgi?artid=2249588&tool=pmcentrez&rendertype=abstract
16. UNFPA. Preventing HIV and unintended pregnancies: strategic framework 2011–2015. 2012.
17. Tugwell P, Petticrew M, Kristjansson E, Welch V, Ueffing E, Waters E, Brockhoff J, Bonnefoy J, Morgan A, Doohan E, Kelly M P. Assessing equity in systematic reviews: realising the recommendations of the Commission on Social Determinants of Health. Bmj. 2010;341:c4739. http://dx.doi.org/10.1136/bmj.c4739.
18. StataCorp LP. STATA/SE [Internet]. College Station, Texas, United States: StataCorp LP; 2013. Available from: www.stata.com
19. Carr-hill R, Chalmers-dixon P. The Public Health Observatory Handbook of Health Inequalities Measurement. Lin J, editor. 2005.
20. Wagstaff A, Paci P, Van Doorslaer E. On the measurement of inequalities in health. Soc Sci Med. 1991;33:545–57.
21. WHO. Health inequality monitoring with a special focus on low- and middle-income countries. Luxembourg: WHO Press; 2013.
22. Bambara C. Health inequalities and welfare state regimes: theoretical insights on a public health "puzzle". J Epidemiol Community Health. 2011;65:740–5.
23. Mackenbach J, Kunst A. Measuring the magnitude of socio-economic inequalities in health: an overview of available measures illustrated with two examples from Europe. Soc Sci Med. 1997;44:757–71.
24. Ernstsen L, Strand BH, Nilsen SM, Espnes GA, Krokstad S. Trends in absolute and relative educational inequalities in four modifiable ischaemic heart disease risk factors: repeated cross-sectional surveys from the Nord-Trøndelag Health Study (HUNT) 1984–2008. BMC Public Health [Internet]. BioMed Central Ltd; 2012;12:266. Available from: http://www.pubmedcentral.nih.gov/articlerender.fcgi?artid=3434116&tool=pmcentrez&rendertype=abstract
25. Asada Y. On the choice of absolute or relative inequality measures. Milbank Q. 2010;88:616–22.
26. Kunst A, Mackenbach J. Measuring socioeconomic inequalities in health. Copenhagen: World Health Organization Regional Office for Europe; 2000.
27. Wacholder S. Binomial regression in GLIM: estimating risk ratios and risk differences. Am J Epidemiol. 1986;123:174–84.

28. Barros AJD, Hirakata VN. Alternatives for logistic regression in cross-sectional studies: an empirical comparison of models that directly estimate the prevalence ratio. BMC Med. Res. Methodol. [Internet]. 2003;3:21. Available from: http://www.pubmedcentral.nih.gov/articlerender.fcgi?artid=521200&tool=pmcentrez&rendertype=abstract. Accessed 5 July 2016
29. Khang Y, Yun S, Lynch J. Monitoring trends in socioeconomic health inequalities: it matters how you measure. BMC Publ Heal. 2008;8:66. doi:10.1186/1471-2458-8-66.
30. Spiegelman D, Hertzmark E. Easy SAS calculations for risk or prevalence ratios and differences. Am J Epidemiol. 2005;162:199–200.
31. Wagstaff A. Socioeconomic inequalities in child mortality: comparisons across nine developing countries. Bull. World Health Organ. [Internet]. 2000; 78:19–29. Available from: http://www.pubmedcentral.nih.gov/articlerender.fcgi?artid=2560599&tool=pmcentrez&rendertype=abstract
32. Zou G. A modified Poisson regression approach to prospective studies with binary data. Am J Epidemiol. 2004;159:702–6.
33. Kakwani N, Wagstaff A, van Doorslaer E. Socioeconomic inequalities in health: measurement, computation and statistical inference. J Econ. 1997;77:87–103.
34. Business Day Live. North West departments put under administratio. 2015;
35. Corruption Watch. The sickness in E Cape Health Department. 2016.
36. National Department of Health South Africa. Saving Mothers 2008–2010 Fifth Report on Confidential Enquiries into Maternal Deaths in South Africa [Internet]. 2012. Available from: http://www.doh.gov.za/docs/reports/2012/savingmothersshort.pdf. Accessed 9 July 2016
37. Centre for Health Policy. Mapping maternal health research in low-middle income (LMIC) countries. Johannesburg, South Africa; 2014.
38. National Department of Health SA. South African National AIDS Council. Clinical guidelines: PMTCT (Prevention of Mother-to-Child Transmission). 2010. 2010.
39. Goga A, Dinh T, Jackson D, SAPMTCTE study group. Evaluation of the effectiveness of the national prevention of mother-to-child transmission (PMTCT) programme measured at six weeks postpartum in South Africa. 2010.
40. Hoffman R, Black V, Technau K. Effects of highly active antiretroviral therapy duration and regimen on risk for mother-to-child transmission of HIV in Johannesburg, South Africa. J Acquir Immune Defic Syndr. 2010;54:35–41.
41. Okonji J, Zeh C, Weidle P. CD4, viral load response, and adherence among antiretroviral-naive breast-feeding women receiving triple antiretroviral prophylaxis for prevention of mother-to-child transmission of HIV in Kisumu. Kenya J Acquir Immune Defic Syndr. 2012;61:249–57.
42. Scorgie F, Blaauw D, Dooms T, Coovadia A, Black V. "I get hungry all the time": experiences of poverty and pregnancy in an urban healthcare setting in South Africa. Glob Heal. 2015;11:37. doi:10.1186/s12992-015-0122-z.
43. DSD SASSA and UNICEF. The South African Child Support Grant Impact Assessment: Evidence from a survey of children, adolescents and their households [Internet]. Pretoria; 2012. Available from: http://www.unicef.org/southafrica/resources_10737.html. Accessed 11 Aug 2016
44. Murray M, Hunter B, Bisht R, Ensor T, Bick D. Demand-side financing measures to increase maternal health service utilisation and improve health outcomes: a systematic review of evidence from low- and middle-income countries. JBI Libr Syst Rev. 2012;10:4165–567.
45. UK Department for International Development and Bill and Melinda Gates Foundation. London Summit on Family Planning. 2012.
46. WHO. Strategic approaches to the prevention of HIV infection in infants: report of a WHO meeting, Morges, Switzerland, 20–22 March 2002. 2003 [Internet]. 2003. Available from: http://www.who.int/hiv/pub/mtct/en/StrategicApproachesE.pdf. Accessed 10 July 2016
47. Jylha M. What is self-rated health and why does it predict mortality? Towards a unified conceptual model. Soc Sci Med. 2009;69:307–16.
48. Bailis D, Segall A, Chipperfield J. Two views of self-rated general health status. Soc Sci Med. 2003;56:203–17.
49. Dowd J, Todd M. Does self-reported health bias the measurement of health inequalities in U.S. Adults? evidence using anchoring vignettes from the health and retirement study. J Gerontol B Psychol Sci Soc Sci. 2011;66:478–89.
50. Mnyani C, Simango A, Murphy J, Chersich M, McIntyre J. Patient factors to target for elimination of mother-to-child transmission of HIV. Glob Heal. 2014;10:36.

Permissions

All chapters in this book were first published in P&C, by BioMed Central; hereby published with permission under the Creative Commons Attribution License or equivalent. Every chapter published in this book has been scrutinized by our experts. Their significance has been extensively debated. The topics covered herein carry significant findings which will fuel the growth of the discipline. They may even be implemented as practical applications or may be referred to as a beginning point for another development.

The contributors of this book come from diverse backgrounds, making this book a truly international effort. This book will bring forth new frontiers with its revolutionizing research information and detailed analysis of the nascent developments around the world.

We would like to thank all the contributing authors for lending their expertise to make the book truly unique. They have played a crucial role in the development of this book. Without their invaluable contributions this book wouldn't have been possible. They have made vital efforts to compile up to date information on the varied aspects of this subject to make this book a valuable addition to the collection of many professionals and students.

This book was conceptualized with the vision of imparting up-to-date information and advanced data in this field. To ensure the same, a matchless editorial board was set up. Every individual on the board went through rigorous rounds of assessment to prove their worth. After which they invested a large part of their time researching and compiling the most relevant data for our readers.

The editorial board has been involved in producing this book since its inception. They have spent rigorous hours researching and exploring the diverse topics which have resulted in the successful publishing of this book. They have passed on their knowledge of decades through this book. To expedite this challenging task, the publisher supported the team at every step. A small team of assistant editors was also appointed to further simplify the editing procedure and attain best results for the readers.

Apart from the editorial board, the designing team has also invested a significant amount of their time in understanding the subject and creating the most relevant covers. They scrutinized every image to scout for the most suitable representation of the subject and create an appropriate cover for the book.

The publishing team has been an ardent support to the editorial, designing and production team. Their endless efforts to recruit the best for this project, has resulted in the accomplishment of this book. They are a veteran in the field of academics and their pool of knowledge is as vast as their experience in printing. Their expertise and guidance has proved useful at every step. Their uncompromising quality standards have made this book an exceptional effort. Their encouragement from time to time has been an inspiration for everyone.

The publisher and the editorial board hope that this book will prove to be a valuable piece of knowledge for researchers, students, practitioners and scholars across the globe.

List of Contributors

Bakar Fakih, Abdallah Mkopi, Ali M. Ali, Godfrey Mbaruku and Mwifadhi Mrisho
Ifakara Health Institute, Dar es Salaam, Tanzania

Kate Ramsey
Ifakara Health Institute, Dar es Salaam, Tanzania
Columbia University Mailman School of Public Health, 722 W 168th St, New York, NY 10032, USA

Azzah A. S. Nofly and Ali O. Ali
Intergrated Reproductive and Child Health Program - Zanzibar Ministry of Health, Zanzibar, Tanzania

Ali Hassan
Ministry of Health, Health Sector Program Support, DANIDA-Zanzibar, Zanzibar, Tanzania

Theopista John Kabuteni
Maternal, Newborn and Child Health, World Health Organisation, Dar es Salaam, Tanzania

Firew Ayalew, Gizachew Eyassu, Negash Seyoum, Alemnesh Tekleberhan, Hannah Gibson and Ephrem Daniel
Jhpiego Ethiopia, Addis Ababa, Ethiopia

Jos van Roosmalen
Athena Institute, VU University, Amsterdam, The Netherlands

Eva Bazant and Young Mi Kim
Jhpiego, 1615 Thames St # 200, Baltimore, MD 21231, USA

Jelle Stekelenburg
Department of Health Sciences, Global Health, University Medical Centre Groningen, University of Groningen, Groningen, The Netherlands
Department of Obstetrics and Gynecology, Leeuwarden Medical Centre, Leeuwarden, The Netherlands

Asha S. George
South African Research Chair in Health Systems, Complexity and Social Change, School of Public Health, University of the Western Cape, Private Bag X17, Bellville 7535, South Africa
Health Systems Program, Department of International Health, Johns Hopkins School of Public Health, 615 North Wolfe Street, Baltimore, MD 21205, USA

Casey Branchini
Health Systems Program, Department of International Health, Johns Hopkins School of Public Health, 615 North Wolfe Street, Baltimore, MD 21205, USA

Sonila M. Tomini
UNU MERIT, Boschstraat, 246211, AX, Maastricht, The Netherlands

Choolwe Muzyamba
UNU MERIT, Boschstraat, 246211, AX, Maastricht, The Netherlands
A9 Marshlands Village, Lusaka, Zambia

Wim Groot and Milena Pavlova
Department of Health Services Research. Room 0.073, Maastricht University, Duboisdomein 30, 6229, GT, Maastricht, The Netherlands

Md Tariqujjaman
Centre for Universal Health Coverage, Health Systems and Population Studies Division, International Centre for Diarrhoeal Disease Research, 68 Shahid Tajuddin Ahmed Sharani, Mohakhali, Dhaka 1212, Bangladesh

Herfina Y. Nababan
Centre for Universal Health Coverage, Health Systems and Population Studies Division, International Centre for Diarrhoeal Disease Research, 68 Shahid Tajuddin Ahmed Sharani, Mohakhali, Dhaka 1212, Bangladesh
Nossal Institute for Global Health, Melbourne School of Population and Global Health, the University of Melbourne, 333 Exhibition Street, Melbourne, Victoria 3004, Australia

Rubana Islam
Centre for Universal Health Coverage, Health Systems and Population Studies Division, International Centre for Diarrhoeal Disease Research, 68 Shahid Tajuddin Ahmed Sharani, Mohakhali, Dhaka 1212, Bangladesh
School of Public Health & Community Medicine, Faculty of Medicine, University of New South Wales, Sydney, Australia

Shabnam Mostari and Malabika Sarker
James P. Grant School of Public Health, BRAC University, 68 Shahid Tajuddin Ahmed Sharani, Mohakhali, Dhaka 1212, Bangladesh

Mohammad Tajul Islam
Japan International Cooperation Agency (JICA), 3rd Floor, Bay's Galleria, 57 Gulshan Avenue (CWS-A19), Gulshan-1, Dhaka 1212, Bangladesh

Corrina Moucheraud
Department of Health Policy and Management, UCLA Fielding School of Public Health, 650 Charles E Young Dr S, Los Angeles, CA 90095, USA

Sameer Timilsina, Pujan Bhusal and Deepak Sharma
Department of Physiology, Chitwan Medical College, Tribhuwan University, Bharatpur-13, Chitwan 42, Nepal

Sirisa Karki and Gita Paudel
Department of Pharmacology, Chitwan Medical College, Tribhuwan University, Bharatpur-13, Chitwan, Nepal

Aajeevan Gautam
Department of Anatomy, Chitwan Medical College, Tribhuwan University, Bharatpur-13, Chitwan, Nepal

C. M. Gitobu
Institute of Tropical and Infectious Diseases (UNITID), University of Nairobi, Nairobi, Kenya

P. B. Gichangi
Department of Human Anatomy, University of Nairobi, Nairobi, Kenya
Department of Obstetrics and Gynecology, University of Ghent, Ghent, Belgium

W. O. Mwanda
Department of Human Pathology, University of Nairobi, Nairobi, Kenya

Aschenaki Z. Kea
REACH Ethiopia, Hawassa, Ethiopia

Olivia Tulloch and Sally Theobald
Liverpool School of Tropical Medicine, Liverpool, UK

Daniel G. Datiko
REACH Ethiopia, Hawassa, Ethiopia
Liverpool School of Tropical Medicine, Liverpool, UK

Maryse C. Kok
Royal Tropical Institute, 1090, HA, Amsterdam, The Netherlands

Tensae Tadesse Mekonnen
Department of Midwifery, Tseda Health Science College, Gondar, Ethiopia

Gizachew Assefa Tessema
Department of Reproductive Health, Institute of Public Health, University of Gondar, Gondar, Ethiopia
School of Public Health, The University of Adelaide, Adelaide, Australia

Zelalem Birhanu Mengesha
Department of Reproductive Health, Institute of Public Health, University of Gondar, Gondar, Ethiopia
Centre for Health Research, Western Sydney University, Sydney, Australia

Katherine Tumlinson
Department of Maternal and Child Health, Gillings School of Global Public Health, University of North Carolina at Chapel Hill, Chapel Hill, USA

Ying Ji, Shenglan Liu, Yang Shen and Chun Chang
Department of Social Medicine and Health Education, School of Public Health, Peking University, Beijing, China

Xiaoping Zhao
Service Center for Immigrant of National Health and Family Planning Commission of China, Beijing, China

Zhili Wang
China Population and Development Research Center, Beijing, China

Rebecca Garcia
The School of Healthcare Practice, University of Bedfordshire, Putteridge Bury, Hitchin Road, Luton, Luton LU2 8LE, England

Nasreen Ali and Gurch Randhawa
The Institute For Health Research, University of Bedfordshire, Putteridge Bury, Hitchin Road, Luton, Luton LU2 8LE, England

Malcolm Griffiths
Luton & Dunstable University Hospital NHS Foundation Trust, Lewsey Rd, Luton LU4 0DZ, England

Jacek Smereka and Lukasz Terpilowski
Department of Emergency Medical Service, Laboratory of Experimental Medicine and Innovative Technology, Wroclaw Medical University, Wroclaw, Poland

Lukasz Szarpak
Faculty of Medicine, Lazarski University, 43 Swieradowska Str., 02-662 Warsaw, Poland

Kurt Ruetzler and Yehoshua Schacham
Department of Outcomes Research, Anesthesiology Institute, Cleveland Clinic, Cleveland, OH, USA

Adam Smereka
Department of Clinic of Gastroenterology and Hepatology, Wroclaw Medical University, Wroclaw, Poland

Marek Dabrowski
Chair and Department of Medical Education, Poznań University of Medical Sciences, Poznan, Poland

Marzena Terpilowska
Division of Neonatology, Department of Pediatrics, Faculty of Health Sciences, Wroclaw Medical University, Wroclaw, Poland

Ishag Adam
Faculty of Medicine, University of Khartoum, Khartoum, Sudan

Jacqueline E. W. Broerse
Athena Institute, Faculty of Science, Vrije Universiteit Amsterdam, De Boelelaan 1085, 1081 HV Amsterdam, The Netherlands

Roselyter Monchari Riang'a
School of Arts and Social Sciences, Moi University, Eldoret, Kenya
Athena Institute, Faculty of Science, Vrije Universiteit Amsterdam, De Boelelaan 1085, 1081 HV Amsterdam, The Netherlands

Anne Kisaka Nangulu
School of Arts and Social Sciences, Moi University, Eldoret, Kenya
Commission for University Education, Red Hill Road, off Limuru Road, Gigiri, Nairobi, Kenya

Henry Chikadaya, Mugove Gerald Madziyire and Stephen P. Munjanja
Department of Obstetrics and Gynaecology, University of Zimbabwe College of Health Sciences, Central Hospital, Southerton, Harare, Zimbabwe

Guadalupe González-Mata
Department of Health Sciences, University of Jaen, Campus de Las Lagunillas s n Edificio B3, 23071 Jaén, Spain

Juan Miguel Martínez-Galiano and Miguel Delgado-Rodríguez
Department of Health Sciences, University of Jaen, Campus de Las Lagunillas s n Edificio B3, 23071 Jaén, Spain
CIBER de Epidemiología y Salud Pública (CIBERESP), Jaén, Spain

Carmen Amezcua-Prieto, Inmaculada Salcedo-Bellido and Aurora Bueno-Cavanillas
CIBER de Epidemiología y Salud Pública (CIBERESP), Jaén, Spain
Department of Preventive Medicine and Public Health, University of Granada, Granada, Spain
Biosanitary Research Institute Granada (IBS-Granada), Granada, Spain

Maria Raisa Jessica V. Aquino
Primary Care Unit, Department of Public Health and Primary Care, University of Cambridge, Cambridge, UK

Ellinor K. Olander and Rosamund M. Bryar
Centre for Maternal and Child Health Research, School of Health Sciences, City, University of London, London, UK

Amanual Getnet Mersha
Department of Gynecology and Obstetrics, School of Medicine, College of Medicine and Health Sciences, University of Gondar, Gondar, Ethiopia

Andrea Solnes Miltenburg
Institute of Health and Society, Department of Community Medicine and Global Health, Faculty of Medicine, University of Oslo, Oslo, Norway
Women Centered Care Project, a project of the African Woman Foundation, Magu, Mwanza Region, Tanzania

Richard Forget Kiritta
Department of Obstetrics and Gynaecology, Sekotoure Regional Referral Hospital, Mwanza, Mwanza Region, Tanzania

Thabea Benedicto Bishanga
Magu District Council, Magu, Mwanza Region, Tanzania

Jos van Roosmalen
Department of Obstetrics, Leiden University Medical Center, Leiden, The Netherlands
Athena Institute, VU University, Amsterdam, The Netherlands

Jelle Stekelenburg
Department of Obstetrics and Gynaecology, Leeuwarden Medical Centre, Henri Dunantweg 2, 8934 AD Leeuwarden, The Netherlands
Department of Health Sciences, Community and Occupational Medicine, Global Health, University Medical Centre Groningen/University of Groningen, Antonius Deusinglaan 1, AD Groningen, The Netherlands

Ajesh George
Collaboration for Oral Health Outcomes, Research Translation and Evaluation (COHORTE) Research Group, Western Sydney University, South Western Sydney Local Health District, Ingham Institute Applied Medical Research, University of Sydney, Liverpool BC, Locked Bag 7103, Liverpool, NSW 1871, Australia

Hannah G. Dahlen
School of Nursing & Midwifery, Western Sydney University, Ingham Institute Applied Medical Research, Parramatta 2150, Australia

Anthony Blinkhorn
Faculty of Dentistry, University of Sydney, Sydney 2006, Australia

Shilpi Ajwani and Sameer Bhole
Sydney Local Health District Oral Health Services, Sydney Dental Hospital, University of Sydney, Sydney 2010, Australia

Sharon Ellis
Antenatal Services, Camden and Campbelltown Hospitals, South Western Sydney Local Health District, Campbelltown 2560, Australia

Anthony Yeo
School of Nursing & Midwifery, Western Sydney University, Parramatta 2150, Australia

Emma Elcombe
Western Sydney University, University of New South Wales, Ingham Institute Applied Medical Research, Liverpool 2170, Australia

Ayesha Sadozai
Centre for Applied Nursing Research, Western Sydney University, South Western Sydney Local Health District, Ingham Institute Applied Medical Research, Liverpool 1871, Australia

Maree Johnson
Faculty of Health Sciences, Australian Catholic University, Ingham Institute Applied Medical Research, Sydney 2060, Australia

Vicki Flenady and Aleena M. Wojcieszek
Mater Research Institute, The University of Queensland (MRI-UQ), Brisbane, Australia
International Stillbirth Alliance, Bristol, UK

Ingvild Fjeldheim and Ingrid K. Friberg
Department of International Public Health, Norwegian Institute of Public Health, Oslo, Norway

Victoria Nankabirwa
Department of Epidemiology and Biostatics, School of Public Health, College of Health Sciences, Makerere University, Kampala, Uganda
Centre for Intervention Science in Maternal and Child Health (CISMAC), Centre for International health, University of Bergen, Bergen, Norway

Mahima Venkateswaran
Department of International Public Health, Norwegian Institute of Public Health, Oslo, Norway
Centre for Intervention Science in Maternal and Child Health (CISMAC), Centre for International health, University of Bergen, Bergen, Norway

J. Frederik Frøen
International Stillbirth Alliance, Bristol, UK
Department of International Public Health, Norwegian Institute of Public Health, Oslo, Norway
Centre for Intervention Science in Maternal and Child Health (CISMAC), Centre for International health, University of Bergen, Bergen, Norway

Robert Pattinson
Medical Research Council, University of Pretoria, Pretoria, South Africa

Jacqueline Ho
Penang Medical College and Penang Hospital, Penang, Malaysia

Jiji Matthews
Christian Medical College, Vellore, Tamil Nadu, India

Aurora Bermudez Ortega
The Australian Nurse Family Partnership Program National Program Centre, Abt Australia, Brisbane, Australia

Doris Chou, Lale Say and Garret Mehl
Department of Reproductive Health and Research, World Health Organization, Geneva, Switzerland

Tesera Bitew
Department of Psychiatry, College of Health Sciences School of Medicine, Addis Ababa University, Addis Ababa, Ethiopia
Department of Psychology, College of Social Science and Humanities, Debre Markos University, Debre Markos, Ethiopia

Charlotte Hanlon
Department of Psychiatry, College of Health Sciences School of Medicine, Addis Ababa University, Addis Ababa, Ethiopia
Global Mental Health, Centre for Global Mental Health, Health Services and Population Research Department, Institute of Psychiatry, King's College London, London, UK

Eskinder Kebede
Department of Obstetrics and Gynecology, College of Health Sciences, Addis Ababa University, Addis Ababa, Ethiopia

Girmay Medhin
Aklilu Lemma Institute of Pathobiology, Addis Ababa University, Addis Ababa, Ethiopia

Abebaw Fekadu
Department of Psychiatry, College of Health Sciences School of Medicine, Addis Ababa University, Addis Ababa, Ethiopia
Center for Innovative Drug Development and Therapeutic Trials for Africa (CDT-Africa), Addis Ababa University, Addis Ababa, Ethiopia
Department of Psychological Medicine, Centre for Affective Disorders, Institute of Psychiatry, Psychology and Neuroscience, King's College London, London, UK

Njeri Wabiri and Ntabozuko Dwane
Epidemiology and Strategic Information Unit, Human Sciences Research Council, Pretoria, South Africa

Matthew Chersich and Helen Rees
Wits Reproductive Health and HIV Institute, Faculty of Health Sciences, University of the Witwatersrand, Johannesburg, South Africa

Olive Shisana
Evidence Based Solutions, Cape Town, South Africa
Department of Psychiatry and Mental Health, University of Cape Town, Cape Town, South Africa

Duane Blaauw
Centre for Health Policy, School of Public Health, Faculty of Health Sciences, University of the Witwatersrand, Johannesburg, South Africa

Index

O

P

Q

R

S

T

U

W

www.ingramcontent.com/pod-product-compliance
Lightning Source LLC
LaVergne TN
LVHW080718210926
848485LV00003B/485